Advanced Imaging and Therapy in Neuro-Oncology

Egesta Lopci · Luigi Mansi

Editors

Advanced Imaging and Therapy in Neuro-Oncology

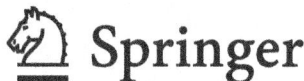 Springer

Editors
Egesta Lopci
Nuclear Medicine Unit
IRCCS-Humanitas Research Hospital
Rozzano, Milano, Italy

Luigi Mansi
Interuniversity Research Center for
Sustainable Development (CIRPS)
Section Health and Development
Napoli, Italy

ISBN 978-3-031-59343-7   ISBN 978-3-031-59341-3   (eBook)
https://doi.org/10.1007/978-3-031-59341-3

This Springer imprint is published by the registered company Springer Nature Switzerland AG
The registered company address is: Gewerbestrasse 11, 6330 Cham, Switzerland

If disposing of this product, please recycle the paper.

Foreword

It brings me great pleasure to introduce this comprehensive publication: *Advanced Imaging and Therapy in Neuro-Oncology*. As we reflect on the past years, it is evident that the landscape of neuro-oncology has undergone remarkable transformations, with breakthroughs in imaging technologies and therapeutic strategies reshaping the way we understand and approach brain tumours.

This compilation comprises a series of chapters authored by distinguished experts and thought leaders in the field, each offering unique insights into the multifaceted realm of neuro-oncology. The breadth of topics covered in this book attests to the interdisciplinary nature of the field, exploring advancements in brain tumour classification, state-of-the-art imaging techniques, and novel therapeutic modalities.

The journey begins with an exploration of the rapidly evolving landscape of brain tumour classification. The first chapter delves into the complexities of advancements in this crucial area, presents the latest developments that hold the potential to redefine our understanding of the diverse spectrum of brain tumours. As we delve deeper into the classification, we lay the foundation for more precise and personalized approaches to diagnosis and treatment.

The subsequent chapter discusses the pivotal role of conventional and advanced magnetic resonance imaging techniques. From anatomical details to functional insights, this section presents an overview of an imaging modality that is instrumental in guiding clinical decisions and fostering a deeper understanding of brain architecture.

Positron emission tomography (PET) emerges as a powerful tool for the evaluation of brain tumours, ranging from the conventional FDG to the more specific amino acid tracers. This journey through the evolution of PET imaging reveals the dynamic landscape of molecular imaging, providing clinicians with invaluable information for precise diagnosis and treatment planning.

The surgical realm of brain tumour management is explored in depth from the current state-of-the-art procedures to the frontiers of surgical innovation. Simultaneously, the exploration of future frontiers challenges our understanding of what is possible, hinting at a landscape in which the limits of surgical treatment are continually pushed.

As we transition from surgery to therapeutics, the chapters devoted to current and future drugs for brain tumour treatment provide a panoramic view of pharmaceutical interventions. The landscape of drug development and the promise of novel agents underscore the persistent pursuit of improved outcomes for patients dealing with brain tumours.

Radiation oncology takes centre stage in the subsequent chapters, offering a comprehensive exploration of established techniques and emerging technologies. From conventional radiation therapy to the cutting-edge realm of heavy ion therapy, each chapter sheds light on the evolving landscape of radiation-based treatments, promising enhanced precision and efficacy.

In the ever-expanding arena of diagnostic tools, the exploration of new radiopharmaceuticals for brain tumour imaging reflects the relentless pursuit of innovation. These radiopharmaceuticals hold the potential to revolutionize our ability to detect and monitor brain tumours, offering unprecedented insights into their behaviour and response to treatment.

The compilation concludes with an exploration of the incremental role of radiomics and artificial intelligence in shaping the future of neuro-oncology. The transformative potential of these technologies to unravel complex patterns within imaging data promises to usher in a new era of precision medicine.

In closing, *Advanced Imaging and Therapy in Neuro-Oncology* is a testament to the remarkable advances made in recent years. I am confident that this collection will serve as a valuable resource for clinicians, researchers, and students alike, inspiring new advances in the quest to unravel the mysteries of neuro-oncology and improve the lives of people affected by brain tumours.

I extend my heartfelt gratitude to the editors and authors for their meticulous work in crafting this exceptional book in imaging and therapy in neuro-oncology. Happy reading and here's to more years of progress and discovery in the fascinating world of precision medicine and theranostics!

Nuclear Medicine and Diagnostic Imaging Section,   Diana Paez
Division of Human Health,
Department of Nuclear Sciences and Applications
International Atomic Energy Agency,
Vienna, Austria

Preface

Is It Possible to Cure Brain Tumors?

In recent years, research in the battle against cancer has yielded remarkable advancements in various areas, thanks to the potential for earlier and more precise diagnosis, accurate prognostic characterization, and the adoption of new, increasingly effective, sustainable, and personalized therapeutic strategies. However, these advancements have not been equally realized for all types of tumors, including brain tumors, particularly glioblastoma, for which improving outcomes, duration, and quality of life remains very challenging.

In fact, detecting brain tumors on time is highly challenging, except for incidentalomas, as there are currently no widely recommended screening methods for early detection. The initial symptoms of early-stage brain tumors are often fortuitous and difficult to interpret. Similarly, identifying an initial recurrence is not easy due to the presence of many non-specific features that do not distinguish between disease relapse and post-therapeutic changes.

Neuroimaging has made significant advancements with the introduction of revolutionary computerized equipment such as Computed Tomography (CT), Positron Emission Tomography (PET), and Magnetic Resonance Imaging (MRI), which complement invasive radiological methods and electroencephalographic techniques. Since the 1980s, further progress, facilitated by hybrid machines, advanced functional and molecular imaging, technological evolution, artificial intelligence, and new therapeutic approaches, has led to improved classification and characterization of individual cases and the adoption of better overall strategies. This progress is also attributed to the advancement of preclinical and pharmacological research, which has contributed to the development of targeted therapies. However, despite these advancements, gliomas, particularly in patients with glioblastoma, remain challenging to cure, and their prognosis remains grim.

This book is being published during an "interlocutory" phase in the fight against brain tumors. Unlike other types of cancer, personalized therapies that can effectively treat individual patients have not yet been validated. This is in contrast to the progress seen in other types of cancer. As shown by a recent systematic review on personalized therapeutic approaches to glioblastoma, such personalized therapy has not been proven to significantly ameliorate the survival of patients with glioblastoma, and there is currently no therapy ready for regular clinical use. Nevertheless, ongoing endeavors are focused on advancing personalized medicine in the treatment of brain tumors, including glioblastoma, through innovative strategies such as mRNA vaccines and immunotherapies.

The book aims to inform readers about the latest tools for better characterizing primary brain tumors and evaluating response. It also seeks to facilitate the early detection of recurrence and assist surgeons and radiotherapists in performing the most decisive interventions while prioritizing the patient's quality of life. These objectives align with the ongoing evolution of brain tumor imaging, which plays a crucial role in improving preoperative diagnosis, predicting tumor grading and patient prognosis, planning surgery and radiation therapy, and assessing treatment response.

The text also emphasizes the growing necessity for collaboration among experts from various disciplines, enabling the combined use of advanced diagnostic and therapeutic approaches. To assemble the most effective team, it is essential to enlist leading professionals from all relevant fields, creating a balanced blend of experienced authors and vibrant young scientists. These individuals should possess the ability to merge creativity, expertise, culture, and knowledge of the most cutting-edge tools for the adoption and explanation of modern diagnostic and therapeutic techniques.

In our view, this approach represents the most promising way to embrace the future, while maintaining a strong foundation in preclinical research and an understanding of the history of science, which serves as the framework for new discoveries.

Thus, to experts in the pathological and molecular classification of tumors, we have added professionals skilled in the use of PET with new and more established radiotracers, neuroimaging experts, surgeons, oncologists, and radiotherapists. These experts present the latest advancements in their respective fields of expertise.

We are very proud, as coaches of this team, to have among the authors some of the leading international authorities in the most important issues involved.

Our hope is to be able to remove the question mark from our editorial and rewrite a new edition of this book shortly in which the title of our introductory comment would be: "**It is possible to cure brain tumors.**"

P.S.: Egesta Lopci and Luigi Mansi want to thank, for their support, the Palummo family, organizer since 2019 of the Carla Russo Prize, dedicated to the memory of a glioblastoma victim, rewarding the best young researchers contributing in the fight against gliomas. Our purpose, as editors, is to help turn their pain into hope.

Milano, Italy   Egesta Lopci
Napoli, Italy   Luigi Mansi

Contents

Advancements in Brain Tumors Classification

Imran Noorani and Antonio Di Ieva

1.1 Introduction

Brain tumors are a major cause of morbidity and mortality, and some types are highly difficult to treat. Therefore, it is crucial to make an accurate diagnosis of the specific subtype to facilitate optimal treatment, especially in the emerging field of precision medicine.

The diagnosis of brain tumors through histopathological changes alone has been challenged by the variability in interpretation between neuropathologists, leading to discrepancies in the classification of tumor types. The 2021 World Health Organization (WHO) classification for brain tumors builds on the 2016 and previous classifications by leveraging new discoveries in the molecular changes of brain tumors and integrating them with standard histopathology to more accurately define tumor types [1], which is information of paramount importance for patients' treatment and prognostication. In this chapter, we will primarily focus on adult diffuse

gliomas and discuss the latest advances in molecular diagnosis for these tumors.

Gliomas represent the most common intrinsic brain tumor in adults, and their high-grade form has a particularly poor prognosis [2], presenting significant clinical challenges. With the latest WHO classification, tumors are given an integrated diagnosis based not only on histology and grade but also on key molecular features, for example, the mutational status of the isocitrate dehydrogenase (*IDH*) genes. Older children can also develop gliomas, although the incidence is higher in adults. New insights into the molecular differences between adult and pediatric gliomas have led to a separation in the integrated diagnosis of adult and pediatric gliomas in the WHO 2021 classification.

Perhaps one of the most significant advances in the last few decades for the diagnosis of brain tumors was the discovery of the *IDH1* and *IDH2* mutations that likely initiate the development of low-grade gliomas [3]. As such, the presence of an *IDH* mutation is given such importance in the WHO classification that a key brain tumor entity is the *IDH*-mutant glioma. IDH1 and IDH2 are enzymes that convert isocitrate into α-ketoglutarate (α-KG) by oxidative decarboxylation. Mutations in IDH1/2 lead to gain-of-function in their enzyme activity causing intracellular accumulation of the onco-metabolite 2-hydroxyglutarate (2-HG). 2-HG has a similar structure to α-KG, and so competes with the lat-

I. Noorani
National Hospital for Neurology and Neurosurgery, University College London, London, UK
e-mail: imran.noorani@cantab.net

A. Di Ieva (✉)
Computational NeuroSurgery (CNS) Lab and Macquarie Neurosurgery, Macquarie Medical School, Faculty of Medicine, Human and Health Sciences, Macquarie University, Sydney, NSW, Australia
e-mail: antonio.diieva@mq.edu.au

© The Author(s), under exclusive license to Springer Nature Switzerland AG 2024
E. Lopci, L. Mansi (eds.), *Advanced Imaging and Therapy in Neuro-Oncology*,
https://doi.org/10.1007/978-3-031-59341-3_1

ter for enzymes, including propyl-hydroxylases, histone lysine demethylases, and DNA demethylases (chromatin modifiers). As a result, the build-up of 2-HG causes histone and DNA hypermethylation, and potentially glioma initiation. Indeed, the introduction of *Idh1* R132H mutation into immortal astrocytes, in combination with other mutations including loss of *Pten* and *Cdkn2a*, led to glioma formation in mice [4].

Over time, it is thought that low-grade *IDH*-mutant gliomas acquire secondary mutations such as in *TP53* that drive progression into high-grade tumors. On the other hand, *IDH* wild-type gliomas typically contain different mutations, such as *EGFR* amplification and point/indel (i.e., insertion or deletion of bases) mutations, *CDKN2A/B* deletions, telomerase reverse transcriptase (*TERT*) promoter mutations, chromosome 10 loss, and chromosome 7 gain [5, 6]. *CDKN2A* is a tumor suppressor gene in the retinoblastoma (RB) pathway, the deletion of which

has been shown to promote glioblastoma in mouse models in combination with *EGFR* mutations [7]. *TERT* (telomerase reverse transcriptase) promoter mutations lead to abnormal reactivation of telomerase, allowing cells to overcome senescence.

Gliomas in adults are categorized into four types: (1) diffuse gliomas, (2) circumscribed gliomas such as pilocytic astrocytoma, (3) glioneuronal and neuronal tumors, for example, gangliogliomas, and (4) ependymomas [8]. Substantial changes to the WHO classification in 2021 compared to 2016 include the requirement of a wild-type *IDH* for the diagnosis of glioblastoma, the reclassification of the previously so-called *IDH*-mutated glioblastoma to the now-named astrocytoma, *IDH*-mutated grade 4, and also the diagnosis of astrocytomas or oligodendrogliomas requiring an *IDH* mutation. We will now discuss in further detail the molecular pathology of adult diffuse gliomas (Fig. 1.1).

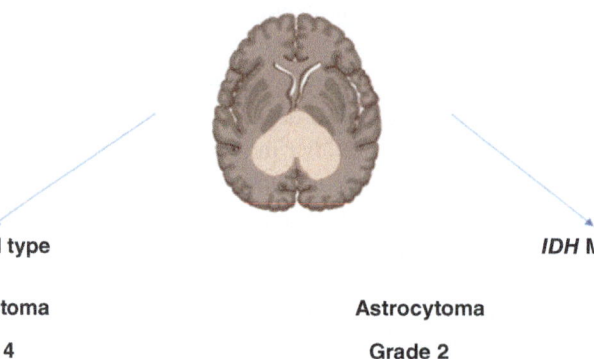

IDH Wild type	*IDH* Mutant	
Glioblastoma	**Astrocytoma**	**Oligodendroglioma**
Grade 4	**Grade 2**	**Grade 2**
Chromosome 7 gain	*ATRX* loss	*1p/19q*
Chromosome 10 loss	*TP53* mutation	*TERT* promoter mutation
EGFR amplification		
CDKN2A/2B Homozygous loss	**Grade 3**	**Grade 3**
TERT promoter mutation	*ATRX* loss	Anaplastic features
ATRX retained	*TP53* mutation	High mitotic index
	Anaplastic features	*CDKN2A/B* Homozygous loss
	High mitotic index	
	Grade 4	
	ATRX loss	
	TP53 mutation	
	CDKN2A/2B Homozygous loss	

Fig. 1.1 The molecular stratification of adult-type diffuse gliomas based on the World Health Organization Classification of Tumors of the Central Nervous System 2021

1.2 *IDH*-Mutant Astrocytomas, Grades 2–4

Astrocytomas with *IDH* mutation (grades 2–4) typically occur in younger adults than *IDH* wild-type gliomas, in the fourth and fifth decades of life. The typical presentation is with seizures, headaches, or neurological deficits. As the name implies, diagnosing this tumor type requires detecting an *IDH1* or *IDH2* mutation. The most common *IDH1* mutation is the *IDH1* R132H point mutation, present in 90% of cases, which can be specifically detected by a commercially available antibody through immunohistochemistry [9]. The other 10% of cases have alternative *IDH1* mutations or *IDH2* mutations, which can be detected through Sanger sequencing of these genes. A debate remains whether *IDH*-mutant astrocytomas may arise from astrocytic precursors, including neural stem cells. The majority of these tumors have *TP53* and *ATRX* loss-of-function mutations, the latter of which causes aberrant telomere lengthening to avoid cellular senescence. These tumors also lack 1p/19q codeletion. Immunohistochemistry can detect the presence of *TP53* and *ATRX* loss-of-function mutations, which is more accessible to most clinical pathology laboratories than next-generation sequencing.

From a histological perspective, grade 2 tumors contain differentiated astrocyte-like tumor cells with moderately increased nuclear atypia and cellularity. The previously called anaplastic astrocytomas are now simply named grade 3 astrocytomas according to the WHO 2021 classification and are histologically defined by increased cellularity, mitoses, and high nuclear atypia. Grade 4 astrocytomas contain the aforementioned features, as well as microvascular proliferation and/or necrosis, which may take the form of the characteristic pseudopalisading necrosis. Cases lacking necrosis or microvascular proliferation but having *CDKN2A* homozygous deletions are also diagnosed as grade 4 astrocytoma if *IDH*-mutant, as these tumors have a particularly poor prognosis [8].

1.3 Oligodendrogliomas, *IDH* Mutant, Grades 2 and 3

This type of tumor typically arises in the fourth or fifth decade of life and usually presents with headaches, seizures, or focal neurological deficits. These brain tumors are thought to arise from oligodendroglial precursor cells. The histologic findings of an oligodendroglioma include a "fried egg" like appearance of tumor cells, where the cells contain large perinuclear halos. Anaplastic cellular morphology predicts a marginally worse prognosis and is suggestive of a grade 3 tumor.

Oligodendrogliomas require a positive *IDH* mutation status for diagnosis. These differ from *IDH*-mutant astrocytomas because oligodendrogliomas must demonstrate on histology that they contain 1p/19q codeletion, which is a clonal early event in the oncogenesis of these tumors. The 1p/19q codeletion can be detected by fluorescence in situ hybridization, array comparative genomic hybridization, or next-generation DNA sequencing. Oligodendrogliomas lack *TP53* and *ATRX* mutations, which can help differentiate them from astrocytomas by immunohistochemistry for these markers [10]. In contrast, *TERT* promoter mutations are common in oligodendrogliomas. If these tumors contain a homozygous *CDKN2A* deletion, then they are categorized as grade 3 oligodendroglioma, as this deletion is associated with a worse prognosis [11]. However, with the new WHO classification, the difference in prognosis between grades 2 and 3 is not substantial, and the overall median survival is 12–15 months.

1.4 *IDH* Wild-Type, Glioblastoma

Glioblastoma is the most common and aggressive type of adult diffuse glioma, with a median survival of only 14 months. It typically occurs in individuals around 65 years old and presents with headaches, seizures, or neurological deficits. Glioblastomas are characterized by a wild-type *IDH* gene and often harbor a chromosome 7 amplification and/or epidermal growth factor receptor (EGFR) focal amplification or mutation,

CDKN2A/B homozygous deletion, *TERT* mutation, and/or chromosome 10 loss. Histopathological features include microvascular proliferation and/or necrosis, and the diagnosis now requires integrated molecular analysis, including immunohistochemistry for *IDH1* R132H mutation. *EGFR* amplification plays a prominent role in driving oncogenesis in glioblastoma and mutations in *EGFR* that lead to constitutive activation of its receptor can drive signaling through the Ras and PI3K/Akt pathways that promote cellular proliferation. While the *EGFRvIII* mutation has been shown to be an early driver mutation in mouse models of glioma [7], in human tumors, *EGFR* amplification may occur at different stages of tumor development and can be a later event in some cases. However, intratumor heterogeneity in the presence of *EGFRvIII*-positive cells and cells with wild-type *EGFR* amplification is a significant challenge in targeted therapy for glioblastoma [12].

The advent of next-generation sequencing has made the existence of intratumoral heterogeneity in glioblastoma much more readily apparent [13]. By performing DNA genomic sequencing from multiple regions within a tumor and at multiple time points, we often observe the presence of different mutations in different samples from the same patient [14]. This intratumoral heterogeneity has been acknowledged as a key driver of glioblastoma evolution and resistance to therapy, representing a major challenge to overcome in order to improve clinical outcomes.

1.4.1 Extrachromosomal DNA Amplifications

Extrachromosomal DNA (ecDNA) is a class of circular DNA located outside of the usual centromeric chromosomes [15–17]. Originally described as double minute chromosomes because of their frequent occurrence in pairs as observed in metaphase spreads, it is now known that only 30% of ecDNA molecules exist in duplets. EcDNA-containing oncogenes are identified in approximately 70% of *IDH* wild-type

glioblastomas, such as EGFR amplifications that are often in the form of ecDNA [18]. The activating mutation *EGFRvIII*, which contains a deletion spanning from exons 2 to 7 of the *EGFR* gene [19], is also often amplified in the form of ecDNA molecules. The importance of ecDNA in glioblastoma cannot be overstated, as it has been identified as a critical mechanism of resistance to targeted therapy, including EGFR-directed therapy, which has failed to improve overall outcomes in glioblastoma. For example, glioblastoma cells containing *EGFRvIII* ecDNA molecules rapidly proliferate, and in the presence of EGFR-targeted inhibitors, the cells rapidly lose *EGFRvIII* copies, leading to resistance to treatment. Upon stopping therapy, *EGFRvIII* ecDNA molecules quickly re-emerge to drive cell proliferation again [17]. Therefore, the presence of ecDNA in cancer has been linked to a poor prognosis [20]. Many different oncogenes in several cancer types have been identified to be present in ecDNA, including not only *EGFR* but also *PDGFRA*, *CDK4*, *CDK6*, and MET in glioblastoma. The key reason for this is that as ecDNA is not present on chromosomes and does not have centromeres, it does not follow Mendelian inheritance patterns. This enables random segregation to mitotic daughter cells, and this uneven distribution of copy number to daughter cells can greatly boost the intratumoral heterogeneity of oncogenic amplifications and accelerate cancer evolution.

The gold standard tool for detecting ecDNA is fluorescence in situ hybridization (FISH), which uses fluorescent probes against targets of interest, such as *EGFR*. In metaphase FISH, the extrachromosomal DNA contents are visualized as separate from the corresponding genomic loci. Newer methods, such as whole-genome sequencing, can predict ecDNA presence based on their circular structure and define their genomic contents. However, these methods are not widely available in clinical laboratories, and novel methods are being developed to detect ecDNA, particularly without fresh surgical glioblastoma tissue [21]. Although not currently used for the classification of brain tumors, ecDNA oncogene presence may facilitate clinical stratification of glioblastoma patients in therapeutic trials, given its association with drug resistance [22].

1.4.2 Transcriptional and Methylation Classes

Although not routinely used in clinical practice, in 2010, Verhaak et al. identified four subtypes of glioblastoma based on their differing transcriptomic profiles: proneural, neural, mesenchymal, and classical [23]. Since then, the neural subtype has been removed from this classification as it was found to represent contamination from non-malignant neural cell lineages and samples of low tumor content [24]. Recently, DNA methylation has also been recognized to be important in the molecular diagnosis of glioblastoma. The integration of transcriptomic signatures and DNA methylation profiles has led to the definition of new molecular subgroups of brain tumors. O6-methylguanine-DNA-methyltransferase (MGMT) promoter methylation is a clinically relevant prognostic biomarker that is also predictive of response to chemotherapy for glioblastoma [25]. Patients whose tumors have *MGMT* promoter methylation have a more favorable prognosis of 23 months median survival and are more likely to respond to temozolomide chemotherapy. In contrast, those without *MGMT* promoter methylation have a poor prognosis of approximately 12 months and are less likely to respond to chemotherapy. Therefore, it is routine clinical practice for *IDH* wild-type glioblastoma tissue to be sent for *MGMT* promoter methylation status as part of the clinical workup.

Several CNS methylation classifiers have been proposed. The molecular neuropathology classifier (MNP) is one of the most widely used classifiers that categorizes various tumor entities based on their methylation profiles, using a reference cohort of around 2800 CNS tumors [26]. One of the primary advantages of the MNP classifier is its objectivity and independence from the user, unlike the purely histopathological classification that has significant inter- and intrauser variability. One study assessing the comparison of meth-

ylation profiling with histological diagnosis of adult brain tumors showed that methylation profiling changed the diagnosis in 25% of cases. The MNP has "methylation super families" of tumors that are named similarly to the WHO 2021 classification (e.g., adult diffuse gliomas and pediatric diffuse gliomas). However, the methylation classifier allows for further sub-stratification of these tumors into multiple classes and subclasses. For example, in the WHO 2021 classification, an adult glioblastoma is not further stratified, but the MNP can further stratify this tumor into six subclasses: RTK 1, RTK 2, mesenchymal subtype, mesenchymal subtype subclass B, primitive neuronal compartment, and posterior fossa subtype. The *IDH*-mutant adult gliomas have methylation types that correspond to the subtypes in the WHO 2021 classification, except for a novel methylation subclass called oligosarcoma *IDH*-mutant that has a mixture of oligodendroglial and sarcomatous features.

Although the MNP (as well as other methylation classifiers) was originally intended for research purposes, it is increasingly being used for clinical diagnostics due to its objectivity and ease of use [27]. Moreover, methylation classifiers have the potential to identify new subtypes of brain tumors, as exemplified by the increased number of subtypes in the MNP compared to the WHO 2021 classification. There are also several examples where subclasses in the methylation classifier have subsequently been added to the WHO classification, such as for medulloblastoma and ependymoma. Knowledge of the methylation classification may also have clinical implications, although this requires further research. For example, a maximal extent of resection was observed to provide a survival benefit in the RTK1 and RTK2 glioblastoma subtypes but not in the mesenchymal subtype [28].

Although most brain tumors can be diagnosed by a combination of histopathology and detection of the characteristic genetic alterations described earlier, methylome profiling can be highly effective for diagnosing tumors with atypical morphology or rare tumor types. Given the requirement for minimal amounts of tissue, methylome profiling is also useful when only small biopsy samples are available for diagnosis and that may be insufficient for other technologies. From a practical point of view, the neuropathologist will pay close attention to the common calibrated score threshold of the methylation profile, which is typically set at 0.84 or 0.90 [29], and suggested diagnoses with a threshold of less than 0.84 should be treated with caution.

1.5 Computational Modeling and Artificial Intelligence in Brain Tumors Classification

Beyond the current gold standard of the histopathology and molecular/genetic analysis of surgical samples of brain tumors, in the last years, computational modeling and Artificial Intelligence (AI) techniques have been investigated for automatic or semi-automatic classification of brain tumors, in neuroimaging and digital neuropathology as well.

For example, extraction and quantification of features from neuroimaging (i.e., radiomics) and histopathology slides (i.e., pathomics) can be used to identify diagnostic, prognostic, and therapeutic biomarkers related to brain tumors [30].

In neuroimaging, deep learning has been used to segment the edges of gliomas' components (i.e., necrotic core, enhancing regions, and perilesional edema) [31]. The combination of deep convolutional neural networks and images' geometric transformation (i.e., spherical coordinates transformation preprocessing of MRIs) has also been proposed to improve the accuracy of the segmentation task even with small datasets [32]. The automatic segmentation of gliomas, along with the use of other techniques and information, can be used for feature extraction, diagnostic inference, molecular markers' prediction [33, 34], and even prognostication (i.e., survival prediction) [35, 36]. Applying the principles of fractal geometry, computational fractal-based analysis has also been shown to be a promising tool for automatic classification of brain tumors in neuroimaging (above all, on ultra-high field, 7 T, MRI) [37, 38], and in neuropathology as well

[39]. Deep learning applied to magnetic resonance images has also been proposed for differentiating glioma recurrence from post-treatment radiation necrosis (i.e., "pseudoprogression"). In radiogenomics, deep learning has also been proposed to predict the genetic status in gliomas, along with other radiological features (e.g., T2-FLAIR mismatch sign in *IDH*-mutant gliomas) [40–42]. IDH status can also be predicted on MRI by means of 2-HG detection on magnetic resonance spectroscopy [43, 44].

In digital neuropathology, *IDH* status can be predicted on histopathology slides of gliomas even before the gold standard immunohistochemistry and genetic sequencing techniques by using deep learning methodologies [45]. In neuropathology, deep learning has also been used to automatically classify gliomas' grades using whole-slide images, with the aim to support pathologists' differential diagnosis and expedite personalized medical care [46].

Although developed as research tools, computational modeling and AI techniques are very promising tools to support differential diagnosis, enhance physicians' decision-making, and improve precision medicine for the management of patients affected by brain tumors. In such a perspective, the neuro-oncology multidisciplinary teams of the future should be supported and augmented by these novel and powerful technologies [47].

1.6 Conclusions and Future Directions

The increasing availability of molecular analysis, including DNA and methylation profiling, and the development and use of new technologies, including computational modeling and AI, have led to significant refinements in the diagnosis of brain tumors, categorizing them into more clinically meaningful entities. As a result, patients with brain tumors can have more accurate prognostication and clearer management pathways. Moving forward, it will be important to understand how intratumoral heterogeneity and the peri-tumoral environment can influence the consistency of such molecular classifications. Radiogenomics, pathomics, and AI-based analyses will eventually be incorporated into the future WHO classification systems. Additionally, since methylation profiling has the potential to broaden the classification of brain tumors, it is important to determine how these profiles can be integrated into clinical practice in a meaningful way. The contribution of the immunosuppressive microenvironment in gliomas and the diversity of immune cell phenotypes will be important to incorporate in future clinical stratification [48, 49], given the interest in trialing immunotherapies, particularly for glioblastoma. Understanding the biology of these tumors, including the presence of extrachromosomal DNA amplifications and how they may impact brain tumor diagnosis and treatment, will be a critical avenue for advancing diagnostic classification and the development of newer treatments.

References

1. Louis DN, Perry A, Wesseling P, et al. The 2021 WHO classification of tumors of the central nervous system: a summary. Neuro Oncol. 2021;23(8):1231–51.
2. Stupp R, Mason WP, van den Bent MJ, et al. Radiotherapy plus concomitant and adjuvant temozolomide for glioblastoma. N Engl J Med. 2005;352(10):987–96.
3. Yan H, Parsons DW, Jin G, et al. IDH1 and IDH2 mutations in gliomas. N Engl J Med. 2009;360(8):765–73.
4. Philip B, Yu DX, Silvis MR, et al. Mutant IDH1 promotes glioma formation in vivo. Cell Rep. 2018;23(5):1553–64.
5. Ceccarelli M, Barthel FP, Malta TM, et al. Molecular profiling reveals biologically discrete subsets and pathways of progression in diffuse glioma. Cell. 2016;164(3):550–63.
6. Eckel-Passow JE, Lachance DH, Molinaro AM, et al. Glioma groups based on 1p/19q, IDH, and TERT promoter mutations in tumors. N Engl J Med. 2015;372(26):2499–508.
7. Noorani I, de la Rosa J, Choi YH, et al. PiggyBac mutagenesis and exome sequencing identify genetic driver landscapes and potential therapeutic targets of EGFR-mutant gliomas. Genome Biol. 2020;21(1):181.
8. Berger TR, Wen PY, Lang-Orsini M, Chukwueke UN. World Health Organization 2021 classification of central nervous system tumors and implications for therapy for adult-type gliomas: a review. JAMA Oncol. 2022;8(10):1493–501.
9. Han S, Liu Y, Cai SJ, et al. IDH mutation in glioma: molecular mechanisms and potential therapeutic targets. Br J Cancer. 2020;122(11):1580–9.
10. Weller M, van den Bent M, Preusser M, et al. EANO guidelines on the diagnosis and treatment of diffuse gliomas of adulthood. Nat Rev Clin Oncol. 2021;18(3):170–86.
11. Appay R, Dehais C, Maurage CA, et al. CDKN2A homozygous deletion is a strong adverse prognosis factor in diffuse malignant IDH-mutant gliomas. Neuro Oncol. 2019;21(12):1519–28.
12. Westphal M, Maire CL, Lamszus K. EGFR as a target for glioblastoma treatment: an unfulfilled promise. CNS Drugs. 2017;31(9):723–35.
13. Brennan CW, Verhaak RG, McKenna A, et al. The somatic genomic landscape of glioblastoma. Cell. 2013;155(2):462–77.
14. Lee JK, Wang J, Sa JK, et al. Spatiotemporal genomic architecture informs precision oncology in glioblastoma. Nat Genet. 2017;49(4):594–9.
15. Shimizu N, Nakamura H, Kadota T, et al. Loss of amplified c-myc genes in the spontaneously differentiated HL-60 cells. Cancer Res. 1994;54(13):3561–7.
16. Shimizu N, Hanada N, Utani K, Sekiguchi N. Interconversion of intra- and extra-chromosomal sites of gene amplification by modulation of gene expression and DNA methylation. J Cell Biochem. 2007;102(2):515–29.
17. Nathanson DA, Gini B, Mottahedeh J, et al. Targeted therapy resistance mediated by dynamic regulation of extrachromosomal mutant EGFR DNA. Science. 2014;343(6166):72–6.
18. deCarvalho AC, Kim H, Poisson LM, et al. Discordant inheritance of chromosomal and extrachromosomal DNA elements contributes to dynamic disease evolution in glioblastoma. Nat Genet. 2018;50(5):708–17.
19. Batra SK, Castelino-Prabhu S, Wikstrand CJ, et al. Epidermal growth factor ligand-independent, unregulated, cell-transforming potential of a naturally occurring human mutant EGFRvIII gene. Cell Growth Differ. 1995;6(10):1251–9.
20. Kim H, Nguyen NP, Turner K, et al. Extrachromosomal DNA is associated with oncogene amplification and poor outcome across multiple cancers. Nat Genet. 2020;52(9):891–7.
21. Noorani I, Luebeck J, Rowan A, Grönroos E, Barbe V, Fabian M, Nicoll JAR, Boche D, Bafna V, Mischel PS, Swanton C. Oncogenic extrachromosomal DNA identification using whole-genome sequencing from formalin-fixed glioblastomas. PMID: 38555024. https://doi.org/10.1016/j.annonc.2024.03.008.
22. Noorani I, Mischel PS, Swanton C. Leveraging extrachromosomal DNA to fine-tune trials of targeted therapy for glioblastoma: opportunities and challenges. Nat Rev Clin Oncol. 2022;19(11):733–43.
23. Verhaak RG, Hoadley KA, Purdom E, et al. Integrated genomic analysis identifies clinically relevant subtypes of glioblastoma characterized by abnormalities

in PDGFRA, IDH1, EGFR, and NF1. Cancer Cell. 2010;17(1):98–110.

24. Wang Q, Hu B, Hu X, et al. Tumor evolution of glioma-intrinsic gene expression subtypes associates with immunological changes in the microenvironment. Cancer Cell. 2017;32(1):42–56 e46.

25. Hegi ME, Diserens AC, Gorlia T, et al. MGMT gene silencing and benefit from temozolomide in glioblastoma. N Engl J Med. 2005;352(10):997–1003.

26. Capper D, Jones DTW, Sill M, et al. DNA methylation-based classification of central nervous system tumours. Nature. 2018;555(7697):469–74.

27. Jaunmuktane Z, Capper D, Jones DTW, et al. Methylation array profiling of adult brain tumours: diagnostic outcomes in a large, single centre. Acta Neuropathol Commun. 2019;7(1):24.

28. Drexler R, Schuller U, Eckhardt A, et al. DNA methylation subclasses predict the benefit from gross total tumor resection in IDH-wildtype glioblastoma patients. Neuro Oncol. 2023;25(2):315–25.

29. Capper D, Stichel D, Sahm F, et al. Practical implementation of DNA methylation and copy-number-based CNS tumor diagnostics: the Heidelberg experience. Acta Neuropathol. 2018;136(2):181–210.

30. Jang K, Russo C, Di Ieva A. Radiomics in gliomas: clinical implications of computational modeling and fractal-based analysis. Neuroradiology. 2020;62(7):771–90.

31. Di Ieva A, Russo C, Liu S, et al. Application of deep learning for automatic segmentation of brain tumors on magnetic resonance imaging: a heuristic approach in the clinical scenario. Neuroradiology. 2021;63(8):1253–62.

32. Russo C, Liu S, Di Ieva A. Spherical coordinates transformation pre-processing in deep convolution neural networks for brain tumor segmentation in MRI. Med Biol Eng Comput. 2022;60(1):121–34.

33. Petrujkic K, Milosevic N, Rajkovic N, et al. Computational quantitative MR image features—a potential useful tool in differentiating glioblastoma from solitary brain metastasis. Eur J Radiol. 2019;119:108634.

34. Jian A, Jang K, Manuguerra M, Liu S, Magnussen J, Di Ieva A. Machine learning for the prediction of molecular markers in glioma on magnetic resonance imaging: a systematic review and meta-analysis. Neurosurgery. 2021;89(1):31–44.

35. Jian A, Liu S, Di Ieva A. Artificial intelligence for survival prediction in brain tumors on neuroimaging. Neurosurgery. 2022;91(1):8–26.

36. Gao Y, Xiao X, Han B, et al. Deep learning methodology for differentiating glioma recurrence from radiation necrosis using multimodal magnetic resonance imaging: algorithm development and validation. JMIR Med Inform. 2020;8(11):e19805.

37. Di Ieva A, God S, Grabner G, et al. Three-dimensional susceptibility-weighted imaging at 7 T using fractal-based quantitative analysis to grade gliomas. Neuroradiology. 2013;55(1):35–40.

38. Di Ieva A, Le Reste PJ, Carsin-Nicol B, Ferre JC, Cusimano MD. Diagnostic value of fractal analysis for the differentiation of brain tumors using 3-tesla magnetic resonance susceptibility-weighted imaging. Neurosurgery. 2016;79(6):839–46.

39. Di Ieva A, Bruner E, Widhalm G, Minchev G, Tschabitscher M, Grizzi F. Computer-assisted and fractal-based morphometric assessment of microvascularity in histological specimens of gliomas. Sci Rep. 2012;2:429.

40. Kihira S, Derakhshani A, Leung M, et al. Multiparametric radiomic model to predict 1p/19q codeletion in patients with IDH-1 mutant glioma: added value to the T2-FLAIR mismatch sign. Cancers (Basel). 2023;15(4):1037.

41. Xu Q, Xu QQ, Shi N, Dong LN, Zhu H, Xu K. A multitask classification framework based on vision transformer for predicting molecular expressions of glioma. Eur J Radiol. 2022;157:110560.

42. Hosseini SA, Hosseini E, Hajianfar G, et al. MRI-based radiomics combined with deep learning for distinguishing IDH-mutant WHO grade 4 astrocytomas from IDH-wild-type glioblastomas. Cancers (Basel). 2023;15(3):951.

43. Choi C, Ganji SK, DeBerardinis RJ, et al. 2-Hydroxyglutarate detection by magnetic resonance spectroscopy in IDH-mutated patients with gliomas. Nat Med. 2012;18(4):624–9.

44. Di Ieva A, Magnussen JS, McIntosh J, Mulcahy MJ, Pardey M, Choi C. Magnetic resonance spectroscopic assessment of isocitrate dehydrogenase status in gliomas: the new frontiers of spectrobiopsy in neurodiagnostics. World Neurosurg. 2020;133:e421–7.

45. Liu S, Shah Z, Sav A, et al. Isocitrate dehydrogenase (IDH) status prediction in histopathology images of gliomas using deep learning. Sci Rep. 2020;10(1):7733.

46. Jose L, Liu S, Russo C, et al. Artificial intelligence-assisted classification of gliomas using whole-slide images. Arch Pathol Lab Med. 2022;147:916.

47. Di Ieva A. AI-augmented multidisciplinary teams: hype or hope? Lancet. 2019;394(10211):1801.

48. Gangoso E, Southgate B, Bradley L, et al. Glioblastomas acquire myeloid-affiliated transcriptional programs via epigenetic immunoediting to elicit immune evasion. Cell. 2021;184(9):2454–2470. e2426.

49. Noorani I, Petty G, Grundy PL, et al. Novel association between microglia and stem cells in human gliomas: a contributor to tumour proliferation? J Pathol Clin Res. 2015;1(2):67–75.

Conventional and Advanced MRI in Neuro-Oncology

2

Patrick L. Y. Tang, Esther A. H. Warnert, and Marion Smits

2.1 Basic Physical Principles of MRI

Since its first development in the 1970s, magnetic resonance imaging (MRI) has revolutionized the field of medical imaging [1]. Its working principle is based on the natural magnetic properties of certain atomic nuclei. Hydrogen atoms, in particular, are commonly exploited in medical imaging due to their abundance in fat and water. The nucleus of a hydrogen atom consists of a single proton, which spins around an internal axis in a process called *precession*. This spin induces a magnetic moment and, to a certain extent, makes the proton mimic the behavior of a small bar magnet, constituted with its own local magnetic field and north and south pole. In a normal state, the rotational axis of the protons is oriented in random directions, but when positioned in a strong external magnetic field, the protons will align with the magnetic field. Once aligned, the application of a specific radiofrequency (RF) pulse can put the protons in an *excited* state, temporarily deflecting them from alignment. When the RF pulse ends, the protons will realign with the magnetic field, this is known as *relaxation*. During this phase, the RF energy absorbed by the protons is re-emitted and transformed into a signal, which can be used to construct an image. This phenomenon is referred to as *Nuclear Magnetic Resonance (NMR)* and serves as the foundation of MRI [2]. NMR eliminates the need for ionizing radiation for medical imaging while providing excellent soft tissue contrast and anatomical detail in three-dimensional space. Within neuro-oncology, MRI has established itself as the

P. L. Y. Tang
Department of Radiology and Nuclear Medicine, Erasmus MC, University Medical Center Rotterdam, Rotterdam, The Netherlands

Brain Tumor Center, Erasmus MC Cancer Institute, University Medical Center Rotterdam, Rotterdam, The Netherlands

Department of Radiotherapy, Erasmus MC Cancer Institute, University Medical Center Rotterdam, Rotterdam, The Netherlands
e-mail: p.l.y.tang@erasmusmc.nl

E. A. H. Warnert
Department of Radiology and Nuclear Medicine, Erasmus MC, University Medical Center Rotterdam, Rotterdam, The Netherlands

Brain Tumor Center, Erasmus MC Cancer Institute, University Medical Center Rotterdam, Rotterdam, The Netherlands
e-mail: e.warnert@erasmusmc.nl

M. Smits (✉)
Department of Radiology and Nuclear Medicine, Erasmus MC, University Medical Center Rotterdam, Rotterdam, The Netherlands

Brain Tumor Center, Erasmus MC Cancer Institute, University Medical Center Rotterdam, Rotterdam, The Netherlands

Medical Delta, Delft, The Netherlands
e-mail: marion.smits@erasmusmc.nl

imaging modality of choice and is routinely acquired to diagnose and monitor disease, support treatment decision-making and treatment planning, and assess therapeutic response. Different aspects of the brain can be visualized by altering the strategy of how RF pulses are applied and collected. Where conventional MRI sequences, like T1- and T2-weighted MRI, provide valuable information on brain structure or the presence of edema, more advanced MRI sequences can reveal microarchitecture and physiological or metabolic changes within the brain.

2.2   Conventional MRI

When a brain tumor is suspected, conventional MRI sequences are commonly used to non-invasively evaluate intracranial pathology: T2-weighted, T2-weighted fluid-attenuated inversion recovery (FLAIR), and T1-weighted MRI before and after administration of a gadolinium-based contrast agent form the diagnostic gold standard for brain tumor detection [3]. These sequences depict variations in tissue density and composition within the brain, enabling radiologists to identify important structures and evaluate the overall integrity of the

brain. Intravenous administration of a gadolinium-based contrast agent can significantly improve the detection of abnormalities, as gadolinium appears as a striking enhancement on T1-weighted MRI. In the healthy brain, the contrast agent is restricted to the vascular system, but when the blood-brain barrier is disrupted, the contrast agent will leak into interstitial tissue and accumulate locally, resulting in atypical enhancement (Fig. 2.1).

Although conventional MRI is unmatched in brain structure assessment and detection of intracranial pathology, it falls short in three critical areas [4, 5]. Reliable non-invasive differentiation of tumor type and grade is not possible with conventional MRI alone, which may result in unnecessary surgical procedures. Additionally, in some brain tumors, such as diffuse gliomas, conventional MRI lacks the ability to reveal the full extent of the tumor. This can jeopardize the success of focal treatments like resection or radiotherapy, often forcing treating clinicians to opt for suboptimal treatment plans. Another limitation of conventional MRI is that it is incapable of reliably differentiating between tumor progression and treatment-related effects. A phenomenon known as *pseudoprogression* shows new or increasing contrast-enhancement and/or T2-weighted hyper-

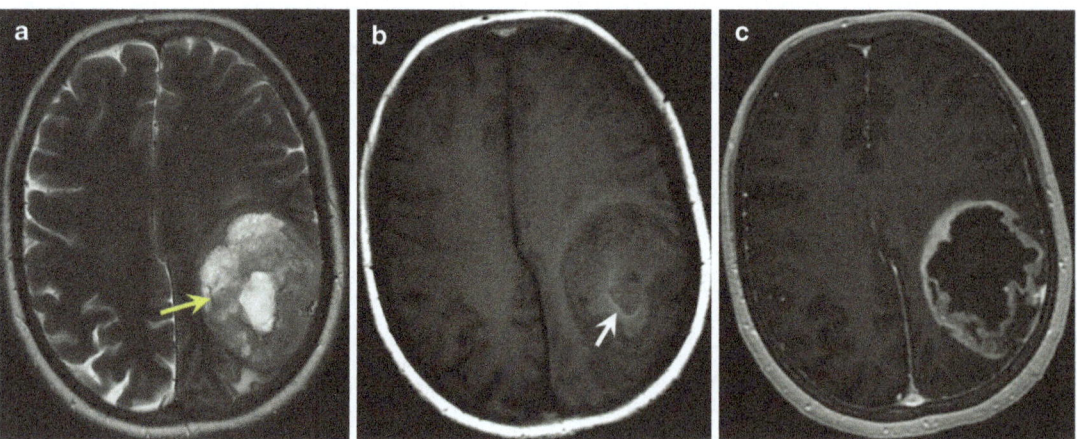

Fig. 2.1 MRI acquisition of a patient with a glioblastoma (female, 53 years old) shows a heterogeneous mass and adjacent vasogenic edema in the left fronto-parietal lobe. The structural MRI-scans exhibit a typical radiological presentation of glioblastoma, and reveal the presence of neovasculature (*yellow arrow*), hypointense on T2-weighted MRI (**a**), and areas of hemorrhage (*white arrow*), hyperintense on pre-contrast T1-weighted MRI (**b**). On post-contrast T1-weighted MRI (**c**), irregular enhancement peripheral to the necrotic center implies leakage of the intravenously administered contrast agent and thus disruption of the blood-brain barrier

intensity after treatment with radio- or chemotherapy, implying progressive disease at first, but eventually subsiding without any therapeutic interaction [6]. The inability of conventional MRI to accurately distinguish pseudoprogression from true tumor progression brings additional complexity to treatment decision-making during follow-up and can contribute to over- or undertreatment of the patient.

The value that conventional MRI brings to the field of neuro-oncology is undisputed, yet there are still pivotal clinical questions that cannot be answered with these techniques alone. Advanced MRI provides a broad range of complementary information and, while still finding its way into clinical practice, may hold the key to unlocking the full potential of MRI for neuro-oncology.

2.3 Advanced MRI

With advanced MRI comes the opportunity to assess microstructural integrity and gauge various physiological and metabolic aspects of the tumor, providing a new dimension of information that may overcome some of the shortcomings of conventional MRI [7–10]. Commonly used advanced MRI techniques, such as diffusion imaging, perfusion MRI, functional MRI (fMRI), susceptibility-weighted imaging (SWI), and proton magnetic resonance spectroscopy (MRS), can improve tumor type and grade prediction, reveal the extent of the tumor in greater detail, and distinguish treatment-related effects from tumor progression with higher precision. In addition, emerging techniques like chemical exchange saturation transfer (CEST) imaging, quantitative blood oxygenation level-dependent (qBOLD)-MRI, ultra-high field MRI, or magnetic resonance (MR) relaxometry, are quickly gaining momentum in the research arena, adding to the arsenal of advanced MRI techniques. When implemented appropriately, advanced MRI has the capability to reshape the landscape of neuro-oncological imaging and pave the way for improved treatment decision-making, focal treatment planning, and, ultimately, patient outcomes.

2.3.1 Diffusion Imaging

Diffusion imaging refers to various MRI techniques that principally explore the Brownian motion of water molecules [11]. The natural random micromovement of water molecules can be confined by the presence of all types of cellular structures. Cell membranes, intracellular organelles, macromolecules, and other tissue compartments can act like barriers and ultimately limit the diffusion of water molecules. In vivo, areas with higher cellular density are typically characterized by hindered diffusion. Additionally, cellular integrity and the presence of macromolecules can alter the water diffusivity.

2.3.1.1 Diffusion-Weighted Imaging

Diffusion-weighted imaging (DWI) is a series of T2-weighted sequences where gradient pulses are applied in a way that water molecules with no net movement between pulse applications are refocused and generate a hyperintense DWI signal [11]. Conversely, net movement of water molecules comes with loss of signal and thus a hypointense DWI signal. This contrast mechanism is key to spatially mapping water molecule diffusion patterns: Areas with hindered diffusion will typically appear bright on DWI, whereas areas with free water motion will appear darker. However, hyperintense DWI signals are not solely attributed to hindered diffusion of water molecules. Because DWI sequences contain T2-weighting, high inherent T2 signal intensities can also appear bright on DWI. This phenomenon is called *T2 shine-through* and can considerably complicate clinical interpretation [12]. To allow differentiation between T2 shine-through and true hindered diffusion, an apparent diffusion coefficient (ADC) map is often derived from DWI that enables an estimation of the diffusion independent of the influence of T2 shine-through (Fig. 2.2). An ADC-map can be calculated by acquiring DWI with two or more different b-values, which determine the degree of diffusion weighting. Typical b-values are 0 and 500–1000 s/mm^2 [3]. Areas with true hindered diffusion will appear bright on DWI and dark on an ADC-map,

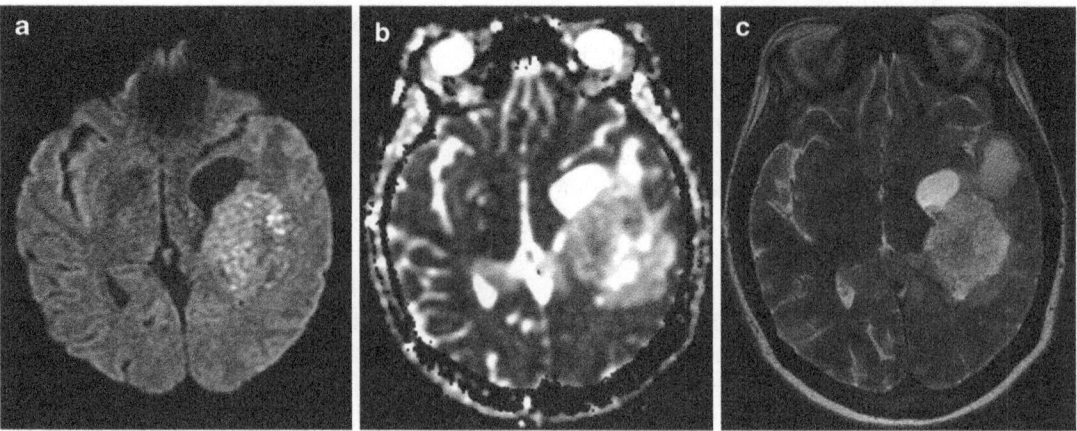

Fig. 2.2 MRI acquisition of a patient (female, 50 years old) with a glioblastoma in the left temporal lobe shows a hyperintense signal on DWI (**a**), which may be suggestive for diffusion restriction. However, no corresponding hypointense signal on the ADC-map (**b**) and a hyperintense signal on the T2-weighted MRI (**c**) indicate that the hyperintensity on DWI is more likely due to T2 shine-through than true diffusion restriction

while T2 shine-through will show a hyperintense signal on both. With the addition of the ADC, DWI has established itself as a reliable MRI technique for assessment of the diffusion and microstructure in the brain.

In clinical practice, DWI is commonly integrated into the brain tumors imaging protocol for assessment of the water diffusivity within and around the lesion. The ADC-map is often only evaluated qualitatively, i.e., through visual inspection [13], but this comes with the pitfall that lesions surrounded by vasogenic edema (bright signal on the ADC-map) may appear dark in contrast, even though no diffusion restriction is present. A simple measurement of ADC within the lesion compared to normal-appearing brain tissue avoids such visual misinterpretation (Fig. 2.3). Additionally, the utilization of the ADC as a quantitative imaging biomarker in neuro-oncology is an active area of research and may further establish DWI as a clinical MRI technique.

Detecting lower ADC values resulting from high tumor cellularity can aid in non-invasive tumor characterization and differentiation between true tumor progression and pseudoprogression. Meningioma, high-grade glioma, primary central nervous system lymphoma (PCNSL), and cerebral metastasis, amongst other brain tumors, can notably increase cellularity, yielding low ADCs. PCNSL, in particular, exhibits relatively high cellular densities with limited extracellular space and may show lower ADC values than metastasis, glioblastoma, or other high-grade glioma [14–19]. Furthermore, assessment of the ADC has been found useful for differentiating between high-grade glioma and solitary metastasis [20], predicting overall survival [21], and distinguishing tumor progression from treatment-related effects [22, 23]. For glioma grading, the ADC may distinguish high-grade from low-grade gliomas in both adult [24–26] and pediatric [27] patients. However, an overlap between observed ADC values complicates grading on the individual level [28, 29]. The overlap is likely due to the fact that necrosis or vasogenic edema typically manifests in high-grade tumors and exhibits increased ADC values. Higher grade brain tumors are generally associated with low ADCs because of their increased cellularity, but the presence of necrosis or edema may cause substantial variations in diffusivity.

Careful quantitative interpretation of the ADC is needed to avoid misinterpretation, and subregion identification or a multiparametric approach may help overcome the limitations resulting from intratumoral heterogeneity. Nonetheless, DWI is widely used due to its qualitative value, with lower ADC-values associated with highly cellular tumors, higher grade, tumor progression, and poor prognosis.

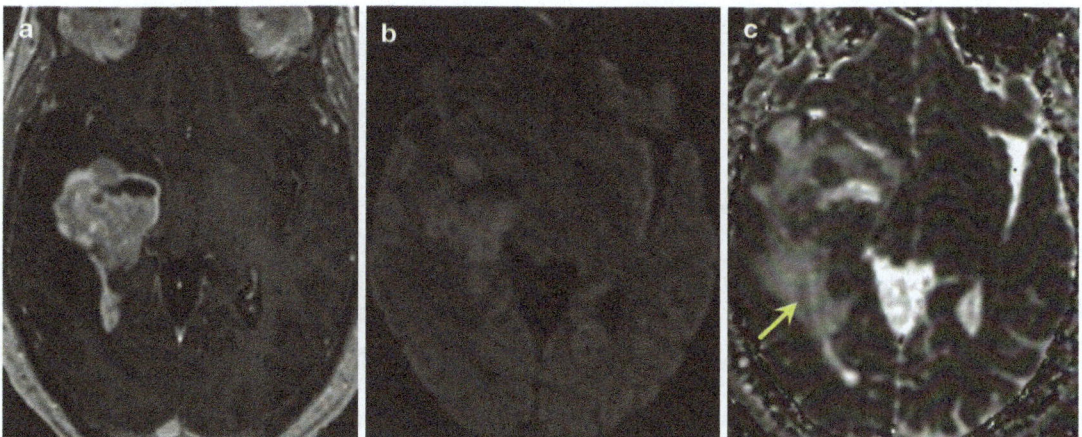

Fig. 2.3 Preoperative MRI acquisition of a patient (male, 62 years old) showed a homogeneously enhancing lesion in the right temporal lobe on post-contrast T1-weighted MRI (**a**). In this case, diffusion imaging may aid in the differential diagnosis, as PCNSL typically exhibits a higher degree of hindered diffusion than glioblastoma. Qualitative interpretation would suggest hyperintensity on DWI (**b**) and corresponding hypointensity on the ADC-map (**c**), implying true hindered diffusion and thus favoring PCNSL as the diagnosis. However, quantitative ADC-measurements revealed that the ADC-ratio between the enhancing lesion (ADC = 903×10^{-6} mm^2/s) and the normal-appearing contralateral side (ADC = 765×10^{-6} mm^2/s) was 1.2, meaning that there was no hindered diffusion. The observed hypointensity on the ADC-map was most likely due to surrounding edema, which appears bright on the ADC-map (*yellow arrow*), making adjacent isointense regions appear hypointense when evaluated qualitatively. Pathological examination later revealed that this lesion was a glioblastoma

2.3.1.2 Diffusion Tensor Imaging

Building on the concept of DWI, diffusion tensor imaging (DTI) is a technique for which data is acquired in six or more directions, allowing the definition of not only the magnitude (estimated through the mean diffusivity or ADC) but also the direction of water diffusion within a voxel [30]. Fractional anisotropy (FA) reflects the directionality of molecular diffusion and ranges from 0 to 1, where 0 represents isotropic diffusion (equal diffusion in all directions) and 1 represents diffusion in a single direction. The FA is one of the main parameters derived from DTI and is used to assess structural connectivity in the brain. In white matter tracts, the diffusivity is preferentially oriented along the tracts, making DTI extremely suitable for fiber tractography (Fig. 2.4).

Measurement of the FA does not majorly enhance tumor type and grade differentiation compared to ADC [20, 31, 32]. However, variations in the peritumoral mean diffusivity and the FA have been observed between high-grade glioma and low-grade glioma or metastasis, empha-sizing DTI's potential to better visualize the extent of the tumor [31, 32]. Diffuse glioma is challenging to treat due to its extensive tumor infiltration, complicating focal treatment planning for surgery and radiotherapy. The integration of DTI into pre-surgical planning, in particular, can contribute to improved localization of eloquent areas, greater extent of resection, and reduced risk for iatrogenic neurological deficits [33, 34].

2.3.1.3 Emerging Diffusion Imaging Techniques

Both DWI and DTI are based on the assumption that water diffusivity follows a Gaussian normal distribution. Although justified for pure liquids, this assumption neglects the in vivo complexities in biological tissue. Diffusion kurtosis imaging (DKI) is an extension of DTI that quantifies non-Gaussian water diffusion and is thought to be more sensitive to microstructural changes than DWI or DTI [35]. Mean kurtosis, the main parameter derived from DKI, shows high diagnostic accuracy for glioma grading, suggesting it

Fig. 2.4 DTI acquistion of a patient (male, 42 years old) with an oligodendroglioma in the right frontal lobe. Bright signal on the FA-map (**a**) indicates areas with highly organized white matter; in this patient, the integrity of nearby white matter tracts is compromised by the tumor. The color-coded orientation map (**b**) reflects the direction of white matter fibers: Red shows left-right oriented fibers (e.g., the splenium or genu of the corpus callosum), blue superior-inferior oriented fibers (e.g., the internal capsule), and green anterior-posterior oriented fibers. Fiber tractography as an overlay of a T1-weighted MRI-scan (**c**) allows visualization of the corticospinal tract

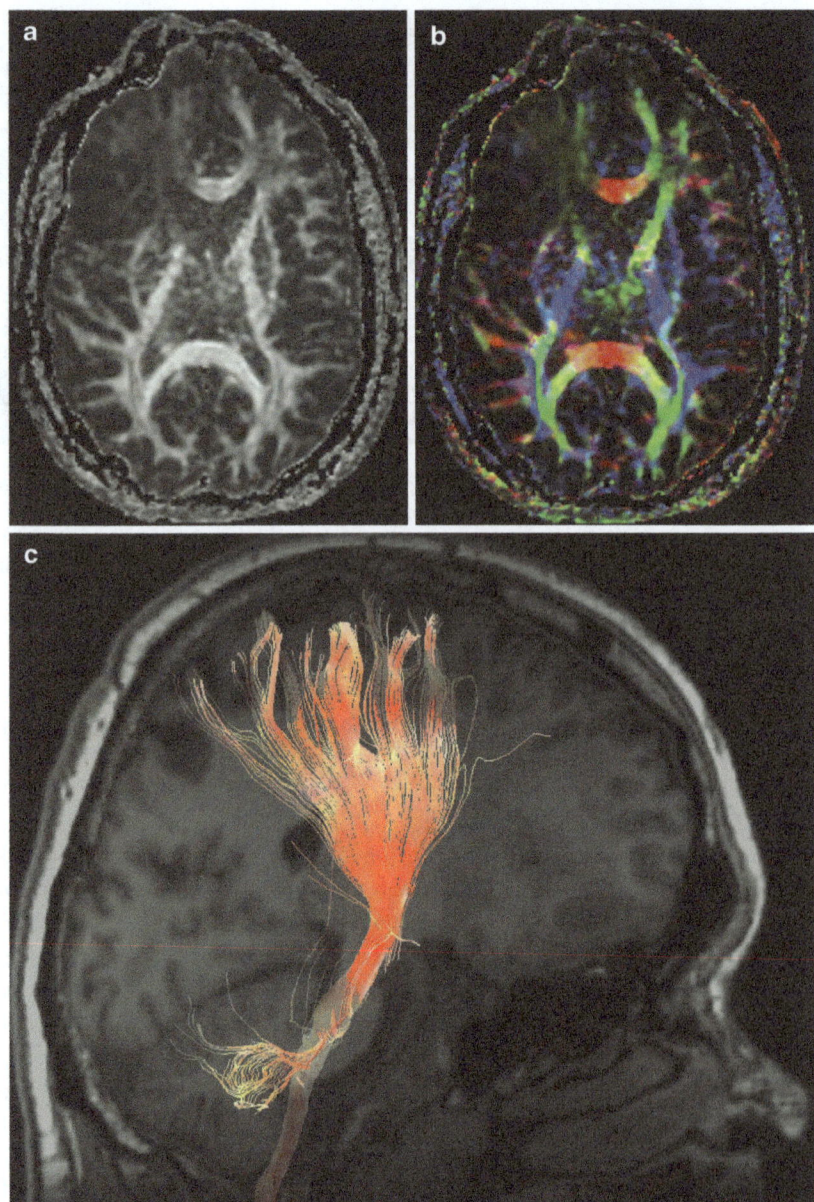

is a promising imaging biomarker for non-invasive tumor grading [36, 37]. DKI, however, is a challenging technique and not yet widely available. Moreover, the majority of published works are carried out with high-field MRI scanners, further hampering adaptation to clinical practice [38]. Additional studies are needed to optimize and standardize kurtosis imaging and confirm initial findings, as well as correlate with other imaging techniques.

Intravoxel incoherent motion (IVIM) imaging is an advanced diffusion imaging technique that enables the simultaneous quantification of diffusion and perfusion characteristics of tissues. IVIM relies on the concept of pseudo-diffusion, where the blood flow in the capillary network mimics a diffusion process [39]. While its role in clinical practice is yet to be established, IVIM has the potential to aid in the grading of gliomas [40].

2.3.2 Perfusion MRI

Perfusion MRI refers to a variety of advanced MRI techniques that probe regional tissue perfusion. Three extensively studied techniques, dynamic susceptibility contrast MRI (DSC-MRI), dynamic contrast-enhanced MRI (DCE-MRI), and arterial spin labeling (ASL), are used in neuro-oncological clinical practice and can provide both qualitative and quantitative measurements of regional hemodynamic conditions in the brain.

2.3.2.1 DSC-MRI

DSC-MRI utilizes rapid imaging to track the first passing of a paramagnetic contrast agent, typically a gadolinium chelate, through a given tissue [41]. The contrast bolus induces a local susceptibility effect, which decreases the signal intensity on T2- and T2*-weighted MRI, a variant of T2-weighted MRI that is highly sensitive to macroscopic magnetic field inhomogeneities [42]. This drop in signal intensity is dependent on the local concentration of the contrast agent, which may serve as a proxy for regional tissue perfusion. By rapidly measuring the signal changes over time during a bolus passage, DSC-MRI enables the voxel-wise computation of various perfusion metrics, including the relative cerebral blood volume (rCBV), usually measured as the ratio between the tumor area and contralateral normal-appearing white matter.

DSC-MRI is the most commonly used MRI technique for perfusion imaging of intracranial tumors [13, 43]. It can be of use for preoperative differential diagnosis and tumor grading. Unlike high-grade glioma, PCNSL is not necessarily characterized by vigorous neovascularization, but rather shows an angiocentric growth pattern with lymphoma cells clustering within and around pre-existing vasculature [44–46]. Correspondingly, PCNSL generally exhibits lower perfusion on DSC-MRI than high-grade glioma [47–49]. Assessment of the peritumoral rCBV can aid in the differentiation between glioma and brain metastasis. Contrary to metastases, gliomas tend to infiltrate into surrounding tissue; an increase in rCBV in the peritumoral region can

therefore be suggestive for glioma [50]. Overall, higher rCBV is associated with higher tumor grade and aggressiveness. The diagnostic accuracy of DSC-MRI for tumor grading, however, may be mediocre in some tumor types, particularly oligodendroglioma [25, 51–53]. Finally, numerous studies have highlighted the potential of DSC-MRI for the distinction of tumor progression from treatment-related effects, demonstrating significantly higher rCBV-values in areas of true tumor recurrence [22, 54–56].

Substantial variations in reported rCBV-values, however, have hampered the path toward universally acknowledged threshold values [13]. The moderate repeatability and reproducibility of rCBV emerge from a mixture of hurdles; variability in internal reference definition, intratumoral heterogeneity, and different approaches for leakage or partial volume corrections have obstructed the search for optimal rCBV cutoff values for specific clinical indications. Because of these hurdles, only recently, a consensus [57] has been published on optimal image acquisition and post-processing for rCBV in high-grade glioma diagnostics, potentially leading to standardized cutoff values in the near future. Nevertheless, DSC-MRI is already widely adopted in both research and clinical practice and has proven its value for perfusion imaging in the brain.

2.3.2.2 DCE-MRI

DCE-MRI is a valuable tool for assessment of the vascular leakiness of a tumor after intravenous administration of a paramagnetic contrast agent. While contrast-enhancement on conventional T1-weighted MRI can imply disruption of the blood-brain barrier, DCE-MRI provides additional information by evaluation of the temporal pattern of enhancement. Through serial T1-weighted MRI acquisition during passage of the contrast agent and the application of a pharmacokinetic model, various DCE metrics can be estimated, reflecting the kinetics of enhancement within the brain. The most commonly studied DCE parameter is the volume transfer constant (K^{trans}), which reflects the efflux rate of a contrast agent from the blood plasma into the extravascular extracellular space (EES) and thus serves as a surrogate for the capillary permeability [58]. Other DCE parameters include the fractional plasma volume (v_p), the fractional volume of the EES (v_e), and the rate constant for reflux of contrast agent from the EES back into the vasculature system (k_{ep}).

Integration of DCE-MRI into clinical practice can help distinguish high-grade glioma from PCNSL [47] or brain metastasis [50]; its diagnostic performance, however, seems to be inferior to other perfusion MRI techniques. Similar to DSC-MRI, DCE-MRI is a promising technique for differentiating treatment-related effects from true tumor progression [22, 55, 56] and stratifying high-grade gliomas from their lower-grade counterparts. The latter is particularly the case when analyzing regions with *hot-spots* rather than a whole lesion approach [59].

The necessity of complex pharmacokinetic models for the estimation of DCE metrics of interest has partially hampered the development of highly reproducible and repeatable quantitative imaging biomarkers [60]. At present, DCE-MRI is not as widely adopted in neuro-oncological clinical practice as DSC-MRI, in part due to its inherently longer scanning times [13, 43]. However, with its better spatial resolution and reduced sensitivity to image artifacts caused by macroscopic magnetic field inhomogeneities, DCE-MRI may be the preferred technique for perfusion analysis in specific situations, like lesions in close proximity to the skull base.

2.3.2.3 ASL

ASL is an MRI technique that exploits the ability of RF pulses to magnetically label blood as it flows into the brain. Labeling, or *"tagging"*, is achieved by applying RF pulses to arterial blood upstream of the region of interest, inverting the longitudinal magnetization of the protons and effectively turning inflowing blood into a natural tracer. This unique concept enables evaluation of cerebral perfusion without the need for intravenous contrast agent administration. There are several methods for labeling; the recommended approach for clinical practice is pseudo-continuous ASL with background suppression, which has now been implemented by all main MRI vendors [61]. Although the spatial resolution of ASL may be inferior to those of other perfusion MRI techniques, its non-invasive nature makes it particularly suitable for the pediatric population and patients in whom intravenous contrast agent administration is contra-indicated. With the addition of a kinetic model, ASL can be used for quantitative mapping of the cerebral blood flow (CBF), typically expressed in *mL/100 g tissue/min* [62].

Due to its high degree of neoangiogenesis, high-grade glioma often demonstrates markedly elevated CBF measurements compared to PCNSL [49, 63] or low-grade glioma [64–66]. The ability to improve preoperative prediction of glioma grade applies to the pediatric population as well, with the exception of diffuse midline gliomas, as they tend to exhibit CBF similar to that of low-grade tumors rather than high-grade tumor subtypes [27, 67]. ASL comes with moderate to high diagnostic value in distinguishing treatment-related effects from glioma recurrence; however, DSC-MRI appears to surpass ASL in terms of diagnostic accuracy [56, 68–70]. Nonetheless, ASL has some advantages over DSC-MRI, including its insensitivity to susceptibility artifacts or other artifacts caused by corrupted permeability or large vessels in the vicinity of the tumor (Fig. 2.5) [71, 72]. Additionally, the unique ability of ASL to probe perfusion without the need for intravenous administration of a contrast agent provides distinctive clinical value in neuro-oncological imaging, particularly for pediatric patients.

2.3.3   fMRI

fMRI relies on the hemodynamic changes within the brain to estimate neuronal activity and localize brain function. When a cluster of neurons becomes activated, the local demand for oxygen rises, resulting in increased blood flow toward that region of the brain. In fMRI, image contrast primarily comes from the blood oxygen level-dependent (BOLD) effect, which reflects changes in deoxygenated hemoglobin [73]. The magnetic susceptibility of hemoglobin differs depending

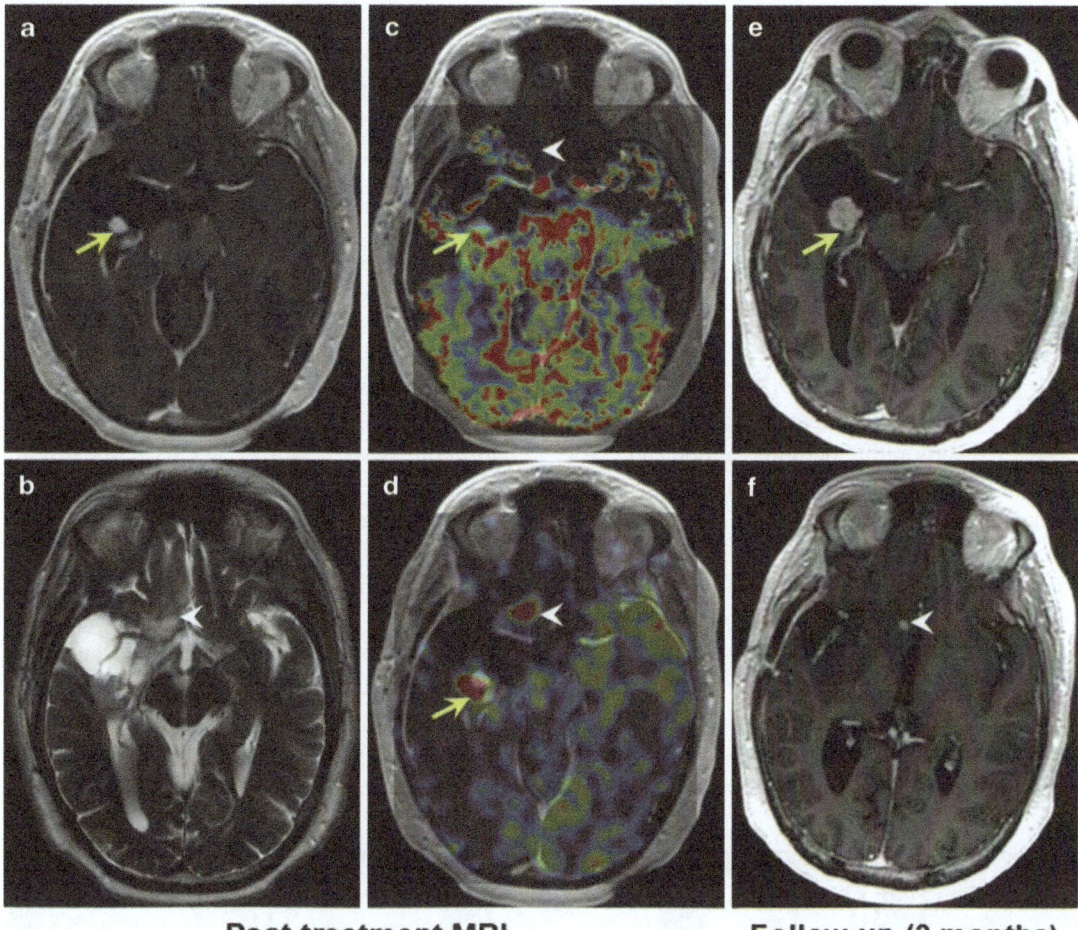

Post-treatment MRI   **Follow-up (3 months)**

Fig. 2.5 Post-treatment acquisition of post-contrast T1-weighted MRI (**a**), T2-weighted MRI (**b**), DSC-MRI (**c**) and ASL (**d**), revealed a contrast-enhancing nodule (*yellow arrow*) in the resection cavity, with increased perfusion both visible on DSC-MRI and ASL. Surrounding signal from large vascular structures, however, limited the detectability of the lesion on DSC-MRI. Furthermore, a non-enhancing lesion (*white arrowhead*) was seen to exhibit high perfusion that was only detectable on ASL. This area could not be assessed on DSC-MRI due to signal dropout from the skull base. Upon 3 month follow-up, both lesions showed tumor progression on post-contrast T1-weighted MRI (**e**, **f**)

on its oxygen state. When oxygen is bound to hemoglobin, the molecule is diamagnetic. After oxygen is released and deoxygenated hemoglobin is formed, it becomes strongly paramagnetic, shortening T2-/T2*-relaxation times and thus decreasing the BOLD signal. In activated areas, the inflow of oxygenated blood is upregulated and brings an amount of oxygen beyond the local demand, causing a drop in the relative concentration of deoxyhemoglobin. During the traditional form of fMRI — task-based fMRI — a patient is asked to perform a specific task, such as finger tapping, or presented with a stimulus, like a flashing checkerboard [74]. Subsequently, mapping of elevated BOLD signals, relative to a baseline condition, can allow identification of the brain regions that are functionally involved with that specific task or stimulus.

In neuro-oncological clinical practice, task-based fMRI is mostly used for surgical planning, providing upfront information on tumor resectability, the locations of eloquent areas, and the optimal interventional approach [13, 75]. A crucial aspect of brain tumor surgery is preserving important brain functions. By preoperatively localizing the language areas and the visual and motor cortex through fMRI (commonly combined with intraoperative electrocortical mapping), the risk of injury to these regions can be minimized [76].

2.3.4 SWI

SWI is a non-invasive MRI technique that enhances magnetic susceptibility differences in tissue by incorporating both magnitude and phase information [77]. The latter is often neglected in other MRI techniques, yet local changes in the precession frequency of protons, reflected by the phase of the T2*-weighted signal, can offer additional and independent information regarding tissue contrast. SWI is particularly useful for enhanced detection of deoxygenated (venous) blood, microhemorrhages, and calcifications [78].

Intratumoral susceptibility signals (ITSS), which are defined as hypointense, linear, or dot-like areas on SWI, may imply the presence of microbleeds or neovasculature within the tumor (Fig. 2.6). A high number of ITSS can indicate a higher tumor grade [79, 80] and an unfavorable molecular profile (IDH1-wildtype and unmethylated MGMT status) in glioma [81]. Assessment of ITSS in metastatic brain disease can yield information about the underlying tumor entity, as intracranial metastatic melanoma often exhibits higher ITSS compared to brain metastasis from breast or lung cancer [82]. Additionally, there has been an increasing interest in contrast-enhanced SWI for high-grade glioma; accumulation of gadolinium-based contrast agent in the highly vascularized peripheral tumor invasion zone can enable enhanced depiction of the tumor border on SWI [83]. By merging the magnitude and phase information of the MRI signal, SWI provides exclusive information that is appreciated in various neurological applications, like settings of trauma and acute neurologic presentations suggestive of stroke [84]. Its clinical value in the field of neuro-oncology, however, is yet to be determined.

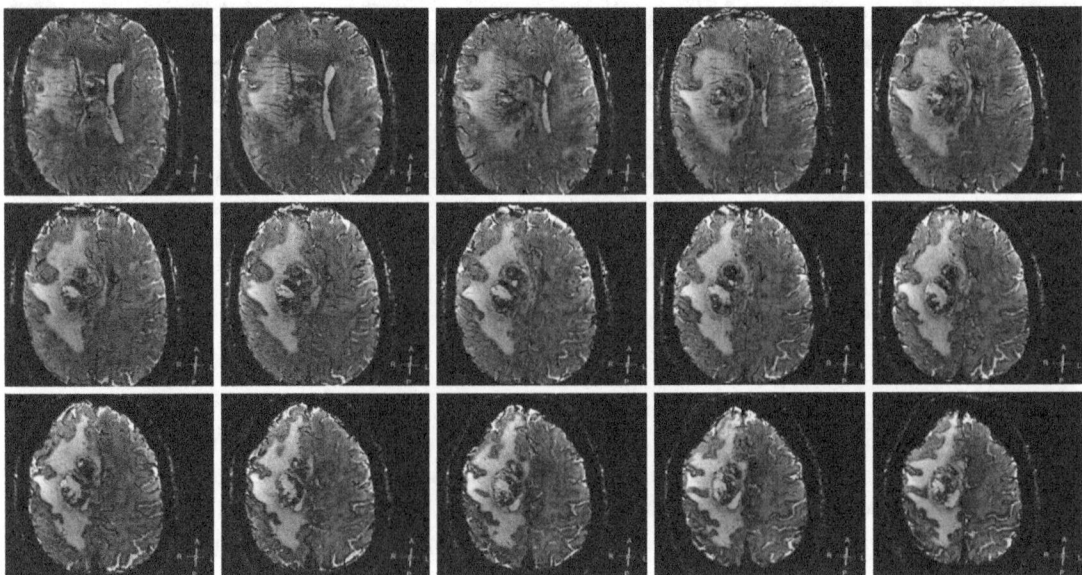

Fig. 2.6 SWI acquisition of a patient (female, 64 years old) with a glioblastoma shows a large amount of ITSS in the lesion on 15 representative slices. Data acquired on a 7 T MRI scanner (Philips Achieva, Best, The Netherlands). (Image courtesy of Bárbara Schmitz-Abecassis, Department of Radiology, Leiden University Medical Center)

2.3.5 Proton MRS

Proton MRS is an MRI technique that probes the metabolic composition of a specific region of interest. The resonance frequencies of protons within different molecules deviate slightly from each other and the free water pool, enabling the detectability of multitudinous metabolites aside from water [85]. As water is present in much greater quantities than other molecules, its overwhelming signal is often suppressed to improve detection of subtle concentrations of various metabolites of interest [86]. Proton MRS can provide unique biochemical details and thus portray the metabolic profile of a lesion. The two most common MRS techniques are single-voxel MRS and MRS imaging (MRSI). In single-voxel MRS, the biochemical composition in a localized region of interest, defined by a single voxel, is examined through an MR spectrum that arranges the detected signals as a function of their relative resonance frequency. Specific resonance frequencies correspond to different metabolites, allowing the determination of various metabolite concentrations within the voxel of interest (Fig. 2.7). Contrary to single-voxel MRS, where the locations of the voxels are specified, MRSI constructs a multi-voxel map of a metabolic parameter of interest by acquiring the MR spectrum for each individual voxel. This allows for visualization of metabolic variations, spatially mapped over a larger volume, and may provide additional information on the metabolic heterogeneity within a tumor.

Within neuro-oncology, frequently examined metabolites include N-acetyl aspartate (NAA), choline (Cho), lactate, mobile lipids, and creatine (Cr) [85]. NAA is a metabolite abundant in healthy neurons and is therefore considered an appropriate marker for their viability. In the MR spectrum of the healthy brain, the NAA peak (at 2.0 ppm) is typically the most prominent; a diminished peak can indicate that the neuronal integrity is compromised [87]. Cho plays a pivotal role as a precursor in several key biochemical processes, including the synthesis of phospholipid components for cell membranes. An elevated peak of choline-containing compounds (at 3.2 ppm) can indicate increased cellular membrane turnover as a result of neoplastic proliferation [88]. Lactate is a marker of anaerobic metabolism and is normally absent in brain tissue. The presence of a lactate peak (at 1.33 ppm) may be associated with the *Warburg effect*, which may indicate a preferential production of lactate during glucose metabolism even in the presence of oxygen, and thus tumor cell metabolism [89, 90]. Similar to lactate, mobile lipids are typically not visible in the spectra of the healthy brain. In the presence of brain pathology, lipid peaks, predominantly arising from methyl and methylene groups (at 0.9 and 1.3 ppm, respectively), can appear and suggest the presence of necrosis or cellular membrane breakdown [91]. Cr or phosphocreatine (at 3.0 ppm) is often present in metabolically active tissue like the brain and considered a marker of intracellular metabolism. As the fluctuation of Cr-levels tends to be limited, it is commonly used as an internal reference for the calculation of metabolite ratios [92]. Apart from the well-known metabolites, detection of the oncometabolite 2-hydroxyglutarate (2-HG) has gained increasing interest and attention in neuro-oncological research. Accumulation of 2-HG is associated with IDH1 mutation; examining the 2-HG peak (at 2.25 ppm) through MRS may provide a noninvasive approach for IDH genotype assessment, although it should be noted that both acquisition and post-processing for its detection are not straightforward due to the low concentration of 2-HG and its partial spectral overlap with other relevant chemical species like glutamate and glutamine [93, 94].

In clinical practice, proton MRS is less frequently adopted in the brain tumor imaging protocol than perfusion MRI to refine preoperative differential diagnosis, aid in tumor grading, or support treatment monitoring [13]. Differentiating between brain tumors and non-neoplastic lesions can be improved with proton MRS, as higher Cho- and lower NAA-levels typically manifest in brain tumors [95–97]. Within adult patients with glioma, increased Cho concentrations have been found to be associated with poorer overall survival and progression-free survival [98].

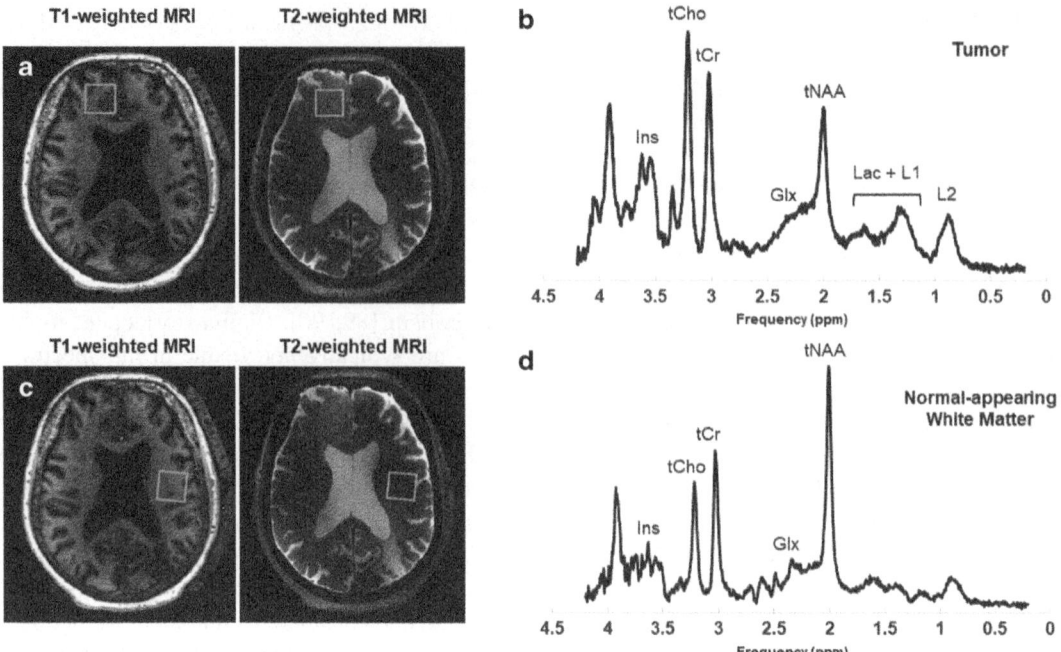

Fig. 2.7 Proton MRS of a patient (female, 76 years old) with a suspected oligodendroglioma. In the tumor region visible on structural MRI (**a**), a voxel of interest (*white square*) has been selected to probe the concentration of various metabolites in an MR spectrum (**b**). As a control, another voxel of interest has been selected in the contra-lateral normal-appearing white matter (**c**), demonstrating a different MR spectrum (**d**). Elevated levels of choline and a diminished NAA peak in the tumor region indicate neoplastic proliferation and disruption of the neuronal integrity, respectively. Dielectric pads were utilized to improve B_1 inhomogeneities (visible on the sides of the head on the T1-weighted MRI-scans). *tNAA:* total *N*-acetyl-aspartate, *Glx:* glutamate + glutamine, *tCr:* total creatine, *tCho:* choline compounds, *Ins:* myo-inositol. Data acquired on a 7 T MRI scanner (Philips Achieva, Best, The Netherlands). (Image courtesy of Bárbara Schmitz-Abecassis, Department of Radiology, Leiden University Medical Center)

Evaluation of Cho/Cr and Cho/NAA ratios and 2-HG concentrations may also help differentiation among tumors or tumor grading, but reliable interpretation of MRS on the individual level can be challenging due to lesion variability, intratumoral heterogeneity, and overlap between tumor types [99–101]. Preoperative proton MRS is therefore mostly used as a third-line diagnostic tool, an adjunct imaging technique that may add confidence to a non-invasive diagnosis based on conventional MRI and clinical presentation. Integrated in follow-up imaging, proton MRS could aid monitoring of disease, as increased Cho/NAA and Cho/Cr ratios are more likely to reflect true tumor recurrence rather than radiation necrosis [22, 54, 102, 103]. However, the timing of imaging should be taken into account; in the early stages following radiation treatment, the MR spectrum may depict metabolic changes sim-ilar to tumor recurrence. These changes can be attributed to radiation-induced inflammation or demyelination rather than true tumor progression [104].

By unraveling the metabolic characteristics of a lesion, proton MRS is a versatile MRI technique in the field of neuro-oncology. It provides complementary information and, particularly in a multiparametric approach, may support clinicians in treatment decision-making.

2.3.6 Emerging Techniques

Although still finding their way into clinical practice, emerging MRI techniques such as CEST imaging, qBOLD-MRI, ultra-high field MRI, and MR relaxometry, can be expected to substantially impact the field of neuro-oncology in the future.

2.3.6.1 CEST Imaging

Similar to proton MRS, CEST imaging leverages the fact that the resonance frequency of a proton can differ slightly depending on its location in a molecule. Specifically, this imaging technique targets certain chemical species that contain protons exchangeable with those of water molecules through *chemical exchange* [105]. To generate contrast in CEST imaging, a range of RF pulses is applied to selectively saturate the exchangeable protons of a chemical species of interest. When chemical exchange occurs with surrounding water molecules, the saturation effect is transferred to the free water pool, resulting in a reduction of the water signal. By repeating this process, the saturation effect accumulates in the free water pool, which can then be detected to indirectly examine the presence of the chemical species of interest. Various types of endogenous protons can be explored with CEST imaging, including those in amide, amine, and hydroxyl bonds. However, the CEST signal is also sensitive to other effects that either affect the chemical exchange rate, such as pH or temperature, or have effects on broad frequency ranges, such as the nuclear Overhauser enhancement from aliphatic and olefinic protons or magnetization transfer effects of semi-solids [106].

Among the different CEST techniques, amide proton transfer weighted (APTw) imaging is the most investigated technique for neuro-oncological application. APTw imaging targets the protons in amides (–NH), which may, in turn, reflect local levels of mobile proteins and peptides. Elevated APTw signal may be indicative of regions with increased Ki-67 expression and cellular proliferation [107–109], higher glioma grade [110], and tumor progression rather than treatment-related effects [111–115]. In vivo assessment of the microenvironment and metabolism through APTw imaging is promising for improved diagnosis and treatment of brain tumors, however, several hurdles are yet to be overcome before clinical implementation of the technique is viable. The exact mechanisms that contribute to the APTw signal, for instance, are still not fully understood. Considerable efforts from the CEST imaging research community to standardize APTw image acquisition for brain tumors have led to a consensus recommendation for the optimal implementation approach [116]. This work encourages both future multicenter and multi-vendor trials and may significantly aid in establishing the clinical value of APTw imaging for clinical practice.

2.3.6.2 qBOLD-MRI

Where task-based fMRI examines the relative BOLD effect to localize brain areas that are associated with specific activity, qBOLD-MRI uses a mathematical model to quantify regional tissue oxygenation [117, 118]. Particularly, the oxygen extraction fraction (OEF), defined as the ratio of oxygen used by brain tissue to oxygen delivered by inflowing blood, is commonly computed and combined with perfusion measurements to estimate in vivo oxygen metabolism (Fig. 2.8) [119]. While its value in clinical practice is yet to be determined [120], qBOLD-MRI shows promise for non-invasive examination of hypoxic regions in brain tumors [121] and may aid in the differentiation of glioblastoma from solitary brain metastasis [122], grading of glioma [123], and prediction of future tumor recurrence [124–127].

2.3.6.3 Ultra-High Field MRI

In clinical practice, MRI examinations are mainly performed at magnetic field strengths of 1.5 or 3.0 Tesla (T). Ultra-high field MRI, at 7.0 T and beyond, has been an active field of research, offering higher signal-to-noise ratios and exquisite spatial resolution (Fig. 2.9) [128]. Techniques such as MRS, CEST, and SWI, in particular, benefit from acquisition at higher field strengths, facilitating the discovery of promising novel MRI biomarkers for neuro-oncology [129]. A myriad of studies have illustrated the potential of ultra-high field MRI for neurological applications; within neuro-oncology, ultra-high field MRI may improve glioma grading, depiction of infiltrative tumor, and assessment of treatment response [130]. As a result, the clinical use of 7.0 T MRI systems for neurological applications was approved by the United States Food and Drug Administration in 2017 [131]. This milestone marks a significant step forward in neuro-

Fig. 2.8 Preoperative MRI acquisition of a patient (female, 68 years old) with multiple intracranial melanoma metastases. On both the post-contrast T1-weighted MRI-scan (**a**) and the skull stripped OEF-map (**b**) derived from qBOLD-MRI, two lesions can be seen in the right parietal and the right frontal lobe

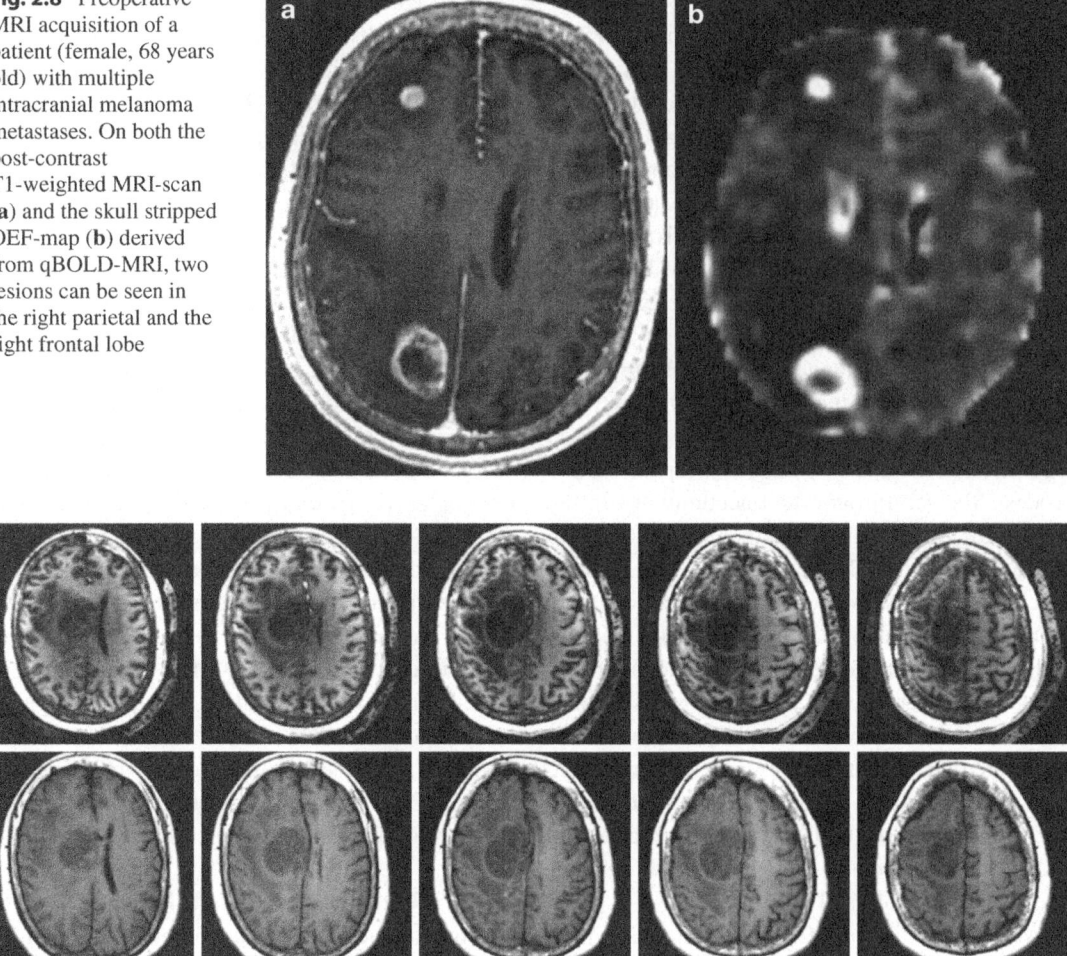

Fig. 2.9 T1-weighted MRI acquisition of a patient (female, 64 years old) with a glioblastoma, scanned on both a 7 T MRI scanner (*top row*)—Philips Achieva, Best, The Netherlands—and a 1.5 T MRI scanner (*bottom row*)—Siemens MAGNETOM Avanto, Erlangen, Germany. Dielectric pads were utilized to improve B_1 inhomogeneities (visible on the sides of the head). (Image courtesy of Bárbara Schmitz-Abecassis, Department of Radiology, Leiden University Medical Center)

oncological imaging, however, further research is needed to fully understand the clinical value of ultra-high field MRI and how to optimize its use to improve patient outcomes.

2.3.6.4 MR Relaxometry

Where conventional T1- and T2-weighted MRI can only be interpreted qualitatively, MR relaxometry enables quantitative mapping of the T1- and T2-relaxation times on which the conventional weighted images are based [132]. The implemen-

tation of relaxometry techniques into clinical practice was formerly hampered by their substantial acquisition times. However, novel approaches for rapid image acquisition, such as MR Fingerprinting (MRF) [133], or eloquent post-processing like synthetic MRI [134], which reconstructs all clinically relevant weighted scans from quantitative maps, are now finding their way to clinical practice. MR relaxometry holds promise for improved depiction of tumor infiltration [135–137] or shortened acquisition times [138] and, although still in its infancy, may open up new possibilities for more accurate brain tumor delineation or reduced patient burden.

2.4 The Future Role of MRI in Neuro-Oncology

Neuro-oncological imaging has advanced toward an era where anatomical imaging is regularly complemented by advanced imaging techniques that provide insights into microstructure, metabolism, and physiology. In addition to conventional MRI, techniques like DWI and DSC-MRI are now routinely acquired to offer enhanced tumor characterization and aid in treatment decision-making. Moreover, preoperative acquisition of DTI and fMRI can assist in the localization of white matter tracts and eloquent areas, respectively, providing valuable information for surgical planning. Further integration of other advanced MRI techniques into the field of neuro-oncology may pave the way toward reliable non-invasive assessment of tumor type and grade, enhanced visualization of tumor infiltration and intratumoral heterogeneity, and accurate differentiation between true tumor progression and treatment-related effects [7–10, 139]. In addition, advanced MRI offers new information that may result in a better general understanding of brain tumor biology and pathophysiology.

Combining different MRI techniques in a multiparametric approach may bring complementary information and overcome some of the technical limitations of individual techniques. The diagnostic performance of multiparametric MRI, however, may not be necessarily better than that from individual approaches [22, 140]. Additionally, a multiparametric approach can be time-consuming and requires local expertise on multiple advanced MRI techniques, making it difficult to adopt in clinical practice. Nevertheless, there is potential for multiparametric MRI, especially with the advent of artificial intelligence like radiomics [141].

The versatility that MRI brings, has led to the development of numerous advanced MRI techniques. While some techniques have already been

adopted in clinical practice, others are still being investigated to determine their added value for neuro-oncology. Effective collaborations between different institutes are essential for establishing consensus recommendations and international guidelines for acquisition and interpretation. With the potential to significantly improve preoperative diagnostics, focal treatment planning, and assessment of treatment response, advanced MRI may, in the near future, reshape the field of neuro-oncological imaging and, ultimately, lead to improved patient outcomes.

References

1. Lauterbur PC. Image formation by induced local interactions: examples employing nuclear magnetic resonance. Nature. 1973;242(5394):190–1. https://doi.org/10.1038/242190a0.
2. Bloch F, Hansen WW, Packard M. Nuclear induction. Phys Rev. 1946;69(3–4):127. https://doi.org/10.1103/PhysRev.69.127.
3. Ellingson BM, Bendszus M, Boxerman J, Barboriak D, Erickson BJ, Smits M, et al. Consensus recommendations for a standardized brain tumor imaging protocol in clinical trials. Neuro Oncol. 2015;17(9):1188–98. https://doi.org/10.1093/neuonc/nov095.
4. Yan PF, Yan L, Zhang Z, Salim A, Wang L, Hu TT, et al. Accuracy of conventional MRI for preoperative diagnosis of intracranial tumors: a retrospective cohort study of 762 cases. Int J Surg (London, England). 2016;36(Pt A):109–17. https://doi.org/10.1016/j.ijsu.2016.10.023.
5. Langen KJ, Galldiks N, Hattingen E, Shah NJ. Advances in neuro-oncology imaging. Nat Rev Neurol. 2017;13(5):279–89. https://doi.org/10.1038/nrneurol.2017.44.
6. Wen PY, Macdonald DR, Reardon DA, Cloughesy TF, Sorensen AG, Galanis E, et al. Updated response assessment criteria for high-grade gliomas: response assessment in neuro-oncology working group. J Clin Oncol. 2010;28(11):1963–72. https://doi.org/10.1200/jco.2009.26.3541.
7. Henriksen OM, Del Mar Á-TM, Figueiredo P, Hangel G, Keil VC, Nechifor RE, et al. High-grade glioma treatment response monitoring biomarkers: a position statement on the evidence supporting the use of advanced MRI techniques in the clinic, and the latest bench-to-bedside developments. Part 1: perfusion and diffusion techniques. Front Oncol. 2022;12:810263. https://doi.org/10.3389/fonc.2022.810263.
8. Booth TC, Wiegers EC, Warnert EAH, Schmainda KM, Riemer F, Nechifor RE, et al. High-grade

glioma treatment response monitoring biomarkers: a position statement on the evidence supporting the use of advanced MRI techniques in the clinic, and the latest bench-to-bedside developments. Part 2: spectroscopy, chemical exchange saturation, multiparametric imaging, and radiomics. Front Oncol. 2021;11:811425. https://doi.org/10.3389/fonc.2021.811425.

9. Hirschler L, Sollmann N, Schmitz-Abecassis B, Pinto J, Arzanforoosh F, Barkhof F, et al. Advanced MR techniques for preoperative glioma characterization: part 1. J Magn Reson Imaging. 2023;57:1655. https://doi.org/10.1002/jmri.28662.

10. Hangel G, Schmitz-Abecassis B, Sollmann N, Pinto J, Arzanforoosh F, Barkhof F, et al. Advanced MR techniques for preoperative glioma characterization: part 2. J Magn Reson Imaging. 2023;57:1676. https://doi.org/10.1002/jmri.28663.

11. Bammer R. Basic principles of diffusion-weighted imaging. Eur J Radiol. 2003;45(3):169–84. https://doi.org/10.1016/s0720-048x(02)00303-0.

12. Le Bihan D, Poupon C, Amadon A, Lethimonnier F. Artifacts and pitfalls in diffusion MRI. J Magn Reson Imaging. 2006;24(3):478–88. https://doi.org/10.1002/jmri.20683.

13. Thust SC, Heiland S, Falini A, Jäger HR, Waldman AD, Sundgren PC, et al. Glioma imaging in Europe: a survey of 220 centres and recommendations for best clinical practice. Eur Radiol. 2018;28(8):3306–17. https://doi.org/10.1007/s00330-018-5314-5.

14. Guo AC, Cummings TJ, Dash RC, Provenzale JM. Lymphomas and high-grade astrocytomas: comparison of water diffusibility and histologic characteristics. Radiology. 2002;224(1):177–83. https://doi.org/10.1148/radiol.2241010637.

15. Kitis O, Altay H, Calli C, Yunten N, Akalin T, Yurtseven T. Minimum apparent diffusion coefficients in the evaluation of brain tumors. Eur J Radiol. 2005;55(3):393–400. https://doi.org/10.1016/j.ejrad.2005.02.004.

16. Ahn SJ, Shin HJ, Chang JH, Lee SK. Differentiation between primary cerebral lymphoma and glioblastoma using the apparent diffusion coefficient: comparison of three different ROI methods. PLoS One. 2014;9(11):e112948. https://doi.org/10.1371/journal.pone.0112948.

17. Makino K, Hirai T, Nakamura H, Kuroda JI, Shinojima N, Uetani H, et al. Differentiating between primary central nervous system lymphomas and glioblastomas: combined use of perfusion-weighted and diffusion-weighted magnetic resonance imaging. World Neurosurg. 2018;112:e1–6. https://doi.org/10.1016/j.wneu.2017.10.141.

18. Neska-Matuszewska M, Bladowska J, Sąsiadek M, Zimny A. Differentiation of glioblastoma multiforme, metastases and primary central nervous system lymphomas using multiparametric perfusion and diffusion MR imaging of a tumor core and a peritumoral zone-searching for a practical approach. PLoS

One. 2018;13(1):e0191341. https://doi.org/10.1371/journal.pone.0191341.

19. Zhang S, Wang J, Wang K, Li X, Zhao X, Chen Q, et al. Differentiation of high-grade glioma and primary central nervous system lymphoma: multiparametric imaging of the enhancing tumor and peritumoral regions based on hybrid (18)F-FDG PET/MRI. Eur J Radiol. 2022;150:110235. https://doi.org/10.1016/j.ejrad.2022.110235.

20. Suh CH, Kim HS, Jung SC, Kim SJ. Diffusion-weighted imaging and diffusion tensor imaging for differentiating high-grade glioma from solitary brain metastasis: a systematic review and meta-analysis. AJNR Am J Neuroradiol. 2018;39(7):1208–14. https://doi.org/10.3174/ajnr.A5650.

21. Zulfiqar M, Yousem DM, Lai H. ADC values and prognosis of malignant astrocytomas: does lower ADC predict a worse prognosis independent of grade of tumor? A meta-analysis. AJR Am J Roentgenol. 2013;200(3):624–9. https://doi.org/10.2214/ajr.12.8679.

22. van Dijken BRJ, van Laar PJ, Holtman GA, van der Hoorn A. Diagnostic accuracy of magnetic resonance imaging techniques for treatment response evaluation in patients with high-grade glioma, a systematic review and meta-analysis. Eur Radiol. 2017;27(10):4129–44. https://doi.org/10.1007/s00330-017-4789-9.

23. Yu Y, Ma Y, Sun M, Jiang W, Yuan T, Tong D. Meta-analysis of the diagnostic performance of diffusion magnetic resonance imaging with apparent diffusion coefficient measurements for differentiating glioma recurrence from pseudoprogression. Medicine. 2020;99(23):e20270. https://doi.org/10.1097/md.0000000000020270.

24. Zhang L, Min Z, Tang M, Chen S, Lei X, Zhang X. The utility of diffusion MRI with quantitative ADC measurements for differentiating high-grade from low-grade cerebral gliomas: evidence from a meta-analysis. J Neurol Sci. 2017;373:9–15. https://doi.org/10.1016/j.jns.2016.12.008.

25. Suh CH, Kim HS, Jung SC, Choi CG, Kim SJ. Imaging prediction of isocitrate dehydrogenase (IDH) mutation in patients with glioma: a systemic review and meta-analysis. Eur Radiol. 2019;29(2):745–58. https://doi.org/10.1007/s00330-018-5608-7.

26. Wang QP, Lei DQ, Yuan Y, Xiong NX. Accuracy of ADC derived from DWI for differentiating high-grade from low-grade gliomas: systematic review and meta-analysis. Medicine. 2020;99(8):e19254. https://doi.org/10.1097/md.0000000000019254.

27. Hales PW, d'Arco F, Cooper J, Pfeuffer J, Hargrave D, Mankad K, et al. Arterial spin labelling and diffusion-weighted imaging in paediatric brain tumours. Neuroimage Clin. 2019;22:101696. https://doi.org/10.1016/j.nicl.2019.101696.

28. Kono K, Inoue Y, Nakayama K, Shakudo M, Morino M, Ohata K, et al. The role of diffusion-weighted

imaging in patients with brain tumors. AJNR Am J Neuroradiol. 2001;22(6):1081–8.

29. Fan GG, Deng QL, Wu ZH, Guo QY. Usefulness of diffusion/perfusion-weighted MRI in patients with non-enhancing supratentorial brain gliomas: a valuable tool to predict tumour grading? Br J Radiol. 2006;79(944):652–8. https://doi.org/10.1259/bjr/25349497.

30. Mori S, Zhang J. Principles of diffusion tensor imaging and its applications to basic neuroscience research. Neuron. 2006;51(5):527–39. https://doi.org/10.1016/j.neuron.2006.08.012.

31. Jiang R, Du FZ, He C, Gu M, Ke ZW, Li JH. The value of diffusion tensor imaging in differentiating high-grade gliomas from brain metastases: a systematic review and meta-analysis. PLoS One. 2014;9(11):e112550. https://doi.org/10.1371/journal.pone.0112550.

32. Miloushev VZ, Chow DS, Filippi CG. Meta-analysis of diffusion metrics for the prediction of tumor grade in gliomas. AJNR Am J Neuroradiol. 2015;36(2):302–8. https://doi.org/10.3174/ajnr.A4097.

33. Dimou S, Battisti RA, Hermens DF, Lagopoulos J. A systematic review of functional magnetic resonance imaging and diffusion tensor imaging modalities used in presurgical planning of brain tumour resection. Neurosurg Rev. 2013;36(2):205–14; discussion 14. https://doi.org/10.1007/s10143-012-0436-8.

34. Manan AA, Yahya N, Idris Z, Manan HA. The utilization of diffusion tensor imaging as an image-guided tool in brain tumor resection surgery: a systematic review. Cancers. 2022;14(10) https://doi.org/10.3390/cancers14102466.

35. Jensen JH, Helpern JA, Ramani A, Lu H, Kaczynski K. Diffusional kurtosis imaging: the quantification of non-gaussian water diffusion by means of magnetic resonance imaging. Magn Reson Med. 2005;53(6):1432–40. https://doi.org/10.1002/mrm.20508.

36. Falk Delgado A, Nilsson M, van Westen D, Falk Delgado A. Glioma grade discrimination with MR diffusion kurtosis imaging: a meta-analysis of diagnostic accuracy. Radiology. 2018;287(1):119–27. https://doi.org/10.1148/radiol.2017171315.

37. Abdalla G, Dixon L, Sanverdi E, Machado PM, Kwong JSW, Panovska-Griffiths J, et al. The diagnostic role of diffusional kurtosis imaging in glioma grading and differentiation of gliomas from other intra-axial brain tumours: a systematic review with critical appraisal and meta-analysis. Neuroradiology. 2020;62(7):791–802. https://doi.org/10.1007/s00234-020-02425-9.

38. Marrale M, Collura G, Brai M, Toschi N, Midiri F, La Tona G, et al. Physics, techniques and review of neuroradiological applications of diffusion kurtosis imaging (DKI). Clin Neuroradiol. 2016;26(4):391–403. https://doi.org/10.1007/s00062-015-0469-9.

39. Le Bihan D. What can we see with IVIM MRI? NeuroImage. 2019;187:56–67. https://doi.org/10.1016/j.neuroimage.2017.12.062.

40. Li WF, Niu C, Shakir TM, Chen T, Zhang M, Wang Z. An evidence-based approach to assess the accuracy of intravoxel incoherent motion imaging for the grading of brain tumors. Medicine. 2018;97(45):e13217. https://doi.org/10.1097/md.0000000000013217.

41. Shiroishi MS, Castellazzi G, Boxerman JL, D'Amore F, Essig M, Nguyen TB, et al. Principles of T2 *-weighted dynamic susceptibility contrast MRI technique in brain tumor imaging. J Magn Reson Imaging. 2015;41(2):296–313. https://doi.org/10.1002/jmri.24648.

42. Chavhan GB, Babyn PS, Thomas B, Shroff MM, Haacke EM. Principles, techniques, and applications of T2*-based MR imaging and its special applications. Radiographics. 2009;29(5):1433–49. https://doi.org/10.1148/rg.295095034.

43. Manfrini E, Smits M, Thust S, Geiger S, Bendella Z, Petr J, et al. From research to clinical practice: a European neuroradiological survey on quantitative advanced MRI implementation. Eur Radiol. 2021;31(8):6334–41. https://doi.org/10.1007/s00330-020-07582-2.

44. Schlegel U, Schmidt-Wolf IG, Deckert M. Primary CNS lymphoma: clinical presentation, pathological classification, molecular pathogenesis and treatment. J Neurol Sci. 2000;181(1–2):1–12. https://doi.org/10.1016/s0022-510x(00)00385-3.

45. Bhagavathi S, Wilson JD. Primary central nervous system lymphoma. Arch Pathol Lab Med. 2008;132(11):1830–4. https://doi.org/10.5858/132.11.1830.

46. Grommes C, DeAngelis LM. Primary CNS lymphoma. J Clin Oncol. 2017;35(21):2410–8. https://doi.org/10.1200/jco.2017.72.7602.

47. Xu W, Wang Q, Shao A, Xu B, Zhang J. The performance of MR perfusion-weighted imaging for the differentiation of high-grade glioma from primary central nervous system lymphoma: a systematic review and meta-analysis. PLoS One. 2017;12(3):e0173430. https://doi.org/10.1371/journal.pone.0173430.

48. Wu Y, Den Z, Lin Y. Accuracy of susceptibility-weighted imaging and dynamic susceptibility contrast magnetic resonance imaging for differentiating high-grade glioma from primary central nervous system lymphomas: meta-analysis. World Neurosurg. 2018;112:e617–23. https://doi.org/10.1016/j.wneu.2018.01.098.

49. Suh CH, Kim HS, Jung SC, Park JE, Choi CG, Kim SJ. MRI as a diagnostic biomarker for differentiating primary central nervous system lymphoma from glioblastoma: a systematic review and meta-analysis. J Magn Reson Imaging. 2019;50(2):560–72. https://doi.org/10.1002/jmri.26602.

50. Suh CH, Kim HS, Jung SC, Choi CG, Kim SJ. Perfusion MRI as a diagnostic biomarker for

differentiating glioma from brain metastasis: a systematic review and meta-analysis. Eur Radiol. 2018;28(9):3819–31. https://doi.org/10.1007/s00330-018-5335-0.

51. Delgado AF, Delgado AF. Discrimination between glioma grades II and III using dynamic susceptibility perfusion MRI: a meta-analysis. AJNR Am J Neuroradiol. 2017;38(7):1348–55. https://doi.org/10.3174/ajnr.A5218.

52. Liang J, Liu D, Gao P, Zhang D, Chen H, Shi C, et al. Diagnostic values of DCE-MRI and DSC-MRI for differentiation between high-grade and low-grade gliomas: a comprehensive meta-analysis. Acad Radiol. 2018;25(3):338–48. https://doi.org/10.1016/j.acra.2017.10.001.

53. van Santwijk L, Kouwenberg V, Meijer F, Smits M, Henssen D. A systematic review and meta-analysis on the differentiation of glioma grade and mutational status by use of perfusion-based magnetic resonance imaging. Insights Imaging. 2022;13(1):102. https://doi.org/10.1186/s13244-022-01230-7.

54. Chuang MT, Liu YS, Tsai YS, Chen YC, Wang CK. Differentiating radiation-induced necrosis from recurrent brain tumor using MR perfusion and spectroscopy: a meta-analysis. PLoS One. 2016;11(1):e0141438. https://doi.org/10.1371/journal.pone.0141438.

55. Patel P, Baradaran H, Delgado D, Askin G, Christos P, John Tsiouris A, et al. MR perfusion-weighted imaging in the evaluation of high-grade gliomas after treatment: a systematic review and meta-analysis. Neuro Oncol. 2017;19(1):118–27. https://doi.org/10.1093/neuonc/now148.

56. Wang L, Wei L, Wang J, Li N, Gao Y, Ma H, et al. Evaluation of perfusion MRI value for tumor progression assessment after glioma radiotherapy: a systematic review and meta-analysis. Medicine. 2020;99(52):e23766. https://doi.org/10.1097/md.0000000000023766.

57. Boxerman JL, Quarles CC, Hu LS, Erickson BJ, Gerstner ER, Smits M, et al. Consensus recommendations for a dynamic susceptibility contrast MRI protocol for use in high-grade gliomas. Neuro Oncol. 2020;22(9):1262–75. https://doi.org/10.1093/neuonc/noaa141.

58. Khalifa F, Soliman A, El-Baz A, Abou El-Ghar M, El-Diasty T, Gimel'farb G, et al. Models and methods for analyzing DCE-MRI: a review. Med Phys. 2014;41(12):124301. https://doi.org/10.1118/1.4898202.

59. Okuchi S, Rojas-Garcia A, Ulyte A, Lopez I, Ušinskienė J, Lewis M, et al. Diagnostic accuracy of dynamic contrast-enhanced perfusion MRI in stratifying gliomas: a systematic review and meta-analysis. Cancer Med. 2019;8(12):5564–73. https://doi.org/10.1002/cam4.2369.

60. Shukla-Dave A, Obuchowski NA, Chenevert TL, Jambawalikar S, Schwartz LH, Malyarenko D, et al. Quantitative imaging biomarkers alliance (QIBA) recommendations for improved precision of DWI and DCE-MRI derived biomarkers in multicenter oncology trials. J Magn Reson Imaging. 2019;49(7):e101–21. https://doi.org/10.1002/jmri.26518.

61. Alsop DC, Detre JA, Golay X, Günther M, Hendrikse J, Hernandez-Garcia L, et al. Recommended implementation of arterial spin-labeled perfusion MRI for clinical applications: a consensus of the ISMRM perfusion study group and the European consortium for ASL in dementia. Magn Reson Med. 2015;73(1):102–16. https://doi.org/10.1002/mrm.25197.

62. Ferré JC, Bannier E, Raoult H, Mineur G, Carsin-Nicol B, Gauvrit JY. Arterial spin labeling (ASL) perfusion: techniques and clinical use. Diagn Interv Imaging. 2013;94(12):1211–23. https://doi.org/10.1016/j.diii.2013.06.010.

63. You G, Wu H, Lei B, Wan X, Chen S, Zheng N. Diagnostic accuracy of arterial spin labeling in differentiating between primary central nervous system lymphoma and high-grade glioma: a systematic review and meta-analysis. Expert Rev Anticancer Ther. 2022;22(7):763–71. https://doi.org/10.1080/14737140.2022.2082948.

64. Kong L, Chen H, Yang Y, Chen L. A meta-analysis of arterial spin labelling perfusion values for the prediction of glioma grade. Clin Radiol. 2017;72(3):255–61. https://doi.org/10.1016/j.crad.2016.10.016.

65. Falk Delgado A, De Luca F, van Westen D, Falk DA. Arterial spin labeling MR imaging for differentiation between high- and low-grade glioma-a meta-analysis. Neuro Oncol. 2018;20(11):1450–61. https://doi.org/10.1093/neuonc/noy095.

66. Alsaedi A, Doniselli F, Jäger HR, Panovska-Griffiths J, Rojas-Garcia A, Golay X, et al. The value of arterial spin labelling in adults glioma grading: systematic review and meta-analysis. Oncotarget. 2019;10(16):1589–601. https://doi.org/10.18632/oncotarget.26674.

67. Delgado AF, De Luca F, Hanagandi P, van Westen D, Delgado AF. Arterial spin-labeling in children with brain tumor: a meta-analysis. AJNR Am J Neuroradiol. 2018;39(8):1536–42. https://doi.org/10.3174/ajnr.A5727.

68. Wan B, Wang S, Tu M, Wu B, Han P, Xu H. The diagnostic performance of perfusion MRI for differentiating glioma recurrence from pseudoprogression: a meta-analysis. Medicine. 2017;96(11):e6333. https://doi.org/10.1097/md.0000000000006333.

69. Liu Y, Chen G, Tang H, Hong L, Peng W, Zhang X. Systematic review and meta-analysis of arterial spin-labeling imaging to distinguish between glioma recurrence and post-treatment radiation effect. Ann Palliat Med. 2021;10(12):12488–97. https://doi.org/10.21037/apm-21-3319.

70. Zhang J, Wang Y, Wang Y, Xiao H, Chen X, Lei Y, et al. Perfusion magnetic resonance imaging in the differentiation between glioma recurrence and pseudoprogression: a systematic review, meta-analysis

and meta-regression. Quant Imaging Med Surg. 2022;12(10):4805–22. https://doi.org/10.21037/qims-22-32.

71. Wolf RL, Detre JA. Clinical neuroimaging using arterial spin-labeled perfusion magnetic resonance imaging. Neurotherapeutics. 2007;4(3):346–59. https://doi.org/10.1016/j.nurt.2007.04.005.

72. Jahng GH, Li KL, Ostergaard L, Calamante F. Perfusion magnetic resonance imaging: a comprehensive update on principles and techniques. Korean J Radiol. 2014;15(5):554–77. https://doi.org/10.3348/kjr.2014.15.5.554.

73. Ogawa S, Lee TM, Kay AR, Tank DW. Brain magnetic resonance imaging with contrast dependent on blood oxygenation. Proc Natl Acad Sci USA. 1990;87(24):9868–72. https://doi.org/10.1073/pnas.87.24.9868.

74. Logothetis NK. What we can do and what we cannot do with fMRI. Nature. 2008;453(7197):869–78. https://doi.org/10.1038/nature06976.

75. Stopa BM, Senders JT, Broekman MLD, Vangel M, Golby AJ. Preoperative functional MRI use in neurooncology patients: a clinician survey. Neurosurg Focus. 2020;48(2):E11. https://doi.org/10.3171/2019.11.Focus19779.

76. Bogomolny DL, Petrovich NM, Hou BL, Peck KK, Kim MJ, Holodny AI. Functional MRI in the brain tumor patient. Topics Magn Reson Imaging. 2004;15(5):325–35. https://doi.org/10.1097/00002142-200410000-00005.

77. Haacke EM, Xu Y, Cheng YC, Reichenbach JR. Susceptibility weighted imaging (SWI). Magn Reson Med. 2004;52(3):612–8. https://doi.org/10.1002/mrm.20198.

78. Mittal S, Wu Z, Neelavalli J, Haacke EM. Susceptibility-weighted imaging: technical aspects and clinical applications, part 2. AJNR Am J Neuroradiol. 2009;30(2):232–52. https://doi.org/10.3174/ajnr.A1461.

79. Park MJ, Kim HS, Jahng GH, Ryu CW, Park SM, Kim SY. Semiquantitative assessment of intratumoral susceptibility signals using non-contrast-enhanced high-field high-resolution susceptibility-weighted imaging in patients with gliomas: comparison with MR perfusion imaging. AJNR Am J Neuroradiol. 2009;30(7):1402–8. https://doi.org/10.3174/ajnr.A1593.

80. Li X, Zhu Y, Kang H, Zhang Y, Liang H, Wang S, et al. Glioma grading by microvascular permeability parameters derived from dynamic contrast-enhanced MRI and intratumoral susceptibility signal on susceptibility weighted imaging. Cancer Imaging. 2015;15(1):4. https://doi.org/10.1186/s40644-015-0039-z.

81. Kong LW, Chen J, Zhao H, Yao K, Fang SY, Wang Z, et al. Intratumoral susceptibility signals reflect biomarker status in gliomas. Sci Rep. 2019;9(1):17080. https://doi.org/10.1038/s41598-019-53629-w.

82. Schwarz D, Bendszus M, Breckwoldt MO. Clinical value of susceptibility weighted imaging of brain metastases. Front Neurol. 2020;11:55. https://doi.org/10.3389/fneur.2020.00055.

83. Fahrendorf D, Schwindt W, Wölfer J, Jeibmann A, Kooijman H, Kugel H, et al. Benefits of contrast-enhanced SWI in patients with glioblastoma multiforme. Eur Radiol. 2013;23(10):2868–79. https://doi.org/10.1007/s00330-013-2895-x.

84. Haller S, Haacke EM, Thurnher MM, Barkhof F. Susceptibility-weighted imaging: technical essentials and clinical neurologic applications. Radiology. 2021;299(1):3–26. https://doi.org/10.1148/radiol.2021203071.

85. Bertholdo D, Watcharakorn A, Castillo M. Brain proton magnetic resonance spectroscopy: introduction and overview. Neuroimaging Clin N Am. 2013;23(3):359–80. https://doi.org/10.1016/j.nic.2012.10.002.

86. Wilson M, Andronesi O, Barker PB, Bartha R, Bizzi A, Bolan PJ, et al. Methodological consensus on clinical proton MRS of the brain: review and recommendations. Magn Reson Med. 2019;82(2):527–50. https://doi.org/10.1002/mrm.27742.

87. Moffett JR, Ross B, Arun P, Madhavarao CN, Namboodiri AM. N-Acetylaspartate in the CNS: from neurodiagnostics to neurobiology. Prog Neurobiol. 2007;81(2):89–131. https://doi.org/10.1016/j.pneurobio.2006.12.003.

88. Miller BL, Chang L, Booth R, Ernst T, Cornford M, Nikas D, et al. In vivo 1H MRS choline: correlation with in vitro chemistry/histology. Life Sci. 1996;58(22):1929–35. https://doi.org/10.1016/0024-3205(96)00182-8.

89. Warburg O, Wind F, Negelein E. The metabolism of tumors in the body. J Gen Physiol. 1927;8(6):519–30. https://doi.org/10.1085/jgp.8.6.519.

90. Schupp DG, Merkle H, Ellermann JM, Ke Y, Garwood M. Localized detection of glioma glycolysis using edited 1H MRS. Magn Reson Med. 1993;30(1):18–27. https://doi.org/10.1002/mrm.1910300105.

91. Kuesel AC, Sutherland GR, Halliday W, Smith IC. 1H MRS of high grade astrocytomas: mobile lipid accumulation in necrotic tissue. NMR Biomed. 1994;7(3):149–55. https://doi.org/10.1002/nbm.1940070308.

92. Rackayova V, Cudalbu C, Pouwels PJW, Braissant O. Creatine in the central nervous system: from magnetic resonance spectroscopy to creatine deficiencies. Anal Biochem. 2017;529:144–57. https://doi.org/10.1016/j.ab.2016.11.007.

93. Dang L, White DW, Gross S, Bennett BD, Bittinger MA, Driggers EM, et al. Cancer-associated IDH1 mutations produce 2-hydroxyglutarate. Nature. 2009;462(7274):739–44. https://doi.org/10.1038/nature08617.

94. Berrington A, Voets NL, Larkin SJ, de Pennington N, McCullagh J, Stacey R, et al. A comparison of 2-hydroxyglutarate detection at 3 and 7 T with long-TE semi-LASER. NMR Biomed. 2018;31(3) https://doi.org/10.1002/nbm.3886.

95. Hourani R, Brant LJ, Rizk T, Weingart JD, Barker PB, Horská A. Can proton MR spectroscopic and perfusion imaging differentiate between neoplastic and nonneoplastic brain lesions in adults? AJNR Am J Neuroradiol. 2008;29(2):366–72. https://doi.org/10.3174/ajnr.A0810.

96. Lai PH, Weng HH, Chen CY, Hsu SS, Ding S, Ko CW, et al. In vivo differentiation of aerobic brain abscesses and necrotic glioblastomas multiforme using proton MR spectroscopic imaging. AJNR Am J Neuroradiol. 2008;29(8):1511–8. https://doi.org/10.3174/ajnr.A1130.

97. Majós C, Aguilera C, Alonso J, Julià-Sapé M, Castañer S, Sánchez JJ, et al. Proton MR spectroscopy improves discrimination between tumor and pseudotumoral lesion in solid brain masses. AJNR Am J Neuroradiol. 2009;30(3):544–51. https://doi.org/10.3174/ajnr.A1392.

98. Shi Y, Liu D, Kong Z, Liu Q, Xing H, Wang Y, et al. Prognostic value of choline and other metabolites measured using (1)H-magnetic resonance spectroscopy in gliomas: a meta-analysis and systemic review. Metabolites. 2022;12(12) https://doi.org/10.3390/metabo12121219.

99. Wang Q, Zhang H, Zhang J, Wu C, Zhu W, Li F, et al. The diagnostic performance of magnetic resonance spectroscopy in differentiating high-from low-grade gliomas: a systematic review and meta-analysis. Eur Radiol. 2016;26(8):2670–84. https://doi.org/10.1007/s00330-015-4046-z.

100. Suh CH, Kim HS, Jung SC, Choi CG, Kim SJ. 2-Hydroxyglutarate MR spectroscopy for prediction of isocitrate dehydrogenase mutant glioma: a systemic review and meta-analysis using individual patient data. Neuro Oncol. 2018;20(12):1573–83. https://doi.org/10.1093/neuonc/noy113.

101. Wang L, Chen G, Dai K. Hydrogen proton magnetic resonance spectroscopy (MRS) in differential diagnosis of intracranial tumors: a systematic review. Contrast Media Mol Imaging. 2022;2022:7242192. https://doi.org/10.1155/2022/7242192.

102. Zhang H, Ma L, Wang Q, Zheng X, Wu C, Xu BN. Role of magnetic resonance spectroscopy for the differentiation of recurrent glioma from radiation necrosis: a systematic review and meta-analysis. Eur J Radiol. 2014;83(12):2181–9. https://doi.org/10.1016/j.ejrad.2014.09.018.

103. Aseel A, McCarthy P, Mohammed A. Brain magnetic resonance spectroscopy to differentiate recurrent neoplasm from radiation necrosis: a systematic review and meta-analysis. J Neuroimaging. 2023;33(2):189–201. https://doi.org/10.1111/jon.13080.

104. Estève F, Rubin C, Grand S, Kolodié H, Le Bas JF. Transient metabolic changes observed with proton MR spectroscopy in normal human brain after radiation therapy. Int J Radiat Oncol Biol Phys. 1998;40(2):279–86. https://doi.org/10.1016/s0360-3016(97)00714-1.

105. Wu B, Warnock G, Zaiss M, Lin C, Chen M, Zhou Z, et al. An overview of CEST MRI for non-MR physicists. EJNMMI Phys. 2016;3(1):19. https://doi.org/10.1186/s40658-016-0155-2.

106. Jones KM, Pollard AC, Pagel MD. Clinical applications of chemical exchange saturation transfer (CEST) MRI. J Magn Reson Imaging. 2018;47(1):11–27. https://doi.org/10.1002/jmri.25838.

107. Togao O, Yoshiura T, Keupp J, Hiwatashi A, Yamashita K, Kikuchi K, et al. Amide proton transfer imaging of adult diffuse gliomas: correlation with histopathological grades. Neuro Oncol. 2014;16(3):441–8. https://doi.org/10.1093/neuonc/not158.

108. Su C, Liu C, Zhao L, Jiang J, Zhang J, Li S, et al. Amide proton transfer imaging allows detection of glioma grades and tumor proliferation: comparison with Ki-67 expression and proton MR spectroscopy imaging. AJNR Am J Neuroradiol. 2017;38(9):1702–9. https://doi.org/10.3174/ajnr.A5301.

109. Jiang S, Eberhart CG, Zhang Y, Heo HY, Wen Z, Blair L, et al. Amide proton transfer-weighted magnetic resonance image-guided stereotactic biopsy in patients with newly diagnosed gliomas. Eur J Cancer (Oxford, England: 1990). 2017;83:9–18. https://doi.org/10.1016/j.ejca.2017.06.009.

110. Sotirios B, Demetriou E, Topriceanu CC, Zakrzewska Z. The role of APT imaging in gliomas grading: a systematic review and meta-analysis. Eur J Radiol. 2020;133:109353. https://doi.org/10.1016/j.ejrad.2020.109353.

111. Park JE, Kim HS, Park KJ, Kim SJ, Kim JH, Smith SA. Pre- and posttreatment glioma: comparison of amide proton transfer imaging with MR spectroscopy for biomarkers of tumor proliferation. Radiology. 2016;278(2):514–23. https://doi.org/10.1148/radiol.2015142979.

112. Park JE, Lee JY, Kim HS, Oh JY, Jung SC, Kim SJ, et al. Amide proton transfer imaging seems to provide higher diagnostic performance in post-treatment high-grade gliomas than methionine positron emission tomography. Eur Radiol. 2018;28(8):3285–95. https://doi.org/10.1007/s00330-018-5341-2.

113. Jiang S, Eberhart CG, Lim M, Heo HY, Zhang Y, Blair L, et al. Identifying recurrent malignant glioma after treatment using amide proton transfer-weighted MR imaging: a validation study with image-guided stereotactic biopsy. Clin Cancer Res. 2019;25(2):552–61. https://doi.org/10.1158/1078-0432.Ccr-18-1233.

114. Ma B, Blakeley JO, Hong X, Zhang H, Jiang S, Blair L, et al. Applying amide proton transfer-weighted MRI to distinguish pseudoprogression from true progression in malignant gliomas. J Magn Reson Imaging. 2016;44(2):456–62. https://doi.org/10.1002/jmri.25159.

115. Park YW, Ahn SS, Kim EH, Kang SG, Chang JH, Kim SH, et al. Differentiation of recurrent diffuse glioma from treatment-induced change using amide

proton transfer imaging: incremental value to diffusion and perfusion parameters. Neuroradiology. 2021;63(3):363–72. https://doi.org/10.1007/s00234-020-02542-5.

116. Zhou J, Zaiss M, Knutsson L, Sun PZ, Ahn SS, Aime S, et al. Review and consensus recommendations on clinical APT-weighted imaging approaches at 3T: application to brain tumors. Magn Reson Med. 2022;88(2):546–74. https://doi.org/10.1002/mrm.29241.

117. He X, Yablonskiy DA. Quantitative BOLD: mapping of human cerebral deoxygenated blood volume and oxygen extraction fraction: default state. Magn Reson Med. 2007;57(1):115–26. https://doi.org/10.1002/mrm.21108.

118. Stone AJ, Blockley NP. A streamlined acquisition for mapping baseline brain oxygenation using quantitative BOLD. NeuroImage. 2017;147:79–88. https://doi.org/10.1016/j.neuroimage.2016.11.057.

119. Raichle ME, MacLeod AM, Snyder AZ, Powers WJ, Gusnard DA, Shulman GL. A default mode of brain function. Proc Natl Acad Sci USA. 2001;98(2):676–82. https://doi.org/10.1073/pnas.98.2.676.

120. Li H, Wang C, Yu X, Luo Y, Wang H. Measurement of cerebral oxygen extraction fraction using quantitative BOLD approach: a review. Phenomics (Cham, Switzerland). 2023;3(1):101–18. https://doi.org/10.1007/s43657-022-00081-y.

121. Tóth V, Förschler A, Hirsch NM, den Hollander J, Kooijman H, Gempt J, et al. MR-based hypoxia measures in human glioma. J Neurooncol. 2013;115(2):197–207. https://doi.org/10.1007/s11060-013-1210-7.

122. Heynold E, Zimmermann M, Hore N, Buchfelder M, Doerfler A, Stadlbauer A, et al. Physiological MRI biomarkers in the differentiation between glioblastomas and solitary brain metastases. Mol Imaging Biol. 2021;23(5):787–95. https://doi.org/10.1007/s11307-021-01604-1.

123. Stadlbauer A, Zimmermann M, Kitzwögerer M, Oberndorfer S, Rössler K, Dörfler A, et al. MR imaging-derived oxygen metabolism and neovascularization characterization for grading and IDH gene mutation detection of gliomas. Radiology. 2017;283(3):799–809. https://doi.org/10.1148/radiol.2016161422.

124. Stadlbauer A, Zimmermann M, Doerfler A, Oberndorfer S, Buchfelder M, Coras R, et al. Intratumoral heterogeneity of oxygen metabolism and neovascularization uncovers 2 survival-relevant subgroups of IDH1 wild-type glioblastoma. Neuro Oncol. 2018;20(11):1536–46. https://doi.org/10.1093/neuonc/noy066.

125. Stadlbauer A, Kinfe TM, Eyüpoglu I, Zimmermann M, Kitzwögerer M, Podar K, et al. Tissue hypoxia and alterations in microvascular architecture predict glioblastoma recurrence in humans. Clin Cancer Res. 2021;27(6):1641–9. https://doi.org/10.1158/1078-0432.Ccr-20-3580.

126. Stadlbauer A, Oberndorfer S, Heinz G, Zimmermann M, Kinfe TM, Doerfler A, et al. Hypoxia and microvascular alterations are early predictors of IDH-mutated anaplastic glioma recurrence. Cancers. 2021;13(8) https://doi.org/10.3390/cancers13081797.

127. Stadlbauer A, Heinz G, Oberndorfer S, Zimmermann M, Kinfe TM, Buchfelder M, et al. Physiological MRI of microvascular architecture, neovascularization activity, and oxygen metabolism facilitate early recurrence detection in patients with IDH-mutant WHO grade 3 glioma. Neuroradiology. 2022;64(2):265–77. https://doi.org/10.1007/s00234-021-02740-9.

128. Platt T, Ladd ME, Paech D. 7 Tesla and beyond: advanced methods and clinical applications in magnetic resonance imaging. Investig Radiol. 2021;56(11):705–25. https://doi.org/10.1097/rli.0000000000000820.

129. Ladd ME, Bachert P, Meyerspeer M, Moser E, Nagel AM, Norris DG, et al. Pros and cons of ultra-high-field MRI/MRS for human application. Prog Nucl Magn Reson Spectrosc. 2018;109:1–50. https://doi.org/10.1016/j.pnmrs.2018.06.001.

130. Shaffer A, Kwok SS, Naik A, Anderson AT, Lam F, Wszalek T, et al. Ultra-high-field MRI in the diagnosis and management of gliomas: a systematic review. Front Neurol. 2022;13:857825. https://doi.org/10.3389/fneur.2022.857825.

131. Barisano G, Sepehrband F, Ma S, Jann K, Cabeen R, Wang DJ, et al. Clinical 7 T MRI: are we there yet? A review about magnetic resonance imaging at ultra-high field. Br J Radiol. 2019;92(1094):20180492. https://doi.org/10.1259/bjr.20180492.

132. Cheng HL, Stikov N, Ghugre NR, Wright GA. Practical medical applications of quantitative MR relaxometry. J Magn Reson Imaging. 2012;36(4):805–24. https://doi.org/10.1002/jmri.23718.

133. Ma D, Gulani V, Seiberlich N, Liu K, Sunshine JL, Duerk JL, et al. Magnetic resonance fingerprinting. Nature. 2013;495(7440):187–92. https://doi.org/10.1038/nature11971.

134. Ji S, Yang D, Lee J, Choi SH, Kim H, Kang KM. Synthetic MRI: technologies and applications in neuroradiology. J Magn Reson Imaging. 2022;55(4):1013–25. https://doi.org/10.1002/jmri.27440.

135. Blystad I, Warntjes JBM, Smedby Ö, Lundberg P, Larsson EM, Tisell A. Quantitative MRI for analysis of peritumoral edema in malignant gliomas. PLoS One. 2017;12(5):e0177135. https://doi.org/10.1371/journal.pone.0177135.

136. Blystad I, Warntjes JBM, Smedby Ö, Lundberg P, Larsson EM, Tisell A. Quantitative MRI using relaxometry in malignant gliomas detects contrast enhancement in peritumoral oedema. Sci Rep. 2020;10(1):17986. https://doi.org/10.1038/s41598-020-75105-6.

137. Nöth U, Tichy J, Tritt S, Bähr O, Deichmann R, Hattingen E. Quantitative T1 mapping indicates tumor infiltration beyond the enhancing part of glioblastomas. NMR Biomed. 2020;33(3):e4242. https://doi.org/10.1002/nbm.4242.

138. Tanenbaum LN, Tsiouris AJ, Johnson AN, Naidich TP, DeLano MC, Melhem ER, et al. Synthetic MRI for clinical neuroimaging: results of the magnetic resonance image compilation (MAGiC) prospective, multicenter, multireader trial. AJNR Am J Neuroradiol. 2017;38(6):1103–10. https://doi.org/10.3174/ajnr.A5227.

139. Smits M. MRI biomarkers in neuro-oncology. Nat Rev Neurol. 2021;17(8):486–500. https://doi.org/10.1038/s41582-021-00510-y.

140. Suh CH, Kim HS, Jung SC, Choi CG, Kim SJ. Multiparametric MRI as a potential surrogate endpoint for decision-making in early treatment response following concurrent chemoradiotherapy in patients with newly diagnosed glioblastoma: a systematic review and meta-analysis. Eur Radiol. 2018;28(6):2628–38. https://doi.org/10.1007/s00330-017-5262-5.

141. Zhou M, Scott J, Chaudhury B, Hall L, Goldgof D, Yeom KW, et al. Radiomics in brain tumor: image assessment, quantitative feature descriptors, and machine-learning approaches. AJNR Am J Neuroradiol. 2018;39(2):208–16. https://doi.org/10.3174/ajnr.A5391.

Positron Emission Tomography from FDG to Amino Acid Tracers

3

Arnoldo Piccardo, Valentina Garibotto,
Angelo Castello, Francesco Cicone,
Francesco Giammarile, Luigia Florimonte,
Roberto C. Delgado Bolton, Luigi Mansi,
and Egesta Lopci

3.1 Imaging Brain Tumors with PET

Brain tumors, i.e., tumors of the central nervous system (CNS), include both primary lesions and metastases to the CNS.

Primary CNS tumors are rare tumors, with an approximate incidence of 12 per 100,000 persons per year [1]. The most common malignant primary tumor is glioblastoma (15% of primary CNS tumors), followed by primary CNS lymphomas, while the most common benign tumors are meningiomas (38% of primary CNS tumors).

The latest World Health Organisation (WHO) classification of primary brain tumors published in 2021 classifies gliomas on the basis of their combined genetic and histological characteristics, as first introduced in the 2016 edition, and distinguishes adult-type diffuse gliomas, pediatric-type diffuse low-grade gliomas,

A. Piccardo
Department of Nuclear Medicine, Galliera Hospital, Genoa, Italy
e-mail: arnoldo.piccardo@galliera.it

V. Garibotto
Division of Nuclear Medicine and Molecular Imaging, Geneva University Hospitals, Geneva, Switzerland

NIMTLab, Geneva University, Geneva, Switzerland
e-mail: valentina.garibotto@hcuge.ch

A. Castello · L. Florimonte
Nuclear Medicine Unit, Fondazione IRCCS Ca' Granda, Ospedale Maggiore Policlinico, Milan, Italy
e-mail: angelo.castello@policlinico.mi.it;
luigia.florimonte@policlinico.mi.it

F. Cicone
Department of Experimental and Clinical Medicine, Neuroscience Research Centre, PET/RM Unit, "Magna Graecia" University of Catanzaro, Catanzaro, Italy

Nuclear Medicine Unit, University Hospital "Mater Domini", Catanzaro, Italy
e-mail: cicone@unicz.it

F. Giammarile
Nuclear Medicine and Diagnostic Imaging Section, Division of Human Health, Department of Nuclear Sciences and Applications, International Atomic Energy Agency (IAEA), Vienna, Austria
e-mail: f.giammarile@iaea.org

R. C. Delgado Bolton
Department of Diagnostic Imaging (Radiology) and Nuclear Medicine, University Hospital San Pedro, Centre for Biomedical Research of La Rioja (CIBIR), Logroño, Spain

Servicio Cántabro de Salud, Santander, Spain
e-mail: robertocarlos.delgado@scsalud.es

L. Mansi
Section Health and Development, Interuniversity Research Center for Sustainable Development (CIRPS), Napoli, Italy
e-mail: Luigi.MANSI@unicampania.it

E. Lopci (✉)
Nuclear Medicine Unit, IRCCS-Humanitas Research Hospital, Rozzano, Milano, Italy
e-mail: egesta.lopci@humanitas.it

pediatric-type diffuse high-grade gliomas, and circumscribed astrocytic gliomas [2]. Emphasis is added to the identification of mutations also beyond isocitrate dehydrogenase 1 (IDH1) in diffuse gliomas, especially in young patients below 55 years of age.

Brain metastases are more than ten times more frequent than primary CNS tumors and mainly associated with lung cancer, breast cancer, and melanoma [3].

The routine workup of brain lesions is based on MRI, which is recommended to complement the evaluation of lesions identified during a systemic workup (with CT or PET/CT) for a primary tumor or during the investigations related to the presence of symptoms possibly related to intracerebral masses. MRI shows an excellent tissue contrast and identifies lesion characteristics and extension, including cellularity and tissue infiltration, as well as blood-brain barrier (BBB) leakage evaluating contrast enhancement. Advanced MR imaging includes diffusion tensor imaging and spectroscopy, for example, allowing a multiparametric tissue characterization [4].

There are however a number of specific indications in which molecular imaging might be of help, namely differential diagnosis of benign lesions and post-treatment changes from malignant lesions, biopsy targeting and tumor grading, and the definition of tumor extent in a pre-surgical or pre-radiation therapy setting. One of the main advantages of PET imaging is that the most frequently used radiopharmaceutical influx is independent of the BBB integrity [5].

Among PET radiopharmaceuticals, 2-deoxy-2-[^{18}F]fluoro-D-glucose (2-[^{18}F]FDG) remains by far the most largely used in oncology. The rational for its use is based on the large energy requirement of malignant cells, and brain metastases and high-grade primary brain tumors are no exception. The increased glycolytic metabolism of the cells induces overexpression of GLUT-1 transporters and hexokinase, which determines the increased 2-[^{18}F]FDG uptake and intracellular trapping.

Silent brain lesions can be identified on the brain acquisition during whole body 2-[^{18}F]FDG PET investigations, highlighting the importance of including the whole brain in oncological FDG acquisitions [6].

However, the brain tissue is physiologically characterized by a high density of GLUT-3 transporters on neurons and glial cells, namely astrocytes, determining the high tissue background that limits the applicability of 2-[^{18}F]FDG PET imaging to detect and characterize brain lesions. In addition, some inflammatory lesions in the brain might exhibit high 2-[^{18}F]FDG uptake [7].

This represents an issue mainly for low-grade lesions/tumors, in which FDG uptake is close to or lower than the physiologic uptake by the white matter [8, 9]. The ability of 2-[^{18}F]FDG PET to provide information associated with the grade of brain lesions and an associated worse prognosis and disease progression is thus well established [8, 10, 11]. The association of 2-[^{18}F]FDG uptake and tumor grade could also support its use to select the site for biopsy targeting, as tumor prognosis is obviously guided by its highest grade component. However, the definition of specific thresholds to distinguish high and low-grade gliomas is hindered by the fact that there is a large overlap in 2-[^{18}F]FDG uptake of these two categories [12]. In addition, there are relevant exceptions of low-grade tumors with high 2-[^{18}F]FDG uptake, namely pilocyic astrocytomas [13].

2-[^{18}F]FDG PET is typically positive in case of recurrence of a high-grade tumor (primary tumor or metastases) (Fig. 3.1) while negative in case of post-radiation therapy changes, with variable sensitivity and specificity values reported in the literature [14, 15]. The reference tissue to define positive or negative uptake is usually the normal brain tissue, considering negative lesions with an uptake inferior or equal to the white matter uptake and positive lesions with an uptake higher than the cortex. This clearly leaves a large undetermined range for lesions with an uptake intermediate between white and gray matter that can ultimately be recurrent tumor, radiation necrosis, or a combination of both [12]. Some authors have suggested the use of dual-phase acquisitions for this purpose, with variable intervals between the two phases, ranging from 2 h to more than 5 h, and thus with limited applicability [16].

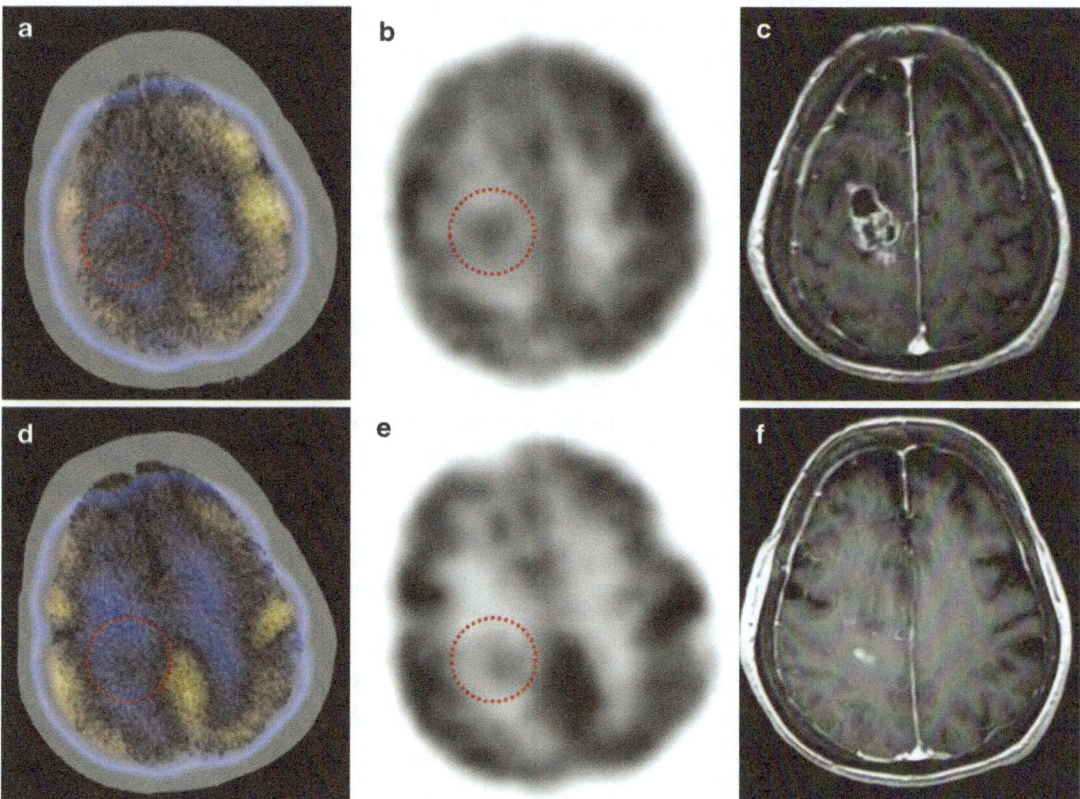

Fig. 3.1 Patient with suspected glioblastoma (GBM) and previous breast cancer investigated with 2-[^{18}F]FDG PET (**a, d**, fused PET/CT; **b, e**, axial PET) and Gd-enhanced MRI (**c, f**). Note the very faint uptake in the right subcorti- cal frontal region highlighted with the red circle (**a, b, d, e**), corresponding to the circumscribed area of enhancement on RMN (**c, f**)

The performance of 2-[^{18}F]FDG PET for this indication has overall been shown to be inferior to other imaging methods, such as amino acid PET and advanced MRI [17].

Finally, 2-[^{18}F]FDG PET might be one of the best molecular imaging modalities for the investigation of suspected primary brain lymphomas. Brain lymphoma is characteristically strongly FDG-avid, and this feature has the potential to distinguish them not only from non-tumoral lesions but also from high-grade gliomas and brain metastases [18]. 2-[^{18}F]FDG PET can also distinguish lymphoma from opportunistic infections in immunocompromised patients, with a better performance than SPECT or MR spectroscopy [19]. 2-[^{18}F]FDG PET can also be of help for the evaluation of the response in primary CNS lymphomas to chemotherapy, namely because of the high negative predictive value of interim 2-[^{18}F]FDG PET, that could thus be of added value in determining the duration for induction therapy, namely in those patients not achieving a complete response on MRI [5]. Importantly, current recommendations from the International Primary CNS Lymphoma Collaborative group recommend a whole-body 2-[^{18}F]FDG PET examination in patients with lymphomatous brain lesions, in order to identify systemic lymphomas [20].

2-[^{18}F]FDG PET imaging can be acquired in static modality, with an acquisition starting 45 min after tracer administration following standard recommendations, or dynamically, with the acquisition starting at injection and lasting 60 min [12, 21].

A dynamic acquisition allows measuring additional parameters, namely the regional metabolic rate (MRglu), which is a more accurate estimate of glucose consumption in the tissue than the standardized uptake value (SUV), which can be assessed with a static acquisition [12]. Discrepancies between SUV and MRglu are mainly observed during and after therapy, as treatments can change the relative equilibrium of the radiopharmaceutical between the circulating and tissular compartments. Thus a dynamic investigation is recommended when testing novel treatments, whose impact on tracer availability is unknown. There is currently no indication in which dynamic scanning for 2-[18F]FDG PET imaging for brain lesions has been proven to be superior to static scanning.

Overall, although 2-[18F]FDG PET has established diagnostic and prognostic abilities in brain tumors with intense 2-[18F]FDG uptake and in the context of tumor recurrence, in current guidelines there is no specific indication in which 2-[18F]FDG PET is preferred over amino acid PET imaging [12, 17, 21, 22].

3.2   The Role of [11C]MET in Primitive and Secondary Brain Tumors

The use of radiolabelled amino acids has emerged as an essential tool for detecting and characterizing brain tumors. Amino acid tracers are particularly accurate for the distinction between tumor recurrence and radiation necrosis, which represents the single most common indication in the clinical management of brain tumor patients. In particular, methyl-11C-L-methionine ([11C]MET) is an example of radiopharmaceuticals utilized for brain tumors imaging, since cancer cells present an overexpressed amino acid transporter systems, resulting in altered tumor vasculature and

tumor cell proliferation [12]. This overexpression allows for radiolabelled amino acids, including [11C]MET, 2-[18F]fluoroethyl)-L-tyrosine ([18F]FET), and 3,4-dihydroxy-6-[18F]fluoro-L-phenylalanine ([18F]DOPA), to achieve a superior target-to-background ratio compared to 2-[18F]FDG in the diagnosis of brain tumors [12, 23, 24].

Methionine uptake primarily occurs through a sodium-independent transporter that facilitates the movement of the amino acid into cells [25]. This transport process is driven by a concentration gradient and is influenced by the amino acid's metabolism within cells, which is directly linked to cellular proliferation. Studies have demonstrated that tumors of various types avidly accumulate methionine [26]. Subsequent to administration, methionine uptake in the brain is generally low, varying depending on the anatomical region and age [27, 28]. This, combined with high tumor uptake, highlights the potential of methionine for imaging brain tumors, offering the prospect of enhanced tumor detection and lesion delineation [29]. The underlying contrast between tumors and normal brain tissue on methionine imaging appears to be attributed to an augmented amino acid transport mechanism. Various subtypes of amino acid transporter systems have been identified, including LAT1, LAT2, and LAT3, each mediating L-transport. Interestingly, one of these subtypes (LAT2) is expressed specifically in tumor cells but not in inflammatory cells [30].

Amino acid brain tumor imaging, comprising [11C]MET, can be employed for various diagnostic and therapeutic purposes [12]. In accordance with the Joint EANM/EANO/RANO practice guidelines/SNMMI procedure standards [12], most common indications for PET imaging in primary brain tumors can be summarized in Table 3.1.

Table 3.1 Principal indications of amino acid PET tracers for imaging primary brain tumors

Timing	Indication
At primary diagnosis	Differentiation of grade III and IV tumors from not neoplastic lesions or grade I and II gliomas
	Prognostication of gliomas
	Definition of the optimal biopsy site (e.g., site of maximum tracer uptake)
	Delineation of tumor extent for surgery and radiotherapy planning
Diagnosis of tumor recurrence	Differentiation of glioma recurrence from treatment-induced changes, e.g., pseudoprogression and radionecrosis
Disease and therapy monitoring	Assessment of response after local or systemic treatment

3.2.1 [^{11}C]MET PET in Primary Gliomas Diagnosis

Numerous studies have assessed the diagnostic accuracy of [^{11}C]MET PET in differentiating presumed gliomas (Fig. 3.2). Overall, sensitivities ranging from 76% to 100% were observed, encompassing both low-grade and high-grade gliomas [31–41]. Notably, sensitivity tended to be lower in studies with a higher proportion of low-grade gliomas. For instance, the study by Herholz et al. exhibiting the lowest sensitivity involved a majority of patients suspected of harboring low-grade gliomas [36]. Alongside the generally satisfactory sensitivities reported, [^{11}C]MET PET has demonstrated remarkable specificity in distinguishing non-tumoral brain lesions from gliomas, ranging from 75% to 100% [32–34, 36, 38, 39, 42, 43]. Nevertheless, false-positive findings have been encountered in certain studies, including necrosis, leucoencephalitis, brain abscesses, hematoma, ischemia, and demyelination.

Of paramount importance to clinicians is the overall diagnostic accuracy, which has only been reported in studies by Herholz et al. [36] (79%), Yamane et al. [43] (81%), and Li et al. [39] (86%). Braun et al. [32] obtained a high positive predictive value of 96% but a low negative predictive value of 43%. Yamane et al. made an important observation by examining the planned therapy prior to the scan and the final treatment following the scan results. In 20 patients with suspected gliomas, the scan outcomes altered the initial management strategy in 63% [43].

Generally, [^{11}C]MET uptake is lower in low-grade gliomas compared to high-grade gliomas, although significant overlap exists between the two groups. Most studies employed a T/N ratio to determine sensitivity and specificity. However, the cut-off ratios employed varied from 1.3 to 2.05 [25, 31, 34, 38, 39] (Table 3.2).

The prevailing opinion among experts is that [^{11}C]MET PET is superior to 2-[^{18}F]FDG PET for imaging brain tumors and metastases. [^{11}C]MET PET offers greater sensitivity compared to 2-[^{18}F]FDG PET, particularly in low-grade gliomas [44]. Observed sensitivity of 100% was reported for [^{11}C]MET PET compared to 40% for 2-[^{18}F]FDG [45].

[^{11}C]MET PET consistently demonstrates superior diagnostic accuracy compared to [^{18}F]FET PET in gliomas, particularly for low-grade gliomas. Studies have reported sensitivities for [^{11}C]MET PET ranging from 76% to 100% in low-grade gliomas, while [^{18}F]FET PET sensitivities typically range from 60% to 80% [31–41]. Additionally, [^{11}C]MET PET is superior to [^{18}F]DOPA PET whose sensitivities range from 70% to 80% [36, 38, 41]. This enhanced

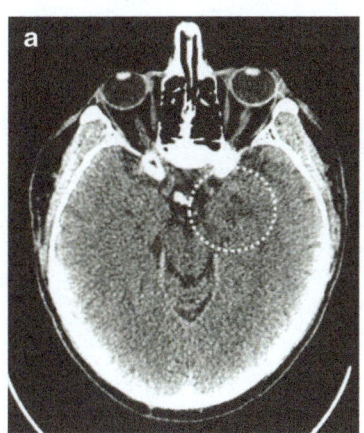 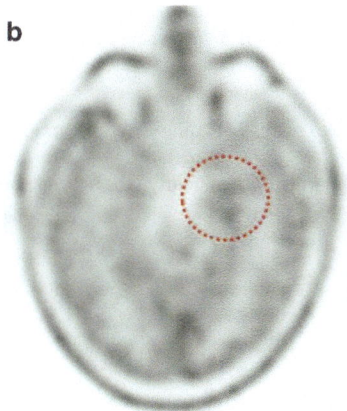 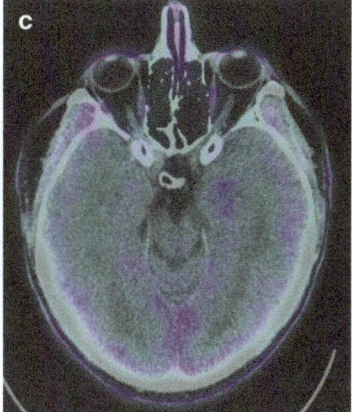

Fig. 3.2 Patient with focal cortical dysplasia on the left temporal lobe, highlighted with the red circle on [^{11}C]MET PET/CT (SUVmax 1.5; SUVratio 1.15): (**a**) axial low-dose CT, (**b**) axial [^{11}C]MET PET, and (**c**) fused PET/CT axial image of the lesion

Table 3.2 Commonly used thresholds for amino acid PET, validated histologically or clinically, according to the clinical question

Clinical indications	Tracers	Variables		Thresholds
Differentiation between neoplastic and non-neoplastic tissue	[^{18}F]FET	TBRmax		2.5
		TBRmean		1.9
	[^{11}C]MET	TBRmax		1.3–1.5
	[^{18}F]DOPA	–		n.a.
Tumor grading (grade I/II versus III/IV glioma)	[^{18}F]FET	TBRmean		1.9–2.0
		TBRmax		2.5–2.7
		TTP		<35 min
		TAC pattern (I, II, III)		Pattern II, III
Tumor extent	[^{18}F]FET	TBR		1.6
	[^{11}C]MET	TBR		1.3
	[^{18}F]DOPA	TBR		2.0
Tumor recurrence	[^{18}F]FET	TBRmean (circular ROI diameter 1.6 cm)		2.0
		TTP		<45 min
	[^{11}C]MET	TBRmax		1.6
	[^{18}F]DOPA	TSRmax		2.1
		TSRmean		1.8
Malignant transformation of grade I/II glioma	[^{18}F]FET	TBRmax		>33% increase
		TBRmean		>13% increase
		TTP change in ROI >1.6 brain		6 min decrease
Differentiation between *early* pseudoprogression and true progression	[^{18}F]FET	TBRmax		2.3
Differentiation between *late* pseudoprogression and true progression	[^{18}F]FET	TBRmax		1.9
		TBRmean		1.9
Identification of responders in treatment response evaluation	[^{18}F]FET	Radiochemotherapy (7–10 days)	TBRmax	>20% decrease
			TBRmean	>5% decrease
		Bevacizumab/irinotecan (4–12 weeks)	BTV	>45% decrease
	[^{11}C]MET	Temozolomide	TBRmax	Stable or decreasing
	[^{18}F]DOPA	Bevacizumab (2 weeks)	BTV	>35% decrease
				<18 mL

TBR tumor to background ratio, *TTP* time to peak, *TAC* time-activity curve, *TSR* tumor to striatum ratio, *ROI* region of interest

Modified from Law I et al. [12] under the terms of the Creative Commons Attribution 4.0 International License (http://creativecommons.org/licenses/by/4.0/)

sensitivity of [^{11}C]MET PET stems from its avid uptake by proliferating cells, which are more prevalent in low-grade gliomas.

3.2.2 Prognosis of Patients with Primary Gliomas

Conventionally accepted prognostic factors for glioma patients include tumor grade, age, performance status, proliferation indices, like Ki-67, and molecular status. In this context, [^{11}C]MET PET has been shown to be an independent prognostic factor in gliomas, while the prognostic value of [^{18}F]FET PET and [^{18}F]DOPA PET is less well-established. Smits et al. observed that patients with high-risk low-grade glioma and high [^{11}C]MET uptake exhibited a poorer prognosis compared to those with high-risk glioma and low [^{11}C]MET uptake, implying the potential of [^{11}C]MET PET for prognostication [25, 46]. Nariai et al. established a significant correlation between survival and pretreatment tumor-to-normal (T/N) ratio [47]. Kim et al. corroborated these findings, concluding that [^{11}C]MET PET acts as an independent prognostic factor and may be employed as a biological prognostic marker [48]. Ribom et al.'s study revealed that baseline [^{11}C]MET PET is a prognostic indicator in low-grade glioma patients, further emphasizing its importance in survival prediction [49]. They also

determined that [^{11}C]MET uptake plays a crucial role in determining survival in astrocytoma and oligodendroglioma patients. Kaschten et al. also supported the prognostic value of [^{11}C]MET PET [50]. However, this study involved a heterogeneous patient population. Only a single study to date has challenged the prognostic significance of [^{11}C]MET PET, suggesting its lack of meaningful prognostic value [25, 51].

3.2.3 Assessment of Tumor Extent, Biopsy, and Radiotherapy Planning

Brain tumors exhibit a heterogeneous distribution of malignancy grades and necrosis within their solid mass. Reliance on MRI alone for biopsy planning can lead to inadequate tissue samples and inaccurate tumor grading. Consequently, advanced imaging techniques are crucial to delineate tumor extent more precisely, identify optimal biopsy targets, and pinpoint areas with heightened recurrence risk [52]. Numerous studies have demonstrated the incremental value of [^{11}C]MET PET in biopsy planning.

It is also well-established that CT and MRI can underestimate the true extent of gliomas in patients, especially in the context of radiotherapy planning [53] (Fig. 3.3). This can lead to an increased risk of radiation necrosis, which can

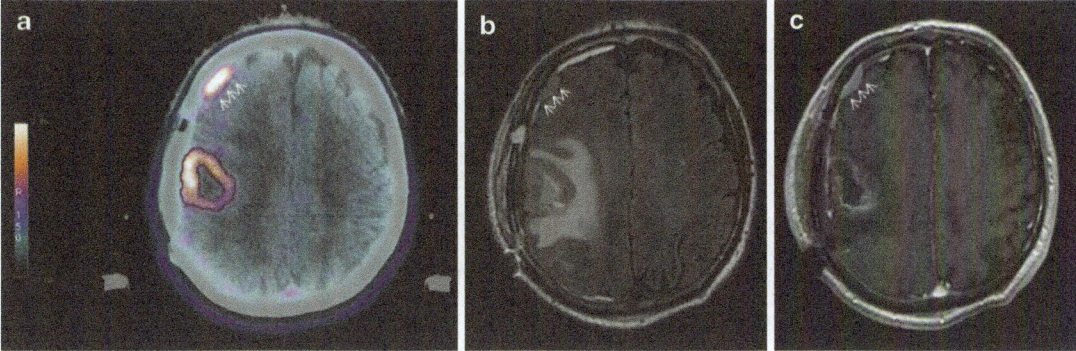

Fig. 3.3 Patient with a diagnosis of glioblastoma (GBM) investigated with [^{11}C]MET PET/CT (**a**), and MRI (**b**, T2w-FLAIR; **c**, Gd-enhanced) before radiotherapy planning. Note the contoured lesion of the right fronto-parietal region (SUVmax 7.2; SUVratio 4.8) presenting with central necrosis. The white arrows indicating the right frontal region highlight the presence of a meningioma

occur in up to 24% of patients [54]. [¹¹C]MET PET has been shown to be superior to other imaging modalities in delineating tumor extent. Pretreatment [¹¹C]MET PET appears to identify areas at highest risk of recurrence, making it a valuable tool for radiation treatment planning [52]. [¹¹C]MET PET significantly improves tumor volume definition in 88% of low-grade and 78% of high-grade gliomas [55]. Multiple studies, involving both low-grade and high-grade tumors, have demonstrated that MET PET is more accurate than CT or MRI in outlining the tumor volume [25]. Voges et al. found that the spatial extent of increased methionine uptake on [¹¹C]MET PET was larger than on CT/MRI images in 67% of cases and equal in 33% [56].

3.2.4 [¹¹C]MET PET in Brain Tumor Recurrence

Challenges arise in distinguishing between recurrent tumors and radiation necrosis in post-treatment/post-irradiation images. CT/MRI patterns can mimic both conditions, as they both involve disruption of the blood-brain barrier. To address this issue, extensive research has been conducted on the use of [¹¹C]MET PET to differentiate between recurrent tumors and radiation necrosis (Fig. 3.4). Comprehensive investigations into the performance of [¹¹C]MET PET for detecting recurrent gliomas have yielded valuable insights. Different T/N cut-off ratios have been employed to establish this association. Tripathi et al. [57] utilized a cut-off ratio of >1.9, achieving high sensitivity and specificity, along with excellent inter-observer agreement. Terakawa et al. [58] achieved optimal sensitivity and specificity utilizing a T/N ratio of 1.58 (by SUVmean). Okamoto et al. [59] observed a statistically significant elevation in the T/N ratio in recurrent tumors (1.98 ± 0.62) compared to radiation necrosis (1.27 ± 0.28), demonstrating its diagnostic value even for small lesions exhibiting a partial volume effect. Yamane et al. [43] reported a change in intended management in 45% of patients following [¹¹C]MET PET evaluation. Van Laere et al. [60] assessed 30 patients with treated gliomas, demonstrating positivity in 28 cases. Inter-observer agree-

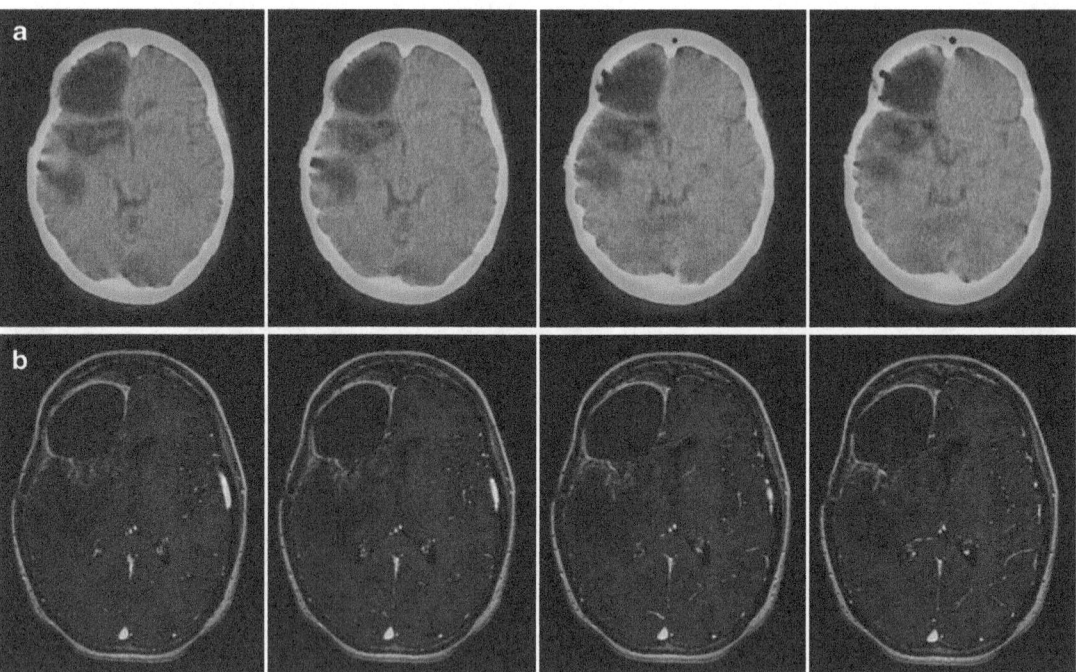

Fig. 3.4 Patient with relapsed glioblastoma (GBM) of the right frontal lobe (SUVmax 3.2; SUVratio 1.7) circumscribed to the posterior portion of the operating cavity (**a**, fused axial PET/CT) as shown also by the Gd-enhanced MRI (**b**)

ment was 100%, and [^{11}C]MET PET emerged as the strongest prognostic predictor in a subgroup of 23 patients with astrocytoma. A meta-analysis of 29 studies [61], involving 899 scans, demonstrated that [^{11}C]MET PET displayed a remarkable level of diagnostic accuracy (AUC = 0.9352) in identifying recurrent tumors, regardless of glioma grade, study design, or reference standard. Specificity and sensitivity were reported to be 0.88 (95% CI: 0.85, 0.91) and 0.85 (95% CI: 0.80, 0.89), respectively, with an area under the curve (AUC) for the summary receiver-operating characteristic curve (SROC) of 0.9352. These findings highlight the effectiveness of [^{11}C]MET PET in accurately detecting recurrent gliomas across diverse clinical scenarios [61–64].

3.2.5 [^{11}C]MET in Secondary Brain Tumors

While contrast-enhanced MRI remains the preferred imaging modality for diagnosing brain metastases, limited literature suggests that [^{11}C]MET PET may play a role in guiding therapy rather than detection [25]. Terakawa et al. [58] found that patients with recurrent metastatic brain tumors exhibited lower T/N ratios compared to those with recurrent gliomas. Grosu et al. [65] corroborated these findings, reporting a mean T/N ratio of 2.6 ± 0.9 in treated glioma patients and 1.8 ± 0.2 in treated metastatic brain tumor patients. Other studies have investigated the ability of [^{11}C]MET PET to differentiate between recurrent metastatic disease and radiation necrosis [65–67]. Similar to gliomas, [^{11}C]MET PET demonstrated its utility in this distinction. Yamane et al. achieved a high diagnostic accuracy for this differentiation in 30 patients with treated metastatic brain tumors (and 88% in 39 patients with treated glioma) [25, 43].

However, depending on where the metastases come from, other radiotracers can also be useful. 2-[^{18}F]FDG is useful in high-grade tumors and tumors with highly increased glucose metabolism, such as melanoma [68, 69]. In brain metastases from neuroendocrine tumors, [^{68}Ga]-DOTA-conjugated somatostatin receptor targeting peptides and [^{18}F]DOPA are the radiotracers of choice [70].

In unknown primary tumors presenting as a brain metastases of unknown primary, 2-[^{18}F]FDG PET provides information not only of the brain metabolism, but is also useful for searching for the primary tumor [68, 71, 72]. In summary, given the high glucose metabolism in the brain, the advantages of [^{11}C]MET over 2-[^{18}F]FDG are clear, thus it should be the radiotracer of choice if readily available. Other radiotracers may present advantages depending on the primary tumor. However, guidelines concur in recommending MRI for the evaluation of secondary brain tumors, as small lesions can go undetected in PET. A multidisciplinary approach is recommended in the management of cancer patients, as has been underlined in clinical guidelines for many solid tumors [73–79]. Finally, the information supplied by different radiotracers and different imaging techniques, including radiomics, may be complementary and could lead to the development of new biomarkers with prognostic impact [80–82].

3.2.6 Advantages and Disadvantages of [^{11}C]MET Imaging

As previously mentioned, [^{11}C]MET is a radiolabelled amino acid that has gained considerable attention for its use in the diagnosis and management of brain tumors, primarily gliomas [12, 83–86]. As an amino acid-based radiopharmaceutical, it provides unique advantages in brain tumor imaging, as well as some limitations that warrant discussion (Table 3.3).

In particular, advantages include:

1. Superior target-to-background ratio: Due to the overexpression of amino acid transporter systems in brain tumor cells, [^{11}C]MET provides a superior target-to-background ratio compared to 2-[^{18}F]FDG [12]. This high contrast allows for the accurate detection of tumor tissue and delineation of tumor margins.
2. Accurate tumor grading: [^{11}C]MET uptake correlates with cell proliferative activity, which can aid in differentiating high-grade

Table 3.3 SWOT (Strength-Weakness-Opportunities-Threats) analysis of [^{11}C]MET for detecting and characterizing brain tumors

Radiopharmaceutical	Strengths	Weaknesses	Opportunities	Threats
Methyl-^{11}C-L-methionine ([^{11}C]MET)	– Superior target-to-background ratio – Accurate tumor grading – Guidance for stereotactic biopsy	– Short half-life (20 min) – Limited specificity – Higher cost and complexity compared to conventional imaging	– Development of new techniques to overcome short half-life – Improved specificity through combination with other imaging agents	– Competition with other radiopharmaceuticals – Limited accessibility due to short half-life and cost

gliomas from histologically benign brain tumors or non-neoplastic lesions. The uptake intensity of [^{11}C]MET is also a reliable prognostic factor for tumor aggressiveness.

3. Guidance for stereotactic biopsy: [^{11}C]MET imaging can be employed to guide stereotactic biopsy, allowing for precise sampling of tumor tissue, which can be vital for accurate histopathological diagnosis.

On the other hand, disadvantages of [^{11}C]MET Imaging comprise:

1. Short half-life: The half-life of ^{11}C is approximately 20 min, which limits the availability and transport of [^{11}C]MET to PET centers in close proximity to a cyclotron facility. This logistical limitation can hinder widespread adoption of [^{11}C]MET imaging in clinical practice.

2. Limited specificity: Although [^{11}C]MET has a high sensitivity for detecting brain tumors, it can also accumulate in non-tumoral tissues and inflammatory lesions, potentially leading to false-positive findings.

3. Cost and complexity: The production and use of [^{11}C]MET PET imaging are more complex and expensive than conventional imaging modalities such as CT and MRI, which may limit its accessibility, especially in resource-limited settings.

In summary, PET/CT with [^{11}C]MET is a state of art technique, well established and widely available for brain tumors. [^{11}C]MET imaging offers several advantages in the diagnosis and management of brain tumors, including superior target-to-background ratios, accurate tumor grading, and guidance for stereotactic biopsy. However, its use is limited by factors such as its short half-life, limited specificity, and higher costs compared to conventional imaging modalities. Future research should focus on addressing these limitations to improve the clinical utility of [^{11}C]MET in brain tumor imaging. In particular, PET/MR represents an ideal alternative technique; it combines two modalities that are mandatory in the diagnostic process of brain tumors and it avoids exposure to CT-radiation.

3.3 The Role of [^{18}F]FET in Neuro-Oncology

Magnetic resonance imaging (MRI) is still considered the first imaging method for detecting both primary brain tumors and brain metastases (BM), due to its soft-tissue contrast, high spatial resolution, as well as wide availability. Nevertheless, although new advanced MRI sequences have been developed (e.g., perfusion-weighted imaging, MR spectroscopy, and MR-chemical exchange saturation transfer), MRI is not free from weaknesses, particularly to distinguish between true progression and treatment-related changes [87, 88]. To overcome these limitations, PET imaging with radiolabelled amino acids has received great impulse in the last years. [^{11}C]C-methyl-methionine ([^{11}C]-MET), O-(2-[^{18}F]F-fluoroethyl)-L-tyrosine ([^{18}F]FET), and 3,4-dihydroxy-6-[^{18}F]F-L-phenylalanine ([^{18}F]-DOPA), the three most widely used amino acid tracers in clinical routine, are internalized into tumor cells by L1- and L2-transporters that are overexpressed in gliomas and BM due to increased protein synthesis [82, 89]. As a consequence, images are characterized by lower physiological brain uptake with a better tumor-to-background contrast and, potentially, a better diagnostic performance. Furthermore, radiolabelled amino acids can pass without the need of blood–brain barrier disruption. Therefore, the Response Assessment in Neuro-Oncology (RANO) Working Group encourages the use of PET imaging with radiolabelled amino acids at all glioma stages, as well as in patients with BM [17, 22]. Due to labelling to long half-life ^{18}F, imaging with [^{18}F]FET has almost completely replaced other amino acid tracers, including [^{11}C]MET, for studying brain lesions. Moreover, [^{18}F]FET is an artificial amino acid which is not metabolized, accumulating only transitorily into the cells. This aspect allows to perform dynamic PET acquisition up to 50 min from injection, leading to extract temporal pattern parameters of [^{18}F]FET uptake, such as time-activity curve (TAC), time to peak (TTP), as well as their slope [90–92]. Another advantage includes its favorable synthesis and elevated stability due to an efficient nucleophilic reaction, as well as a lower uptake in the inflammatory cells.

In the following paragraphs, we will focus on the current role of molecular imaging with [^{18}F] FET in different clinical scenarios, as well as its potential clinical applications in the next future.

3.3.1 Brain Gliomas Diagnosis

In a recent meta-analysis, counting more than 450 patients with primary brain tumors of different WHO grades, [^{18}F]FET demonstrated a pooled sensitivity and specificity of 82% and 76%, respectively, for detecting malignant lesions. Of note, semi-quantitative analysis identified a mean tumor-to-brain ratio (TBRmean) of 1.6 and a maximum tumor-to-brain ratio (TBRmax) of 2.1 as better cut-off to discriminate between neoplastic and non-neoplastic lesions [93]. On the other hand, Rapp et al. [94] showed a high specificity of 92%, while the sensitivity

was only 57%, in 174 patients with suspicious brain tumors. However, a TBRmax value of 2.5 achieved a positive predictive value of 98% for differentiating neoplastic lesions from non-neoplastic ones (Fig. 3.5).

Despite [^{18}F]FET PET confirms a valuable diagnostic accuracy, neuro-pathologic tissue examination is mandatory for the final diagnosis, taking into account that increased [^{18}F]FET uptake may also occur in non-neoplastic lesions such as brain ischemia, abscess, inflammatory lesions secondary to multiple sclerosis, or epilepsy [95]. Finally, it has been demonstrated that approximately 20–30% of patients with WHO grade 2 gliomas and isocitrate dehydrogenase (IDH) mutation have no [^{18}F]FET uptake [96].

3.3.2 Evaluation of Tumor Extent

One of the main limitations of MRI regards the correct identification of non-enhancing gliomas [7]. Indeed, several studies have demonstrated that radiolabeled amino acid uptake is better correlated with neuro-pathologic findings than standard MRI. Moreover, there were significant differences in terms of size, overlap, and spatial correlation of tumor volumes between contrast-enhanced MRI and [^{18}F]FET uptake both in newly diagnosed and recurrent brain tumors [97–99]. This implies a potential impact of [^{18}F] FET PET/CT to guide diagnostic and therapeutic procedures, such as biopsy or radiotherapy target volume delineation [100–102].

3.3.3 Glioma Prognosis

While gadolinium-enhanced volumes on MRI have failed to demonstrate a survival advantage, patients with significant volume reduction by [^{18}F]FET PET had longer overall survival (OS). Of note, after adjuvant radiotherapy with concomitant temozolamide, a 20% decrease of TBRmax was associated with an OS of 16.1 compared to 9.3 months of non-responder patients [103]. Likewise, metabolic tumor volume (MTV) and TBRmax predicted longer OS as early as after two cycles of chemotherapy

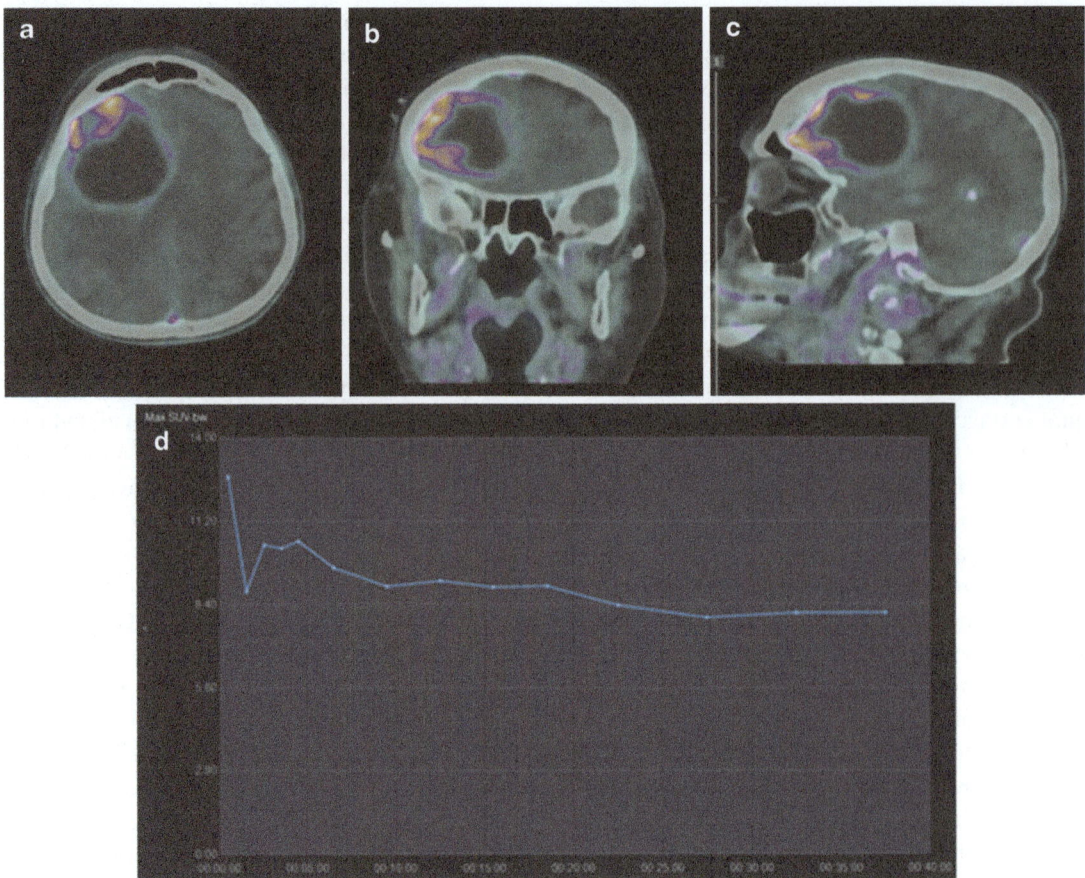

Fig. 3.5 [^{18}F]FET PET/CT of a 80-year-old patient with newly diagnosis of IDH–wild-type glioblastoma. (**a**–**c**) Axial, coronal, and sagittal fused images showed metabolically active lesions as identified by increased amino acid uptake (TBRmax 7.8). (**d**) TAC profile, characterizing by an early peak (<20 min) followed by a rapid descend, suggesting a high-grade lesion

with temozolamide [104]. Furthermore, TBRmax, TBRmean, and MTV have been found useful to assess early response to bevacizumab plus lomustine in patients with progressive glioblastoma [105] as well as to identify pseudo-response. [^{18}F]FET also seems helpful for identifying pseudo-response, a typical phenomenon observed during therapy with bevacizumab, a humanized anti-angiogenic drug, which induces false persistent non-enhancing lesions at MRI [106, 107]. Recently, regorafenib a small-molecule multi-kinase inhibitor has been introduced in the clinical practice of glioblastoma recurrence. Similar to alkylating molecules, it can determine equivocal MRI findings, while [^{18}F]FET has been suggested to be suitable for evaluating response to regorafenib [108, 109].

An example of response assessment during chemotherapy in a patient with a progressive glioblastoma is shown in Fig. 3.6.

3.3.4 Tumor Recurrence and Differential Diagnosis with Treatment-Related Changes

One of the main indications to perform [^{18}F]FET PET/CT or PET/MRI is in case of suspected recurrence or progression of disease by conventional MRI, requested in approximately 50% of glioma patients [110]. Regarding static [^{18}F]FET parameters, a cut-off value of TBRmax ranging

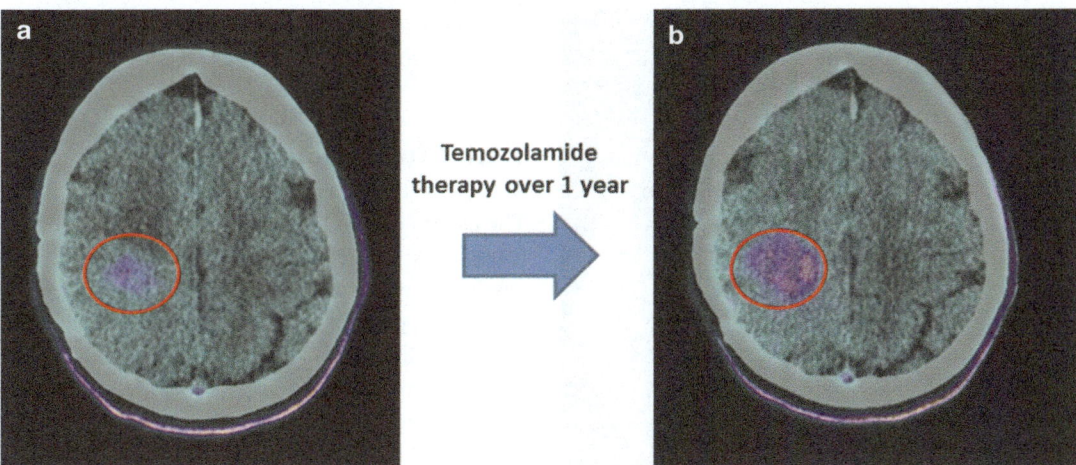

Temozolamide
therapy over 1 year

Fig. 3.6 A 54-year-old woman with history of anaplastic astrocytoma on the right fronto-parietal lobe who had undergone neurosurgery followed by radiotherapy and chemotherapy. Almost 2 years after temozolomide, the first [¹⁸F]FET PET/CT showed (**a**) a small area of increased uptake suggestive for relapse, while TAC profile suggested a low-grade lesion. Therefore the patient continued temozolomide for 1 year when a new [¹⁸F]FET PET/CT (**b**) showed further increased uptake of the abovementioned lesion (TBRmax 4.3 vs 3.1), indicating disease progression. The patient switched to regorafenib

from 1.9 to 2.3 has shown a sensitivity of 91% and a specificity of 84%, with an area under the curve (AUC) of 0.92. Moreover, TBRmean with a cut-off value between 1.8 and 2.3 has demonstrated a sensitivity and specificity of 80% and 87%, respectively, with an AUC of 0.91. On the other hand, curve pattern type II (i.e., early peak below 20 min followed by a plateau) or III (i.e., early peak followed by a constant descend) as well as slope of the TAC in the late phase (cut-off value of 0.2–0.32 SUV/h) showed a sensitivity and specificity of 72% and 78%, respectively, and 0.81 of AUC. Likewise, TTP with a cut-off value of 20–35 min achieved a sensitivity and specificity that ranged from 64% to 83% and 63% to 81%, respectively [110–120].

In conclusion, the correct discrimination between treatment-related changes and tumor recurrence is of primary importance. Indeed, erroneous evaluation may lead either to a premature interruption of effective therapy or to an overestimation of results.

3.3.5 Evaluation of Brain Metastases

As above mentioned, the RANO Working Group recommends the use of radiolabelled amino acids also in patients with BM, due to the high expression of amino acid transporters in these patients. For example, the German group has shown that almost all BM (40%) had a high [¹⁸F] FET uptake compared to normal brain parenchyma [121].

Regarding the potential application of [¹⁸F] FET PET for differentiation of radiation necrosis from BM relapse after radiosurgery, both static and dynamic parameters have shown high sensitivity and specificity of 80% and 90%, respectively [91, 92, 122]. In addition, a recent meta-analysis, including the three main amino acid radiotracers and almost 400 patients, confirmed the elevated diagnostic accuracy of amino acid PET with a pooled sensitivity and specificity were 82% and 84%, respectively [123].

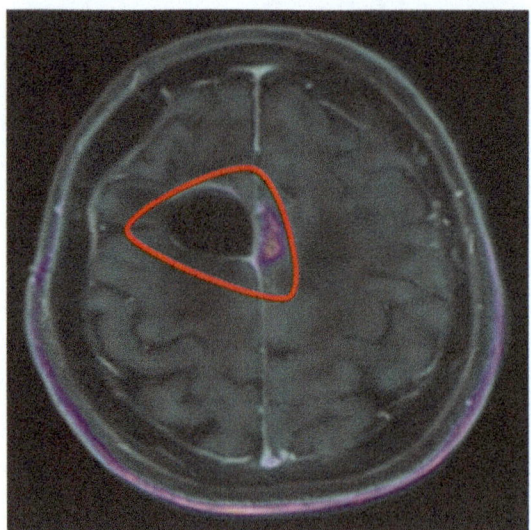

Fig. 3.7 Fused [¹⁸F]FET PET/MRI of a 47-year-old patient with recurrent brain metastasis from lung cancer. The metabolically active lesion was identified by increased uptake of amino acid radiotracer (TBRmax 3.8). Note how the contrast-enhancing tumor on MRI around surgical cavity exceeds metabolically active tumor on [¹⁸F]FET PET

Finally, in the era of immunotherapy with checkpoint inhibitor, few studies have highlighted the potential role of [¹⁸F]FET PET to detect pseudo-progression in patients with BM from melanoma or lung cancer [124, 125].

Figure 3.7 illustrates a case of brain metastases.

3.4 [18F]Fluoro-ʟ-Phenylalanine ([¹⁸F]DOPA) in Brain Tumors

The amino acid radiopharmaceuticals currently available for PET imaging share a similar mechanism of intracellular uptake mediated by the sodium-independent large neutral amino acid transporters LAT1 and LAT2, overrepresented on tumor cells [126, 127]. Differently from other amino acid radiopharmaceuticals, the 3,4-dihydroxy-6-[¹⁸F]fluoro-ʟ-phenylalanine ([¹⁸F]DOPA) is a substrate for the aromatic amino acid decarboxylase and, consequently, a marker of dopaminergic and serotoninergic activity in cerebral structures,

such as basal ganglia and raphe nuclei, respectively [128, 129].

3.4.1 Tumor Volume Delineation

The usefulness of [¹⁸F]DOPA PET for tumor delineation was tested by biopsy-controlled studies in newly diagnosed and recurrent gliomas (Fig. 3.8). In a mixed population of 10 patients with cerebral glioma at diagnosis, Pafundi et al. showed a better accuracy for tumor delineation with [¹⁸F]DOPA PET compared with contrast-enhanced MRI, which might have relevant implications for surgical and radiotherapy planning. In particular, the portion of the tumor showing the highest PET uptake extended beyond contrast-enhancement in a significant proportion of cases, whereas it was always confined within the radiological abnormalities seen in T2/FLAIR sequences [130]. The same group performed another biopsy-controlled, prospective study on 13 patients with suspected recurrence of glioma, confirming that PET has increased sensitivity and specificity for recurrent tumor over MRI [131]. An independent research group carried out a prospective, biopsy-controlled study on 16 treatment-naïve patients with various glioma grade, showing a significant impact of [¹⁸F]DOPA on high-grade tumor volume delineation in about one-third of patients. The addition of [¹⁸F]DOPA PET to multimodal MRI, including PWI, significantly increased sensitivity, thereby improving the accuracy of tumor detection [132]. It has been estimated that the high physiological basal ganglia radiopharmaceutical uptake may interfere with tumor delineation in about 12–13% of patients with glioma [133, 134]. In these cases, tumor delineation based on MRI is essential.

The ability of [¹⁸F]DOPA PET to non-invasively predict the tumor molecular characteristics included in the most recent WHO classifications of cerebral gliomas has been addressed with conflicting results [135–137]. Although, promising findings in that context came from recent reports based on [¹⁸F]DOPA PET radiomics [138, 139], however, their potential clinical impact has yet to be demonstrated.

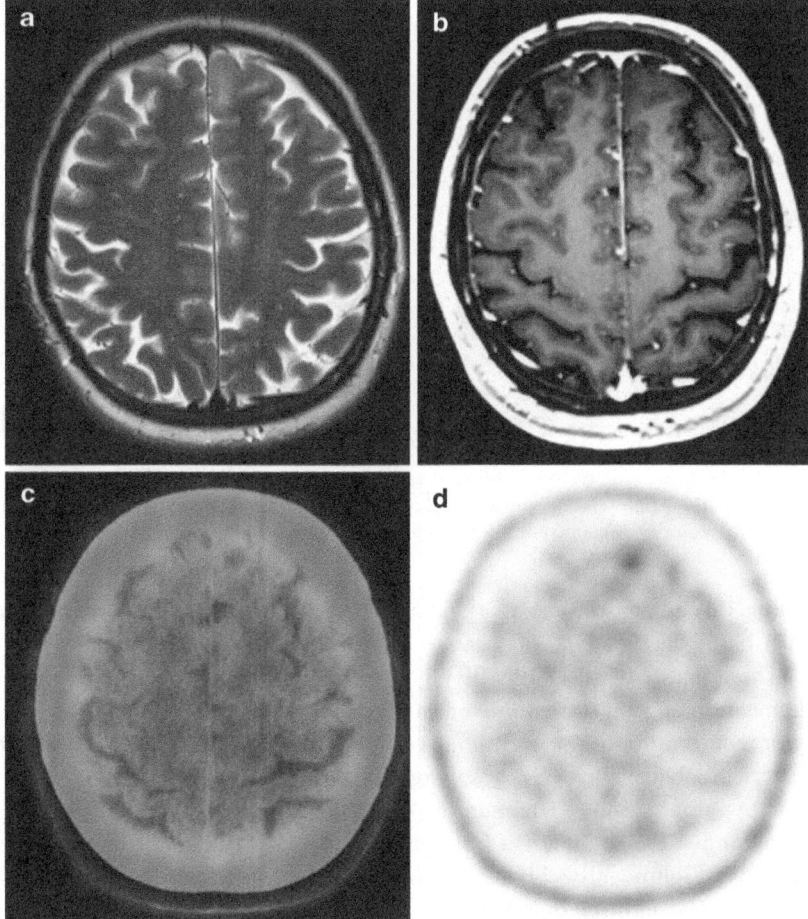

Fig. 3.8 Patient with low-grade glioma (LGG), namely an astrocytoma grade II, 1p/19q codeleted, MGMT methylated, IDH1 mutated marginally visible on MRI in the left frontal para-sagittal region (**a**, T2-weighted; **b**, Gd-enhanced), while defined as a faint focal spot (SUVmax 2, SUVratio 1.8) on [^{18}F]DOPA PET images (**c**, fused PET/CT; **d**, axial PET)

3.4.2 Detection of Tumor Recurrence

Similarly to other radiolabelled amino acid analogs available for PET imaging, [^{18}F]DOPA is most often used in the recurrence setting, owing to its high accuracy for the differential diagnosis between tumor recurrence and treatment-related changes (Fig. 3.9). In a relatively large cohort of 110 patients with suspected high-grade tumor recurrence, Herrmann et al. demonstrated a diagnostic accuracy of 82% for the correct classification of treatment-related changes. Interestingly, visual and semiquantitative PET evaluations were performed equally in this study, and [^{18}F]DOPA PET was strongly predictive of progression-free survival (PFS) [140]. Even better performances were reported by another group

in a similar setting, although on smaller cohorts, suggesting a correlation between the results of [^{18}F]DOPA PET and overall survival (OS) [141, 142].

3.4.3 Radiotherapy Planning

The benefit of adding [^{18}F]DOPA PET to conventional radiotherapy planning of gliomas is under investigation. In 19 patients with newly diagnosed gliomas undergoing radiation treatment, Kosztyla et al. confirmed that gross tumor volumes (GTV) identified by [^{18}F]DOPA PET are larger than those obtained with MRI. Nevertheless, 11 out of 12 (91%) recurrences available for image analysis were observed outside the PET GTV, and most of them (82%) were included

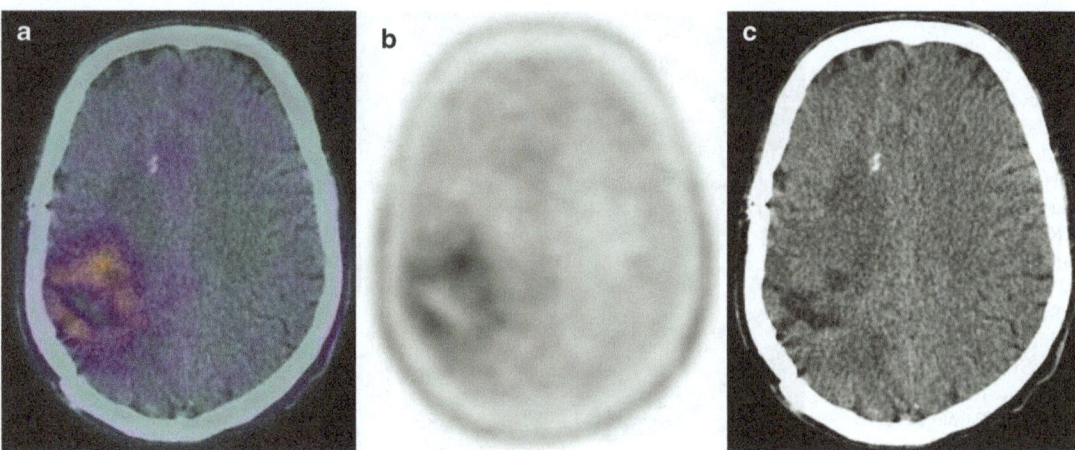

Fig. 3.9 Patient with relapsed diffused glioma of the right parietal lobe presenting with moderate uptake in the peripheral zone of the operating cavity on [^{18}F]DOPA PET/CT (SUVmax 1.9; SUVratio 2.37): (**a**) fused PET/CT axial image, (**b**) axial [^{18}F]DOPA PET, and (**c**) low-dose CT

within the 2-cm isotropic margin added to the MRI-based GTV [143].

The impact of [^{18}F]DOPA PET-guided target delineation on PFS was evaluated in 20 patients with recurrent high-grade gliomas compared to historical controls receiving salvage systemic therapy alone [144]. The authors reported a promising 85% 3-month PFS for irradiated patients, significantly higher than historical controls. The addition of [^{18}F]DOPA to standard therapy planning based on contrast-enhanced T1 sequences resulted in 43% median GTV increase with no apparent additional toxicity. No failures were observed within the PET GTV [144].

The results of a phase II study using [^{18}F]DOPA PET to guide radiotherapy dose-escalation in 75 patients with newly diagnosed glioblastoma were recently published [145]. The regions of highest [^{18}F]DOPA uptake (i.e., >2.0 tumor-to-normal brain ratio) were targeted to receive 76 Gy in a simultaneous integrated boost, and clinical outcomes were compared with those of historical prospective cohorts. The authors showed longer PFS for the MGMT unmethylated patients and longer OS for the MGMG methylated patients in the study cohort compared with historical controls [145]. Taken together, these preliminary data showed that [^{18}F]DOPA PET can be safely and effectively used to inform radiotherapy treatment planning and is worth further investigations.

3.4.4 Treatment Monitoring

Repeated amino acid PET imaging can be used to detect malignant progression of gliomas followed up conservatively or for treatment monitoring. Lately, the PET RANO criteria have been proposed as a framework structured to implement PET imaging into clinical research and clinical routine [146]. The PET technique allows for the simultaneous evaluation of changes in tumor metabolism and tumor volume, which may be particularly advantageous over conventional MRI [147]. Oughourlian et al. retrospectively evaluated 27 patients with WHO grade II glioma who underwent at least two [^{18}F]DOPA PET scans over a mean time of 1.3 years, showing the rate of [^{18}F]DOPA uptake changes to be the only independent predictor of OS, thereby suggesting that the addition of longitudinal amino acid PET to conventional MRI in this group of patients may provide prognostically relevant information [148]. Changes on MTV, not tumor uptake changes, as measured by repeated [^{18}F]DOPA PET, were highly predictive of OS and PFS in 30 patients with recurrent high-grade gliomas undergoing bevacizumab therapy in a study from the same group [149].

3.5 Role of Amino Acid PET Tracer in Pediatric Glioma

Brain gliomas represent the most common malignancies of the central nervous system (CNS) in the pediatric age. Their clonal origin, biological aggressiveness, and growth patterns present relevant variations, ranging from low-grade to highly malignant, and may present a diffusely infiltrating or a more circumscribed growth pattern [150–154].

The WHO classification includes into pediatric low-grade gliomas (pLGG) those with grade 1 or 2. The pilocytic astrocytoma, which is a circumscribed tumor originating from astrocytes, is the most frequently occurring one, while diffuse pLGG, mixed glioneuronal as well as pure neuron-derived tumor are rare entities.

Conversely, the most frequent cause of morbidity and mortality related to CNS tumors is represented by grade 3 and 4 forms (pediatric high-grade gliomas or pHGG), which can affect the cerebral hemispheres as well as the midline structures including the brain stem (the pons represents the most commonly affected localization), the thalamus and the medulla spinalis [153]. In the setting of pHGG, the presence of gene sequence anomalies plays a key role in staging the tumoral behavior; particularly, the H3K27 alteration identifies a grade IV tumor according to the WHO classification, independently of the histological origin [153]. Diffusely-growing tumors of glial cells arising from the pons (diffuse intrinsic pontine gliomas or DIPG) are prevalently (85%) characterized by this genetic feature and are linked with a dire prognosis since they can be treated with radiotherapy only, with very short survival following relapse or progression (<1 year) [155].

Managing pediatric gliomas require a multidisciplinary approach; even in the best of settings, it remains a challenging task. Surgery represents the ideal therapeutic modality since it often represents the only true curative approach. Whenever a full excision is not feasible (be it due to the size of the neoplasm or the infiltration of vital brain structures) a debulking approach may be considered, as a way to obtain histological information and to relieve the patients' symptoms. Thereafter, adjuvant treatment (cytotoxic therapy, targeted molecules, and external beam radiation therapy) can be attempted. This three-way approach was and remains the staple of the treatment of a variety of pediatric brain tumors [156].

Due to the complexity of the surgical and radiotherapy methods, sensitive and reliable imaging procedures are needed; these methods are key in enabling the surgeon to plan the procedure as well as to guide the setup of effective radiotherapy protocols while sparing toxicity. To this purpose, morphological non-invasive imaging is indispensable; the prevalence of soft tissue with similar contrast in the CNS area implies the use of magnetic resonance imaging (MRI). This technique is able to visualize many aspects of tumoral biology in a reliable way, including edema, compression of nearby structures, central necrosis, areas of vascular/blood-brain barrier damage, and enhancement. However, MRI is not without limitations: it is unable to stratify the tumors according to their type and grade. In some instances, MRI might underestimate the disease extension. Finally, one of the most important weaknesses of this method is the incapacity to tell apart the presence of residual disease after treatment from changes caused by the therapy (i.e., "pseudoprogression" or "pseudoresponse"), especially in the earliest phases after surgery/radiotherapy.

Multi-parameter MRI might be able to overcome these issues since it can make use of dedicated sequences to gain information on the metabolic processes of these tumors. However, adding further sequences causes significant prolongation of the procedure duration (potentially limiting the patients' compliance or implying the need for longer sedation). Moreover, there is a relevant lack of standardization of these methods (optimal sequence, scan, and reconstruction parameters), which in turn hinders their clinical application. Image-based biomarkers of tumoral metabolism have been an unmet need for decades.

In recent years, there has been a surge in the use of so-called molecular imaging, i.e. the in vivo visualization of metabolic processes through radiolabelled molecules. Particularly, PET has continuously and significantly improved over the years and now allows for fast and high-resolution visualization of many pathophysiological processes with a minimal absorbed dose. Imaging of brain neoplasms is performed mainly through the use of amino acid labeled compounds, such as L-amino acid [¹¹C]MET [¹⁸F]FET and [¹⁸F]DOPA that show a very high contrast between tumor and background uptake. Furthermore, these tracers can be used independently of the blood-brain barrier status and tumoral vascularization [157, 158]. Indeed, these three tracers have similar uptake mechanisms depending on specific aminoacid transport system and very similar pathological distribution [21] and can be all proposed as an effective alternatives to each other.

Recent practice guidelines about the role of aminoacid PET tracers in pediatric gliomas identified the principal clinical indication of this imaging procedure at staging, post-therapy restaging, and follow-up (Table 3.4) [21].

Considering the higher prevalence of low-grade glioma in pediatric patients when com-

Table 3.4 Common indication of amino acid PET in pediatric gliomas

Clinical indication	At the time of diagnosis	At restaging and follow-up
1	Differentiation between neoplastic and non-neoplastic lesions	Differential diagnosis between relapse and pseudo-progression
2	Glioma grading/ DIPG biological behavior	Restaging after radiotherapy and cytotoxic treatments
3	Identification of metabolically active areas to guide biopsies	Assessment of tumor grading when the occurrence of a de-differentiation is suspected
4	Delineation of glioma extent before surgery and radiation therapy	Identification of residual disease after treatment for the planning of complemental approaches
5	Prognostication	

pared with adults, the need for an affective diagnostic tool able to evaluate the biological activity and aggressiveness of the tumor is highly required. In this setting, amino acid PET imaging has its main clinical indications. This is particularly true in case of lesions with infiltrative pattern and low or inhomogeneous contrast enhancement on MRI for which a precise grading assessment often is challenging.

Although amino acid PET has lower sensitivity than MRI in differentiating pediatric non-neoplastic lesions from supratentorial infiltrative gliomas [159], PET imaging in children with infiltrative astrocytomas correlates reliably with WHO tumor grade and outcome [159]. At the same time it has been proved that in pediatric patients with H3K27M-mutant and wild-type DMG, PET with aminoacid tracers (i.e., [¹⁸F]-DOPA) can be the only imaging tool able to show significant differences in terms of uptake between H3K27M-mutant and wild-type lesions, when compared with MRI modalities. This finding confirms its important role in non-invasively evaluating the H3K27M mutation status that is associated with disease progression and outcome regardless of any histology profile [160].

Even in DIPGs at the time of first diagnosis, [¹⁸F]DOPA PET imaging, considering static parameters of target to contralateral striatum ratio (TSR), was an independent predictor of overall survival, and importantly the area with the highest uptake corresponded to tumoral components with more aggressive biological behavior, less sensitive to first-line treatment with chemotherapy/radiotherapy [161].

Regarding interpretation of the images, although the static semiquantitative uptake parameters as TSR and TBR are important for the discrimination between neoplastic a non-neoplastic brain lesion and grading (Table 3.5), an adequate co-registration with recent MRI should be always performed. Indeed, this first step is the cornerstone for a correct interpretation and recognition of PET findings.

In the case of brain lesion on MRI, any detectable uptake may be considered suspicious and, in

Table 3.5 Commonly used TBR thresholds for amino acid PET in pediatric gliomas

Clinical indication	Amino acid tracer	Method	Threshold	Reference
Differentiation between neoplastic a non-neoplastic brain lesion	[^{18}F]FET	Maximum tumor-to-background ratio	1.6	[162]
	[^{11}C]MET	Maximum tumor-to-background ratio	1–1.5	[163–165]
	[^{18}F]DOPA	Maximum tumor-to-background ratio	1	[159, 166]
Tumor grading	[^{18}F]FET	Time-activity curve shape	N.A.	[167]
	[^{11}C]MET	N.R.	N.R.	
	[^{18}F]DOPA	Maximum tumor-to-background ratio	1	[159, 166]
Prognostic value	[^{18}F]FET	Maximum tumor-to-background ratio and dynamic curve shape	1.6	[162, 167]
	[^{11}C]MET	SUVmax	3	[168]
	[^{18}F]DOPA	Maximum tumor-to-background ratio	1	[159, 166]
Tumor relapse	[^{18}F]FET	Maximum tumor-to-background ratio	1.6	[162]
	[^{11}C]MET	SUVmax	3	[168]
	[^{18}F]DOPA	Not available	Not available	Not available

N.R. not reported, *N.A.* not applicable

this setting, no TBR threshold has been proposed. What is important to recognize first is the MRI pattern of the lesion and differentiate between suspected gliomas with diffuse infiltrative pattern vs. gliomas with a more circumscribed pattern of growth [21].

Supratentorial diffuse infiltrative pattern without contrast enhancement on MRI and lack of uptake or faint uptake on PET is mainly associated with pediatric low-grade gliomas (pLGGs) (Fig. 3.10). In this case, pediatric high-grade gliomas (pHGGs) may be excluded, although some midline gliomas are characterized by low uptake. Low uptake pattern may also exclude oligodendrogliomas (very infrequent in pediatric) which often show intense uptake [21].

On the contrary, when diffuse infiltrative lesions with intense uptake are detected, pHGGs should be always suspected (Fig. 3.10). This pattern is often associated with inhomogeneous contrast enhancement on MRI.

Brain lesions are more likely non-neoplastic when show a more circumscribed growth pattern

lack of contrast enhancement on MRI and lack or faint uptake on PET images [21].

In the case of circumscribed growth patterns, intense tracer uptake on PET and contrast enhancement on MRI may often be associated with pLGG (e.g., pilocytic astrocytomas or gangliogliomas) [169, 170].

Dynamic parameters can be also of great help in grading assessments, being able to add valuable information to static images. In this setting, [^{18}F]FET was the most used aminoacid PET tracer [167, 171]. Indeed, its time-activity curves (TACs) with an early peak ($\leq$20 min), followed by a plateau or by a rapid decline are associated with pHHG [21]. On the other hand, TACs pattern characterized by a rapid intake phase with subsequent further accumulation without any decreasing phases over time is associated with pLGG [21].

More recently, also the role of dynamic parameters of [^{18}F]DOPA PET/CT in pediatric gliomas has been investigated and, as for [^{18}F]FET, the accumulation TAC shape was more common in pLGG than in pHGG [172].

Fig. 3.10 pLGG with infiltrative growth pattern and characterized by lack of tracer uptake on [^{18}F]DOPA PET coregistered with MRI (**a**). pHHG with diffuse infiltrative pattern and intense and inhomogeneous tracer uptake on [^{18}F]DOPA PET coregistered with MRI (**b**)

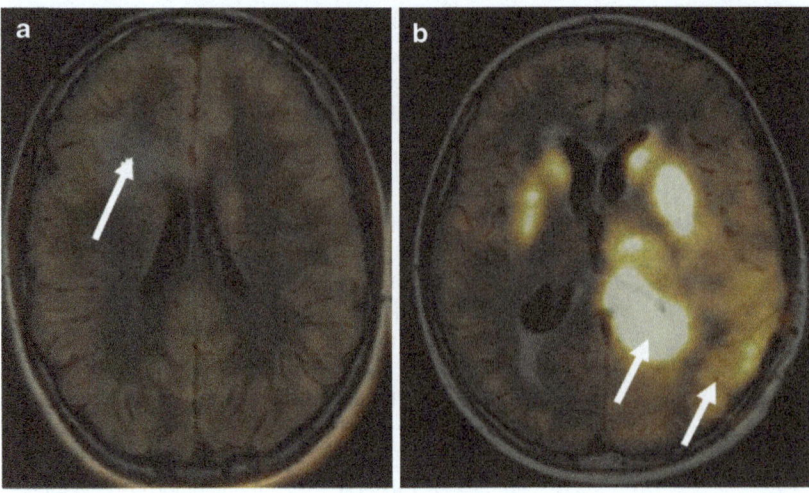

The second most common indication for using aminoacid PET tracers is the differentiation of glioma recurrence from treatment-induced changes. In these patients, particularly in those treated with antiangiogenic agents, PET is able to identify areas of pseudoresponse and non-enhancing tumor progression [106]. In this setting, both semi quantification of static PET images and assessment of dynamic parameters (i.e. TACs) are very useful in identifying disease relapse. Indeed, recurrence of pHGGs is often associated with intense uptake and high TBR (Table 3.5). At the same time, an early peak followed by a plateau or rapid decline is the TACs pattern of pHGGs relapse [21].

References

1. Ostrom QT, Cioffi G, Gittleman H, Patil N, Waite K, Kruchko C, Barnholtz-Sloan JS. CBTRUS statistical report: primary brain and other central nervous system tumors diagnosed in the United States in 2012-2016. Neuro Oncol. 2019;21(Suppl 5):v1–v100.
2. Osborn AG, Louis DN, Poussaint TY, Linscott LL, Salzman KL. The 2021 World Health Organization classification of tumors of the central nervous system: what neuroradiologists need to know. AJNR Am J Neuroradiol. 2022;43(7):928–37.
3. Ostrom QT, Wright CH, Barnholtz-Sloan JS. Brain metastases: epidemiology. Handb Clin Neurol. 2018;149:27–42.
4. Cecchin D, Garibotto V, Law I, Goffin K. PET imaging in neurodegeneration and neuro-oncology: variants and pitfalls. Semin Nucl Med. 2021;51(5):408–18.
5. Verger A, Kas A, Darcourt J, Guedj E. PET imaging in neuro-oncology: an update and overview of a rapidly growing area. Cancers (Basel). 2022;14(5):1103.
6. Pietrzak A, Marszalek A, Kunikowska J, Piotrowski T, Medak A, Pietrasz K, Wojtowicz J, Cholewinski W. Detection of clinically silent brain lesions in [18F]FDG PET/CT study in oncological patients: analysis of over 10,000 studies. Sci Rep. 2021;11(1):18293.
7. Langen KJ, Galldiks N, Hattingen E, Shah NJ. Advances in neuro-oncology imaging. Nat Rev Neurol. 2017;13(5):279–89.
8. Borgwardt L, Hojgaard L, Carstensen H, Laursen H, Nowak M, Thomsen C, Schmiegelow K. Increased fluorine-18 2-fluoro-2-deoxy-D-glucose (FDG) uptake in childhood CNS tumors is correlated with malignancy grade: a study with FDG positron emission tomography/magnetic resonance imaging coregistration and image fusion. J Clin Oncol. 2005;23(13):3030–7.
9. Mertens K, Acou M, Van Hauwe J, De Ruyck I, Van den Broecke C, Kalala JP, D'Asseler Y, Goethals I. Validation of 18F-FDG PET at conventional and delayed intervals for the discrimination of high-grade from low-grade gliomas: a stereotactic PET and MRI study. Clin Nucl Med. 2013;38(7):495–500.
10. Kruer MC, Kaplan AM, Etzl MM Jr, Carpentieri DF, Dickman PS, Chen K, Mathieson K, Irving A. The value of positron emission tomography and proliferation index in predicting progression in low-grade astrocytomas of childhood. J Neurooncol. 2009;95(2):239–45.
11. Colavolpe C, Chinot O, Metellus P, Mancini J, Barrie M, Bequet-Boucard C, Tabouret E, Mundler O, Figarella-Branger D, Guedj E. FDG-PET predicts survival in recurrent high-grade gliomas treated with bevacizumab and irinotecan. Neuro Oncol. 2012;14(5):649–57.
12. Law I, Albert NL, Arbizu J, Boellaard R, Drzezga A, Galldiks N, la Fougere C, Langen KJ, Lopci E, Lowe V, McConathy J, Quick HH, Sattler B, Schuster DM, Tonn JC, Weller M. Joint EANM/EANO/RANO

practice guidelines/SNMMI procedure standards for imaging of gliomas using PET with radiolabelled amino acids and [(18)F]FDG: version 1.0. Eur J Nucl Med Mol Imaging. 2019;46(3):540–57.

13. Zukotynski K, Fahey F, Kocak M, Kun L, Boyett J, Fouladi M, Vajapeyam S, Treves T, Poussaint TY. 18F-FDG PET and MR imaging associations across a spectrum of pediatric brain tumors: a report from the pediatric brain tumor consortium. J Nucl Med. 2014;55(9):1473–80.

14. Santra A, Kumar R, Sharma P, Bal C, Kumar A, Julka PK, Malhotra A. F-18 FDG PET-CT in patients with recurrent glioma: comparison with contrast enhanced MRI. Eur J Radiol. 2012;81(3):508–13.

15. Dankbaar JW, Snijders TJ, Robe PA, Seute T, Eppinga W, Hendrikse J, De Keizer B. The use of (18)F-FDG PET to differentiate progressive disease from treatment induced necrosis in high-grade glioma. J Neurooncol. 2015;125(1):167–75.

16. Horky LL, Hsiao EM, Weiss SE, Drappatz J, Gerbaudo VH. Dual phase FDG-PET imaging of brain metastases provides superior assessment of recurrence versus post-treatment necrosis. J Neurooncol. 2011;103(1):137–46.

17. Galldiks N, Langen KJ, Albert NL, Chamberlain M, Soffietti R, Kim MM, Law I, Le Rhun E, Chang S, Schwarting J, Combs SE, Preusser M, Forsyth P, Pope W, Weller M, Tonn JC. PET imaging in patients with brain metastasis-report of the RANO/PET group. Neuro Oncol. 2019;21(5):585–95.

18. Purandare NC, Puranik A, Shah S, Agrawal A, Gupta T, Moiyadi A, Shetty P, Shridhar E, Jalali R, Rangarajan V. Common malignant brain tumors: can 18F-FDG PET/CT aid in differentiation? Nucl Med Commun. 2017;38(12):1109–16.

19. Yang M, Sun J, Bai HX, Tao Y, Tang X, States LJ, Zhang Z, Zhou J, Farwell MD, Zhang P, Xiao B, Yang L. Diagnostic accuracy of SPECT, PET, and MRS for primary central nervous system lymphoma in HIV patients: a systematic review and meta-analysis. Medicine (Baltimore). 2017;96(19):e6676.

20. Barajas RF, Politi LS, Anzalone N, Schoder H, Fox CP, Boxerman JL, Kaufmann TJ, Quarles CC, Ellingson BM, Auer D, Andronesi OC, Ferreri AJM, Mrugala MM, Grommes C, Neuwelt EA, Ambady P, Rubenstein JL, Illerhaus G, Nagane M, Batchelor TT, Hu LS. Consensus recommendations for MRI and PET imaging of primary central nervous system lymphoma: guideline statement from the International Primary CNS Lymphoma Collaborative Group (IPCG). Neuro Oncol. 2021;23(7):1056–71.

21. Piccardo A, Albert NL, Borgwardt L, Fahey FH, Hargrave D, Galldiks N, Jehanno N, Kurch L, Law I, Lim R, Lopci E, Marner L, Morana G, Young Poussaint T, Seghers VJ, Shulkin BL, Warren KE, Traub-Weidinger T, Zucchetta P. Joint EANM/SIOPE/RAPNO practice guidelines/SNMMI procedure standards for imaging of paediatric gliomas using PET with radiolabelled amino acids and [(18)

F]FDG: version 1.0. Eur J Nucl Med Mol Imaging. 2022;49(11):3852–69.

22. Albert NL, Weller M, Suchorska B, Galldiks N, Soffietti R, Kim MM, la Fougere C, Pope W, Law I, Arbizu J, Chamberlain MC, Vogelbaum M, Ellingson BM, Tonn JC. Response assessment in Neuro-Oncology Working Group and European Association for Neuro-Oncology recommendations for the clinical use of PET imaging in gliomas. Neuro Oncol. 2016;18(9):1199–208.

23. Nakajo K, Uda T, Kawashima T, Terakawa Y, Ishibashi K, Tsuyuguchi N, et al. Diagnostic performance of [11C]methionine positron emission tomography in newly diagnosed and untreated glioma based on the revised World Health Organization 2016 classification. World Neurosurg. 2021;148:e471–81. https://doi.org/10.1016/j.wneu.2021.01.012.

24. Giammarile F, Cinotti LE, Jouvet A, Ramackers JM, Saint Pierre G, Thiesse P, et al. High and low-grade oligodendrogliomas (ODG): correlation of amino-acid and glucose uptakes using PET and histological classifications. J Neurooncol. 2004;68:263–74. https://doi.org/10.1023/b:neon.0000033384.43417.82.

25. Glaudemans AW, Enting RH, Heesters MA, Dierckx RA, van Rheenen RW, Walenkamp AM, Slart RH. Value of 11C-methionine PET in imaging brain tumours and metastases. Eur J Nucl Med Mol Imaging. 2013;40(4):615–35.

26. Jager PL, Vaalburg W, Pruim J, de Vries EG, Langen KJ, Piers DA. Radiolabeled amino acids: basic aspects and clinical applications in oncology. J Nucl Med. 2001;42:432–45.

27. Coope DJ, Cizek J, Eggers C, Vollmar S, Heiss WD, Herholz K. Evaluation of primary brain tumors using 11C-methionine PET with reference to a normal methionine uptake map. J Nucl Med. 2007;48:1971–80.

28. Nagata T, Tsuyuguchi N, Uda T, Terakawa Y, Takami T, Ohata K. Examination of 11C-methionine metabolism by the standardized uptake value in the normal brain of children. J Nucl Med. 2011;52:201–5.

29. Moulin-Romsee G, D'Hondt E, de Groot T, Goffin J, Sciot R, Mortelmans L, et al. Non-invasive grading of brain tumours using dynamic amino acid PET imaging: does it work for 11C-methionine? Eur J Nucl Med Mol Imaging. 2007;34:2082–7.

30. van Waarde A, Elsinga PH. Proliferation markers for the differential diagnosis of tumor and inflammation. Curr Pharm Des. 2008;14:3326–39.

31. Becherer A, Karanikas G, Szabo M, Zettinig G, Asenbaum S, Marosi C, et al. Brain tumour imaging with PET: a comparison between [18F]fluorodopa and [11C]methionine. Eur J Nucl Med Mol Imaging. 2003;30:1561–7.

32. Braun V, Dempf S, Weller R, Reske SN, Schachenmayr W, Richter HP. Cranial neuronavigation with direct integration of (11)C methionine positron emission tomography (PET) data—results

of a pilot study in 32 surgical cases. Acta Neurochir (Wien). 2002;144:777–82.

33. Chung JK, Kim YK, Kim SK, Lee YJ, Paek S, Yeo JS, et al. Usefulness of 11C-methionine PET in the evaluation of brain lesions that are hypo- or isometabolic on 18F-FDG PET. Eur J Nucl Med Mol Imaging. 2002;29:176–82.

34. Galldiks N, Kracht LW, Berthold F, Miletic H, Klein JC, Herholz K, et al. [11C]-L-methionine positron emission tomography in the management of children and young adults with brain tumors. J Neurooncol. 2010;96:231–9.

35. Hatakeyama T, Kawai N, Nishiyama Y, Yamamoto Y, Sasakawa Y, Ichikawa T, et al. 11C-methionine (MET) and 18F-fluorothymidine (FLT) PET in patients with newly diagnosed glioma. Eur J Nucl Med Mol Imaging. 2008;35:2009–17.

36. Herholz K, Holzer T, Bauer B, Schroder R, Voges J, Ernestus RI, et al. 11C-methionine PET for differential diagnosis of low-grade gliomas. Neurology. 1998;50:1316–22.

37. Jacobs AH, Thomas A, Kracht LW, Li H, Dittmar C, Garlip G, et al. 18F-fluoro-L-thymidine and 11C-methylmethionine as markers of increased transport and proliferation in brain tumors. J Nucl Med. 2005;46:1948–58.

38. Kracht LW, Miletic H, Busch S, Jacobs AH, Voges J, Hoevels M, et al. Delineation of brain tumor extent with [11C]L-methionine positron emission tomography: local comparison with stereotactic histopathology. Clin Cancer Res. 2004;10:7163–70.

39. Li DL, Xu YK, Wang QS, Wu HB, Li HS. 11C-methionine and 18F-fluorodeoxyglucose positron emission tomography/CT in the evaluation of patients with suspected primary and residual/recurrent gliomas. Chin Med J (Engl). 2012;125:91–6.

40. Massager N, David P, Goldman S, Pirotte B, Wikler D, Salmon I, et al. Combined magnetic resonance imaging- and positron emission tomography-guided stereotactic biopsy in brainstem mass lesions: diagnostic yield in a series of 30 patients. J Neurosurg. 2000;93:951–7.

41. Nuutinen J, Sonninen P, Lehikoinen P, Sutinen E, Valavaara R, Eronen E, et al. Radiotherapy treatment planning and long-term follow-up with [11C] methionine PET in patients with low-grade astrocytoma. Int J Radiat Oncol Biol Phys. 2000;48:43–52.

42. Ullrich RT, Kracht L, Brunn A, Herholz K, Frommolt P, Miletic H, et al. Methyl-L-11C-methionine PET as a diagnostic marker for malignant progression in patients with glioma. J Nucl Med. 2009;50:1962–8.

43. Yamane T, Sakamoto S, Senda M. Clinical impact of (11)C-methionine PET on expected management of patients with brain neoplasm. Eur J Nucl Med Mol Imaging. 2010;37:685–90.

44. Crippa F, Alessi A, Serafini GL. PET with radiolabeled aminoacid. Q J Nucl Med Mol Imaging. 2012;56:151–62.

45. Yamamoto Y, Nishiyama Y, Kimura N, Kameyama R, Kawai N, Hatakeyama T, et al. 11C-acetate PET in the evaluation of brain glioma: comparison with 11C-methionine and 18F-FDG-PET. Mol Imaging Biol. 2008;10:281–7.

46. Smits A, Westerberg E, Ribom D. Adding 11C-methionine PET to the EORTC prognostic factors in grade 2 gliomas. Eur J Nucl Med Mol Imaging. 2008;35:65–71.

47. Nariai T, Tanaka Y, Wakimoto H, Aoyagi M, Tamaki M, Ishiwata K, et al. Usefulness of L-[methyl-11C] methionine-positron emission tomography as a biological monitoring tool in the treatment of glioma. J Neurosurg. 2005;103:498–507.

48. Kim S, Chung JK, Im SH, Jeong JM, Lee DS, Kim DG, et al. 11C-methionine PET as a prognostic marker in patients with glioma: comparison with 18F-FDG PET. Eur J Nucl Med Mol Imaging. 2005;32:52–9.

49. Ribom D, Eriksson A, Hartman M, Engler H, Nilsson A, Langstrom B, et al. Positron emission tomography (11)C-methionine and survival in patients with low-grade gliomas. Cancer. 2001;92:1541–9.

50. Kaschten B, Stevenaert A, Sadzot B, Deprez M, Degueldre C, Del FG, et al. Preoperative evaluation of 54 gliomas by PET with fluorine-18-fluorodeoxyglucose and/or carbon-11-methionine. J Nucl Med. 1998;39:778–85.

51. Ceyssens S, Van Laere K, de Groot T, Goffin J, Bormans G, Mortelmans L. [11C]methionine PET, histopathology, and survival in primary brain tumors and recurrence. AJNR Am J Neuroradiol. 2006;27:1432–7.

52. Lee IH, Piert M, Gomez-Hassan D, Junck L, Rogers L, Hayman J, et al. Association of 11C-methionine PET uptake with site of failure after concurrent temozolomide and radiation for primary glioblastoma multiforme. Int J Radiat Oncol Biol Phys. 2009;73:479–85.

53. Singhal T, Narayanan TK, Jain V, Mukherjee J, Mantil J. 11C-L-methionine positron emission tomography in the clinical management of cerebral gliomas. Mol Imaging Biol. 2008;10:1–18.

54. Giglio P, Gilbert MR. Cerebral radiation necrosis. Neurologist. 2003;9:180–8.

55. Pirotte B, Goldman S, Dewitte O, Massager N, Wikler D, Lefranc F, et al. Integrated positron emission tomography and magnetic resonance imaging-guided resection of brain tumors: a report of 103 consecutive procedures. J Neurosurg. 2006;104:238–53.

56. Voges J, Herholz K, Holzer T, Wurker M, Bauer B, Pietrzyk U, et al. 11C-methionine and 18F-2-fluorodeoxyglucose positron emission tomography: a tool for diagnosis of cerebral glioma and monitoring after brachytherapy with 125I seeds. Stereotact Funct Neurosurg. 1997;69:129–35.

57. Tripathi M, Sharma R, Varshney R, Jaimini A, Jain J, Souza MM, et al. Comparison of F-18 FDG and C-11 methionine PET/CT for the evaluation of recurrent primary brain tumors. Clin Nucl Med. 2012;37:158–63.

58. Terakawa Y, Tsuyuguchi N, Iwai Y, Yamanaka K, Higashiyama S, Takami T, et al. Diagnostic accuracy of 11C-methionine PET for differentiation of recurrent brain tumors from radiation necrosis after radiotherapy. J Nucl Med. 2008;49:694–9.

59. Okamoto S, Shiga T, Hattori N, Kubo N, Takei T, Katoh N, et al. Semiquantitative analysis of C-11 methionine PET may distinguish brain tumor recurrence from radiation necrosis even in small lesions. Ann Nucl Med. 2011;25:213–20.

60. Van Laere K, Ceyssens S, Van Calenbergh F, de Groot T, Menten J, Flamen P, et al. Direct comparison of 18F-FDG and 11C-methionine PET in suspected recurrence of glioma: sensitivity, interobserver variability and prognostic value. Eur J Nucl Med Mol Imaging. 2005;32:39–51.

61. Xu W, Gao L, Shao A, Zheng J, Zhang J. The performance of 11C-methionine PET in the differential diagnosis of glioma recurrence. Oncotarget. 2017;8(53):91030–9.

62. Bag AK, Wing MN, Sabin ND, Hwang SN, Armstrong GT, Han Y, Li Y, Snyder SE, Robinson GW, Qaddoumi I, Broniscer A, Lucas JT, Shulkin BL. 11C-methionine PET for identification of pediatric high-grade glioma recurrence. J Nucl Med. 2022;63(5):664–71.

63. Mattoli MV, Trevisi G, Scolozzi V, Capotosti A, Cocciolillo F, Marini I, Mare V, Indovina L, Caulo M, Saponiero A, et al. Dynamic 11C-methionine PET-CT: prognostic factors for disease progression and survival in patients with suspected glioma recurrence. Cancers. 2021;13(19):4777.

64. Palanichamy K, Chakravarti A. Diagnostic and prognostic significance of methionine uptake and methionine positron emission tomography imaging in gliomas. Front Oncol. 2017;7:257.

65. Grosu AL, Astner ST, Riedel E, Nieder C, Wiedenmann N, Heinemann F, et al. An interindividual comparison of O-(2-[18F]fluoroethyl)-L-tyrosine (FET)- and L-[methyl-11C]methionine (MET)-PET in patients with brain gliomas and metastases. Int J Radiat Oncol Biol Phys. 2011;81:1049–58.

66. Tsuyuguchi N, Sunada I, Iwai Y, Yamanaka K, Tanaka K, Takami T, et al. Methionine positron emission tomography of recurrent metastatic brain tumor and radiation necrosis after stereotactic radiosurgery: is a differential diagnosis possible? J Neurosurg. 2003;98:1056–64.

67. Rottenburger C, Hentschel M, Kelly T, Trippel M, Brink I, Reithmeier T, et al. Comparison of C-11 methionine and C-11 choline for PET imaging of brain metastases: a prospective pilot study. Clin Nucl Med. 2011;36:639–42.

68. Guedj E, Varrone A, Boellaard R, Albert NL, Barthel H, van Berckel B, et al. EANM procedure guidelines for brain PET imaging using [18F]FDG, version 3. Eur J Nucl Med Mol Imaging. 2022;49:632–51.

69. Jiménez-Requena F, Delgado-Bolton RC, Fernández-Pérez C, Gambhir SS, Schwimmer J, Pérez-Vázquez JM, Carreras-Delgado JL. Meta-

analysis of the performance of (18)F-FDG PET in cutaneous melanoma. Eur J Nucl Med Mol Imaging. 2010;37:284–300.

70. Bozkurt MF, Virgolini I, Balogova S, Beheshti M, Rubello D, Decristoforo C, et al. Guideline for PET/CT imaging of neuroendocrine neoplasms with 68Ga-DOTA-conjugated somatostatin receptor targeting peptides and 18F-DOPA. Eur J Nucl Med Mol Imaging. 2017;44:1588–601.

71. Boellaard R, Delgado-Bolton R, Oyen WJ, Giammarile F, Tatsch K, Eschner W, et al. FDG PET/CT: EANM procedure guidelines for tumour imaging: version 2.0. Eur J Nucl Med Mol Imaging. 2015;42:328–54.

72. Delgado-Bolton RC, Fernández-Pérez C, González-Maté A, Carreras JL. Meta-analysis of the performance of 18F-FDG PET in primary tumor detection in unknown primary tumors. J Nucl Med. 2003;44:1301–14.

73. Berghmans T, Lievens Y, Aapro M, Baird AM, Beishon M, Calabrese F, et al. European cancer organisation essential requirements for quality cancer care (ERQCC): lung cancer. Lung Cancer. 2020;150:221–39.

74. Biganzoli L, Cardoso F, Beishon M, Cameron D, Cataliotti L, Coles CE, et al. The requirements of a specialist breast centre. Breast. 2020;51:65–84.

75. Brausi M, Hoskin P, Andritsch E, Banks I, Beishon M, Boyle H, et al. ECCO essential requirements for quality cancer care: prostate cancer. Crit Rev Oncol Hematol. 2020;148:102861.

76. Allum W, Lordick F, Alsina M, Andritsch E, Ba-Ssalamah A, Beishon M, et al. ECCO essential requirements for quality cancer care: oesophageal and gastric cancer. Crit Rev Oncol Hematol. 2018;122:179–93.

77. Wouters MW, Michielin O, Bastiaannet E, Beishon M, Catalano O, Del Marmol V, et al. ECCO essential requirements for quality cancer care: melanoma. Crit Rev Oncol Hematol. 2018;122:164–78.

78. Andritsch E, Beishon M, Bielack S, Bonvalot S, Casali P, Crul M, et al. ECCO essential requirements for quality cancer care: soft tissue sarcoma in adults and bone sarcoma. A critical review. Crit Rev Oncol Hematol. 2017;110:94–105.

79. Beets G, Sebag-Montefiore D, Andritsch E, Arnold D, Beishon M, Crul M, et al. ECCO essential requirements for quality cancer care: colorectal cancer. A critical review. Crit Rev Oncol Hematol. 2017;110:81–93.

80. Delgado Bolton RC, Calapaquí Terán AK, Fanti S, Giammarile F. New biomarkers with prognostic impact based on multitracer PET/CT imaging in neuroendocrine neoplasms: the light leading out of the darkness in challenging tumors. Clin Nucl Med. 2022;47:219–20.

81. Delgado Bolton RC, Calapaquí Terán AK, Fanti S, Giammarile F. The concept of strength through synergy applied to the search of powerful prognostic biomarkers in gastroesophageal cancer: an example

based on combining clinicopathological parameters, imaging-derived sarcopenia measurements, and radiomic features. Clin Nucl Med. 2023;48:156–7.

82. Urso L, Bonatto E, Nieri A, Castello A, Maffione AM, Marzola MC, Cittanti C, Bartolomei M, Panareo S, Mansi L, Lopci E, Florimonte L, Castellani M. The role of molecular imaging in patients with brain metastases: a literature review. Cancers (Basel). 2023;15(7):2184.

83. Lopci E, Riva M, Olivari L, Raneri F, Soffietti R, Piccardo A, Bizzi A, Navarria P, Ascolese AM, Rudà R, Fernandes B, Pessina F, Grimaldi M, Simonelli M, Rossi M, Alfieri T, Zucali PA, Scorsetti M, Bello L, Chiti A. Prognostic value of molecular and imaging biomarkers in patients with supratentorial glioma. Eur J Nucl Med Mol Imaging. 2017;44(7):1155–64.

84. Riva M, Lopci E, Castellano A, Olivari L, Gallucci M, Pessina F, Fernandes B, Simonelli M, Navarria P, Grimaldi M, Rudà R, Castello A, Rossi M, Alfiero T, Soffietti R, Chiti A, Bello L. Lower grade gliomas: relationships between metabolic and structural imaging with grading and molecular factors. World Neurosurg. 2019;126:e270–80.

85. Castello A, Riva M, Fernandes B, Bello L, Lopci E. The role of 11C-methionine PET in patients with negative diffusion-weighted magnetic resonance imaging: correlation with histology and molecular biomarkers in operated gliomas. Nucl Med Commun. 2020;41(7):696–705.

86. Zaragori T, Castello A, Guedj E, Girard A, Galldiks N, Albert NL, Lopci E, Verger A. Photopenic defects in gliomas with amino-acid PET and relative prognostic value: a multicentric 11C-methionine and 18F-FDOPA PET experience. Clin Nucl Med. 2021;46(1):e36–7.

87. Upadhyay N, Waldman AD. Conventional MRI evaluation of gliomas. Br J Radiol. 2011;84(SI2):S107–11.

88. Brindle KM, Izquierdo-García JL, Lewis DY, Mair RJ, Wright AJ. Brain tumor imaging. J Clin Oncol. 2017;35:2432–8.

89. Castello A, Castellani M, Florimonte L, Ciccariello G, Mansi L, Lopci E. PET radiotracers in glioma: a review of clinical indications and evidence. Clin Translat Imaging. 2022;10:535–51.

90. Wang L, Lieberman BP, Ploessl K, Kung HF. Synthesis and evaluation of (1)(8)F labeled FET prodrugs for tumor imaging. Nucl Med Biol. 2014;41:58–67.

91. Galldiks N, Stoffels G, Filss C, et al. The use of dynamic O-(2-18F-fluoroethyl)-l-tyrosine PET in the diagnosis of patients with progressive and recurrent glioma. Neuro Oncol. 2015;17:1293–300.

92. Ceccon G, Lohmann P, Stoffels G, et al. Dynamic O-(2-18F-fluoroethyl)-L-tyrosine positron emission tomography differentiates brain metastasis recurrence from radiation injury after radiotherapy. Neuro Oncol. 2017;19:281–8.

93. Dunet V, Rossier C, Buck A, Stupp R, Prior JO. Performance of 18F-fluoro-ethyltyrosine (18F-FET) PET for the differential diagnosis of primary brain tumor: a systematic review and metaanalysis. J Nucl Med. 2012;53:207–14.

94. Rapp M, Heinzel A, Galldiks N, et al. Diagnostic performance of 18F-FET PET in newly diagnosed cerebral lesions suggestive of glioma. J Nucl Med. 2013;54:229–35.

95. Hutterer M, Ebner Y, Riemenschneider MJ, et al. Epileptic activity increases cerebral amino acid transport assessed by 18F-fluoroethyl-l-tyrosine amino acid PET: a potential brain tumor mimic. J Nucl Med. 2017;58:129–37.

96. Wollring MM, Werner JM, Ceccon G, et al. Clinical applications and prospects of PET imaging in patients with IDH-mutant gliomas. J Neurooncol. 2023;162:481–8.

97. Pauleit D, Floeth F, Hamacher K, et al. O-(2-[18F] fluoroethyl)-L-tyrosine PET combined with MRI improves the diagnostic assessment of cerebral gliomas. Brain. 2005;128:678–87.

98. Verburg N, Koopman T, Yaqub MM, et al. Improved detection of diffuse glioma infiltration with imaging combinations: a diagnostic accuracy study. Neuro Oncol. 2020;22:412–22.

99. Schön S, Cabello J, Liesche-Starnecker F, et al. Imaging glioma biology: spatial comparison of amino acid PET, amide proton transfer, and perfusion-weighted MRI in newly diagnosed gliomas. Eur J Nucl Med Mol Imaging. 2020;47:1468–75.

100. Dissaux G, Dissaux B, Kabbaj OE, et al. Radiotherapy target volume definition in newly diagnosed high-grade glioma using (18)F-FET-PET imaging and multiparametric perfusion MRI: a prospective study (IMAGG). Radiother Oncol. 2020;150:164–71.

101. Hayes AR, Jayamanne D, Hsiao E, et al. Utilizing 18F-fluoroethyltyrosine (FET) positron emission tomography (PET) to define suspected nonenhancing tumor for radiation therapy planning of glioblastoma. Pract Radiat Oncol. 2018;8(4):230–8.

102. Weber DC, Zilli T, Buchegger F, et al. [(18)F] Fluoroethyltyrosine-positron emission tomography-guided radiotherapy for high-grade glioma. Radiat Oncol. 2008;3:44.

103. Galldiks N, Langen KJ, Holy R, et al. Assessment of treatment response in patients with glioblastoma using O-(2-18Ffluoroethyl)-l-tyrosine PET in comparison to MRI. J Nucl Med. 2012;53:1048–57.

104. Ceccon G, Lohmann P, Werner J-M, et al. Early treatment response assessment using 18F-FET PET compared with contrast enhanced MRI in glioma patients after adjuvant temozolomide chemotherapy. J Nucl Med. 2021;62:918–25.

105. Galldiks N, Dunkl V, Ceccon G, et al. Early treatment response evaluation using FET PET compared to MRI in glioblastoma patients at first progression treated with bevacizumab plus lomustine. Eur J Nucl Med Mol Imaging. 2018;45:2377–86.

106. Morana G, Piccardo A, Garre ML, Nozza P, Consales A, Rossi A. Multimodal magnetic resonance imaging and 18F-L-dihydroxyphenylalanine positron

emission tomography in early characterization of pseudoresponse and nonenhancing tumor progression in a pediatric patient with malignant transformation of ganglioglioma treated with bevacizumab. J Clin Oncol. 2013;31:e1–5.

107. Hutterer M, Nowosielski M, Putzer D, et al. O-(2-18F-fluoroethyl)-L-tyrosine PET predicts failure of antiangiogenic treatment in patients with recurrent high-grade glioma. J Nucl Med. 2011;52:856–64.

108. Galldiks N, Werner JM, Tscherpel C, Fink GR, Langen KJ. Imaging findings following regorafenib in malignant gliomas: FET PET adds valuable information to anatomical MRI. Neurooncol Adv. 2019;1:vdz038.

109. Lombardi G, Spimpolo A, Berti S, et al. PET/MR in recurrent glioblastoma patients treated with regorafenib: [18F]FET and DWI-ADC for response assessment and survival prediction. Br J Radiol. 2022;95:20211018.

110. Pyka T, Hiob D, Preibisch C, et al. Diagnosis of glioma recurrence using multiparametric dynamic 18F-fluoroethyl-tyrosine PET-MRI. Eur J Radiol. 2018;103:32–7.

111. Verger A, Filss CP, Lohmann P, et al. Comparison of O-(2-(18)F-fluoroethyl)-l-tyrosine positron emission tomography and perfusion-weighted magnetic resonance imaging in the diagnosis of patients with progressive and recurrent glioma: a hybrid positron emission tomography/magnetic resonance study. World Neurosurg. 2018;113:e727–37.

112. Maurer GD, Brucker DP, Stoffels G, et al. 18F-FETPET imaging in differentiating glioma progression from treatment-related changes: a single-center experience. J Nucl Med. 2020;61(4):505–11.

113. Mihovilovic MI, Kertels O, Hänscheid H, et al. O-(2-(18F) fluoroethyl)-l-tyrosine PET for the differentiation of tumour recurrence from late pseudoprogression in glioblastoma. J Neurol Neurosurg Psychiatry. 2019;90(2):238–9.

114. Kebir S, Fimmers R, Galldiks N, et al. Late pseudoprogression in glioblastoma: diagnostic value of dynamic O-(2-[18F] fluoroethyl)-l-tyrosine PET. Clin Cancer Res. 2016;22(9):2190–6.

115. Werner JM, Stoffels G, Lichtenstein T, et al. Differentiation of treatment-related changes from tumour progression: a direct comparison between dynamic FET-PET and ADC values obtained from DWI MRI. Eur J Nucl Med Mol Imaging. 2019;46(9):1889–901.

116. Kertels O, Mihovilovic MI, Linsenmann T, et al. Clinical utility of different approaches for detection of pseudoprogression in glioblastoma with O-(2-[18F]fluoroethyl)-l-tyrosine PET. Clin Nucl Med. 2019;44(9):695–701.

117. Galldiks N, Dunkl V, Stoffels G, et al. Diagnosis of pseudoprogression in patients with glioblastoma using O-(2-[18F] fluoroethyl)-l-tyrosine PET. Eur J Nucl Med Mol Imaging. 2015;42(5):685–95.

118. Bashir A, Mathilde Jacobsen S, Molby Henriksen O, et al. Recurrent glioblastoma versus late posttreatment changes: diagnostic accuracy of O-(2-[18F]fluoroethyl)-l-tyrosine positron emission tomography (18F-FET-PET). Neuro Oncol. 2019;21(12):1595–606.

119. Celli M, Caroli P, Amadori E, et al. Diagnostic and prognostic potential of 18F-FET PET in the differential diagnosis of glioma recurrence and treatment-induced changes after chemoradiation therapy. Front Oncol. 2021;11:721821.

120. Puranik AD, Rangarajan V, Dev ID, et al. Brain FET PET tumor-to-white mater ratio to differentiate recurrence from post-treatment changes in high-grade gliomas. J Neuroimaging. 2021;31:1211–8.

121. Unterrainer M, Galldiks N, Suchorska B, et al. 18F-FET PET uptake characteristics in patients with newly diagnosed and untreated brain metastasis. J Nucl Med. 2017;58:584–9.

122. Romagna A, Unterrainer M, Schmid-Tannwald C, et al. Suspected recurrence of brain metastases after focused high dose radiotherapy: can [18F]FET-PET overcome diagnostic uncertainties? Radiat Oncol. 2016;11:139.

123. Schlürmann T, Waschulzik B, Combs S, et al. Utility of amino acid PET in the differential diagnosis of recurrent brain metastases and treatment-related changes: a meta-analysis. J Nucl Med. 2023;64(5):816–21.

124. Kebir S, Rauschenbach L, Galldiks N, et al. Dynamic O-(2-[18F]fluoroethyl)-L-tyrosine PET imaging for the detection of checkpoint inhibitor-related pseudoprogression in melanoma brain metastases. Neuro Oncol. 2016;18:1462–4.

125. Galldiks N, Abdulla DSY, Scheffler M, et al. Treatment monitoring of immunotherapy and targeted therapy using 18F-FET PET in patients with melanoma and lung cancer brain metastases: initial experiences. J Nucl Med. 2021;62:464–70.

126. Youland RS, Kitange GJ, Peterson TE, Pafundi DH, Ramiscal JA, Pokorny JL, et al. The role of LAT1 in (18)F-DOPA uptake in malignant gliomas. J Neurooncol. 2013;111:11–8.

127. Habermeier A, Graf J, Sandhöfer BF, Boissel JP, Roesch F, Closs EI. System L amino acid transporter LAT1 accumulates O-(2-fluoroethyl)-L-tyrosine (FET). Amino Acids. 2015;47:335–44.

128. Pavese N, Simpson BS, Metta V, Ramlackhansingh A, Chaudhuri KR, Brooks DJ. [18F]FDOPA uptake in the raphe nuclei complex reflects serotonin transporter availability. A combined [18F]FDOPA and [11C]DASB PET study in Parkinson's disease. Neuroimage. 2012;59(2):1080–4.

129. Moore RY, Whone AL, Brooks DJ. Extrastriatal monoamine neuron function in Parkinson's disease: an 18F-dopa PET study. Neurobiol Dis. 2008;29(3):381–90.

130. Pafundi DH, Laack NN, Youland RS, Parney IF, Lowe VJ, Giannini C, Kemp BJ, Grams MP, Morris JM, Hoover JM, Hu LS, Sarkaria JN, Brinkmann DH. Biopsy validation of 18F-DOPA PET and biodistribution in gliomas for neurosurgical planning and

radiotherapy target delineation: results of a prospective pilot study. Neuro Oncol. 2013;15(8):1058–67.

131. Youland RS, Pafundi DH, Brinkmann DH, Lowe VJ, Morris JM, Kemp BJ, Hunt CH, Giannini C, Parney IF, Laack NN. Prospective trial evaluating the sensitivity and specificity of 3,4-dihydroxy-6-[18F]-fluoro-L-phenylalanine (18F-DOPA) PET and MRI in patients with recurrent gliomas. J Neurooncol. 2018;137(3):583–91.

132. Girard A, Le Reste PJ, Metais A, Carsin Nicol B, Chiforeanu DC, Bannier E, Campillo-Gimenez B, Devillers A, Palard-Novello X, Le Jeune F. Combining 18F-DOPA PET and MRI with perfusion-weighted imaging improves delineation of high-grade subregions in enhancing and non-enhancing gliomas prior treatment: a biopsy-controlled study. J Neurooncol. 2021;155(3):287–95.

133. Cicone F, Filss CP, Minniti G, Rossi-Espagnet C, Papa A, Scaringi C, Galldiks N, Bozzao A, Shah NJ, Scopinaro F, Langen KJ. Volumetric assessment of recurrent or progressive gliomas: comparison between F-DOPA PET and perfusion-weighted MRI. Eur J Nucl Med Mol Imaging. 2015;42(6):905–15.

134. Carideo L, Minniti G, Mamede M, Scaringi C, Russo I, Scopinaro F, Cicone F. 18F-DOPA uptake parameters in glioma: effects of patients' characteristics and prior treatment history. Br J Radiol. 2018;91(1084):20170847.

135. Verger A, Metellus P, Sala Q, Colin C, Bialecki E, Taieb D, Chinot O, Figarella-Branger D, Guedj E. IDH mutation is paradoxically associated with higher 18F-FDOPA PET uptake in diffuse grade II and grade III gliomas. Eur J Nucl Med Mol Imaging. 2017;44(8):1306–11.

136. Cicone F, Carideo L, Scaringi C, Arcella A, Giangaspero F, Scopinaro F, Minniti G. 18F-DOPA uptake does not correlate with IDH mutation status and 1p/19q co-deletion in glioma. Ann Nucl Med. 2019;33(4):295–302.

137. Ginet M, Zaragori T, Marie PY, Roch V, Gauchotte G, Rech F, Blonski M, Lamiral Z, Taillandier L, Imbert L, Verger A. Integration of dynamic parameters in the analysis of 18F-FDopa PET imaging improves the prediction of molecular features of gliomas. Eur J Nucl Med Mol Imaging. 2020;47(6):1381–90.

138. Qian J, Herman MG, Brinkmann DH, Laack NN, Kemp BJ, Hunt CH, Lowe V, Pafundi DH. Prediction of MGMT status for glioblastoma patients using radiomics feature extraction from 18F-DOPA-PET imaging. Int J Radiat Oncol Biol Phys. 2020;108(5):1339–46.

139. Zaragori T, Oster J, Roch V, Hossu G, Chawki MB, Grignon R, Pouget C, Gauchotte G, Rech F, Blonski M, Taillandier L, Imbert L, Verger A. 18F-FDOPA PET for the noninvasive prediction of glioma molecular parameters: a radiomics study. J Nucl Med. 2022;63(1):147–57.

140. Herrmann K, Czernin J, Cloughesy T, Lai A, Pomykala KL, Benz MR, Buck AK, Phelps ME, Chen W. Comparison of visual and semiquantitative analysis of 18F-FDOPA-PET/CT for recurrence detection in glioblastoma patients. Neuro Oncol. 2014;16(4):603–9.

141. Karunanithi S, Sharma P, Kumar A, Khangembam BC, Bandopadhyaya GP, Kumar R, Gupta DK, Malhotra A, Bal C. 18F-FDOPA PET/CT for detection of recurrence in patients with glioma: prospective comparison with 18F-FDG PET/CT. Eur J Nucl Med Mol Imaging. 2013;40(7):1025–35.

142. Karunanithi S, Sharma P, Kumar A, Gupta DK, Khangembam BC, Ballal S, Kumar R, Kumar R, Bal C. Can (18)F-FDOPA PET/CT predict survival in patients with suspected recurrent glioma? A prospective study. Eur J Radiol. 2014;83(1):219–25.

143. Kosztyla R, Chan EK, Hsu F, Wilson D, Ma R, Cheung a, Zhang S, Moiseenko V, Benard F, Nichol A. High-grade glioma radiation therapy target volumes and patterns of failure obtained from magnetic resonance imaging and 18F-FDOPA positron emission tomography delineations from multiple observers. Int J Radiat Oncol Biol Phys. 2013;87(5):1100–6.

144. Breen WG, Youland RS, Giri S, Jacobson SB, Pafundi DH, Brown PD, Hunt CH, Mahajan A, Ruff MW, Kizilbash SH, Uhm JH, Routman DM, Jones JE, Brinkmann DH, Laack NN. Initial results of a phase II trial of 18F-DOPA PET-guided re-irradiation for recurrent high-grade glioma. J Neurooncol. 2022;158(3):323–30.

145. Laack NN, Pafundi D, Anderson SK, Kaufmann T, Lowe V, Hunt C, Vogen D, Yan E, Sarkaria J, Brown P, Kizilbash S, Uhm J, Ruff M, Zakhary M, Zhang Y, Seaberg M, Wan Chan Tseung HS, Kabat B, Kemp B, Brinkmann D. Initial results of a phase 2 trial of 18F-DOPA PET-guided dose-escalated radiation therapy for glioblastoma. Int J Radiat Oncol Biol Phys. 2021;110(5):1383–95.

146. https://pubmed.ncbi.nlm.nih.gov/38181810/.

147. Cicone F, Galldiks N, Papa A, Langen K-J, Cascini GL, Minniti G. Repeated amino acid PET imaging for longitudinal monitoring of brain tumors. Clin Transl Imaging. 2022;10:457–65.

148. Oughourlian TC, Yao J, Schlossman J, Raymond C, Ji M, Tatekawa H, Salamon N, Pope WB, Czernin J, Nghiemphu PL, Lai A, Cloughesy TF, Ellingson BM. Rate of change in maximum 18F-FDOPA PET uptake and non-enhancing tumor volume predict malignant transformation and overall survival in low-grade gliomas. J Neurooncol. 2020;147(1):135–45.

149. Schwarzenberg J, Czernin J, Cloughesy TF, Ellingson BM, Pope WB, Grogan T, Elashoff D, Geist C, Silverman DH, Phelps ME, Chen W. Treatment response evaluation using 18F-FDOPA PET in patients with recurrent malignant glioma on bevacizumab therapy. Clin Cancer Res. 2014;20(13):3550–9.

150. Sturm D, Pfister SM, Jones DTW. Pediatric gliomas: current concepts on diagnosis, biology, and clinical management. J Clin Oncol. 2017;35:2370–7.

151. Paugh BS, Qu C, Jones C, Liu Z, Adamowicz-Brice M, Zhang J, et al. Integrated molecular genetic profiling of pediatric high-grade gliomas reveals key differences with the adult disease. J Clin Oncol. 2010;28:3061–8.
152. Ryall S, Tabori U, Hawkins C. Pediatric low-grade glioma in the era of molecular diagnostics. Acta Neuropathol Commun. 2020;8:1–22.
153. Louis DN, Perry A, Reifenberger G, von Deimling A, Figarella-Branger D, Cavenee WK, et al. The 2016 World Health Organization classification of tumors of the central nervous system: a summary. Acta Neuropathol. 2016;131:803–20.
154. Gajjar A, Bowers DC, Karajannis MA, Leary S, Witt H, Gottardo NG. Pediatric brain tumors: innovative genomic information is transforming the diagnostic and clinical landscape. J Clin Oncol. 2015;33:2986–98.
155. Cohen KJ, Jabado N, Grill J. Diffuse intrinsic pontine gliomas—current management and new biologic insights. Is there a glimmer of hope? Neuro Oncol. 2017;19:1025–34.
156. Pollack IF. Multidisciplinary management of childhood brain tumors: a review of outcomes, recent advances, and challenges. J Neurosurg Pediatr. 2011;8(2):135–48.
157. Peet AC, Arvanitis TN, Leach MO, Waldman AD. Functional imaging in adult and paediatric brain tumours. Nat Rev Clin Oncol. 2012;9(12):700–11.
158. Chen W, Silverman DH, Delaloye S, Czernin J, Kamdar N, Pope W, Satyamurthy N, Schiepers C, Cloughesy T. 18F-FDOPA PET imaging of brain tumors: comparison study with 18F-FDG PET and evaluation of diagnostic accuracy. J Nucl Med. 2006;47(6):904–11.
159. Morana G, Piccardo A, Puntoni M, Nozza P, Cama A, Raso A, Mascelli S, Massollo M, Milanaccio C, Garrè ML, Rossi A. Diagnostic and prognostic value of 18F-DOPA PET and 1H-MR spectroscopy in pediatric supratentorial infiltrative gliomas: a comparative study. Neuro Oncol. 2015;17(12):1637–47.
160. Piccardo A, Tortora D, Mascelli S, Severino M, Piatelli G, Consales A, Pescetto M, Biassoni V, Schiavello E, Massollo M, Verrico A, Milanaccio C, Garrè ML, Rossi A, Morana G. Advanced MR imaging and 18F-DOPA PET characteristics of H3K27M-mutant and wild-type pediatric diffuse midline gliomas. Eur J Nucl Med Mol Imaging. 2019;46(8):1685–94.
161. Morana G, Tortora D, Bottoni G, Puntoni M, Piatelli G, Garibotto F, Barra S, Giannelli F, Cistaro A, Severino M, Verrico A, Milanaccio C, Massimino M, Garrè ML, Rossi A, Piccardo A. Correlation of multimodal 18F-DOPA PET and conventional MRI with treatment response and survival in children with diffuse intrinsic pontine gliomas. Theranostics. 2020;10(26):11881–91.
162. Marner L, Lundemann M, Sehested A, Nysom K, Borgwardt L, Mathiasen R, Wehner PS, Henriksen OM, Thomsen C, Skjøth-Rasmussen J, Broholm H, Østrup O, Forman JL, Højgaard L, Law I. Diagnostic accuracy and clinical impact of [18F]FET PET in childhood CNS tumors. Neuro Oncol. 2021;23(12):2107–16.
163. Pirotte B, Acerbi F, Lubansu A, Goldman S, Brotchi J, Levivier M. PET imaging in the surgical management of pediatric brain tumors. Childs Nerv Syst. 2007;23(7):739–51.
164. Pirotte BJM, Lubansu A, Massager N, Wikler D, Goldman S, Levivier M. Results of positron emission tomography guidance and reassessment of the utility of and indications for stereotactic biopsy in children with infiltrative brainstem tumors. J Neurosurg. 2007;107:392–9.
165. O'Tuama LA, Phillips PC, Strauss LC, Carson BC, Uno Y, Smith QR, et al. Two-phase [11C] l-methionine PET in childhood brain tumors. Pediatr Neurol. 1990;6:163–70.
166. Morana G, Piccardo A, Milanaccio C, Puntoni M, Nozza P, Cama A, et al. Value of 18F-3,4-dihydroxyphenylalanine PET/MR image fusion in pediatric supratentorial infiltrative astrocytomas: a prospective pilot study. J Nucl Med. 2014;55:718.
167. Dunkl V, Cleff C, Stoffels G, Judov N, Sarikaya-Seiwert S, Law I, et al. The usefulness of dynamic O-(2-18F-Fluoroethyl)-L-tyrosine PET in the clinical evaluation of brain tumors in children and adolescents. J Nucl Med. 2015;56:88–92.
168. Lucas JT Jr, Serrano N, Kim H, Li X, Snyder SE, Hwang S, Li Y, Hua CH, Broniscer A, Merchant TE, Shulkin BL. 11C-Methionine positron emission tomography delineates non-contrast enhancing tumor regions at high risk for recurrence in pediatric high-grade glioma. J Neurooncol. 2017;132(1):163–70.
169. Puget S, Alshehri A, Beccaria K, Blauwblomme T, Paternoster G, James S, Dirocco F, Dufour C, Zerah M, Varlet P, Sainte-Rose C. Pediatric infratentorial ganglioglioma. Childs Nerv Syst. 2015;31(10):1707–16.
170. Luo CB, Teng MM, Chen SS, Lirng JF, Guo WY, Lan GY, Chang T. Intracranial ganglioglioma: CT and MRI findings. Kaohsiung J Med Sci. 1997;13(8):467–74.
171. Marner L, Nysom K, Sehested A, Borgwardt L, Mathiasen R, Henriksen OM, Lundemann M, Munck Af Rosenschöld P, Thomsen C, Bøgeskov L, Skjøth-Rasmussen J, Juhler M, Kruse A, Broholm H, Scheie D, Lauritsen T, Forman JL, Wehner PS, Højgaard L, Law I. Early postoperative 18F-FET PET/MRI for pediatric brain and spinal cord tumors. J Nucl Med. 2019;60(8):1053–8.
172. Fiz F, Bini F, Gabriele E, Bottoni G, Garrè M, Marinozzi F, Milanaccio C, Verrico A, Massollo M, Bosio V, Lattuada M, Rossi A, et al. Role of dynamic parameters of 18F-DOPA PET/CT in pediatric gliomas. Clin Nucl Med. 2022;47:517–24.

State of the Art of Surgical Treatment in Brain Tumors

Massimiliano Del Bene, Giovanni Carone, and Francesco DiMeco

Neuro-oncology is rapidly evolving by recognizing in a multidisciplinary synergy the key to improve diagnosis, treatment, and management of nervous system tumor patients. Surgery is a pivotal module in the treatment path, and recent advancements in surgical techniques and technologies have greatly improved outcomes and efficacy.

This chapter provides an overview of the current state of the art of surgical treatment for neuro-oncological diseases. This aim is pursued by reconstructing the surgical workflow, step by step, starting from the planning, including preoperative imaging and neuronavigation, and ending with the instrumental and functional adjuncts that support surgery.

M. Del Bene
Department of Neurosurgery, Fondazione IRCCS
Istituto Neurologico Carlo Besta, Milan, Italy

Department of Experimental Oncology, IEO,
European Institute of Oncology IRCCS, Milan, Italy

G. Carone
Department of Neurosurgery, Fondazione IRCCS
Istituto Neurologico Carlo Besta, Milan, Italy

F. DiMeco (✉)
Department of Neurosurgery, Fondazione IRCCS
Istituto Neurologico Carlo Besta, Milan, Italy

Department of Pathophysiology and Transplantation,
University of Milan, Milan, Italy

Department of Neurological Surgery, Johns Hopkins
Medical School, Baltimore, MD, USA
e-mail: Francesco.DiMeco@istituto-besta.it

4.1 Preoperative Planning for the Guidance of Brain Tumors Resection

The main goal of surgery is to achieve an as complete as possible resection while preserving the patient's functions. It is universally recognized that surgical planning plays a primary role in this effort, indeed the longer the time spent on this phase, the greater the level of confidence a surgeon can experience during surgery. This phase leads to designing the surgical strategy, thus including patient positioning, approach selection, and defining the expected extent of resection (EOR).

4.1.1 Imaging Techniques

The first pillar of presurgical planning is to establish a correct presumptive diagnosis based on multimodal data obtained from pre-operative imaging modalities.

Simplifying, neuroimaging techniques can be classified into two approaches: one structural and one functional [1]. Structural imaging refers to the visualization and analysis of the anatomical features of the brain. This is particularly indicated for lesion localization and characterization under geometric structural properties such as the size and volume of a given structure or the thickness of a cortical area [2, 3]. Functional imaging is used to identify brain areas and underlying brain processes that are associated with a particular cognitive or behavioural task [4, 5].

Regarding structural imaging, the two main techniques that fall into this category are Computed Tomography (CT) and Magnetic Resonance Imaging (MRI). As far as CT, which utilizes highly focused X-ray beams to produce multiple cross-sectional images, it is mainly indicated to understand the relationship between the bone and lesion density and enhance the accuracy of surface matching in the registration phase of neuronavigation [6, 7]. In contrast, MRI offers highly detailed images of the brain and surrounding structures by highlighting anatomical relationships and tissue characteristics useful to guide diagnosis [8]. A technique that is part of structural examinations but conceptually bridges with functional ones is diffusion tensor imaging (DTI), which is capable of reconstructing white matter connections within the brain in detail. By tracking the constrained movement of water molecules in the brain, DTI can reveal the orientation of underlying white matter tracts, allowing for the reconstruction of neural pathways in three dimensions using tractography algorithms [9, 10].

Functional neuroimaging techniques include functional magnetic resonance imaging (fMRI), which highlights the functional areas in the brain associated with cognitive or behavioural tasks by measuring changes in blood flow and oxygen levels. These changes are referred to as the blood oxygen level-dependent (BOLD) response, and the scanner can detect regional changes in this signal [11, 12]. It has to be said that fMRI is an indirect measure of brain activity, unlike neurophysiological techniques such as electroencephalography (EEG), which directly record the brain's electrical activity using electrodes on the scalp. Magnetoencephalography (MEG) is a related technique that measures the magnetic field generated by the electrical activity of neurons, providing better spatial and temporal resolution than EEG [13]. Positron emission tomography (PET) is another form of functional imaging that uses a radioactive tracer to measure energy consumption in the brain, indicating neural activity.

However, PET is costly and limited by the use of a radioactive tracer, making it less practical for repeated scans [14].

In addition, also vascular imaging (with CT, MRI or angiography) can help identify blood vessels feeding the tumor, allowing for safer and more precise surgical planning and execution. They can detect any abnormalities or changes in blood flow caused by the tumor, aiding in diagnosis and monitoring. By providing a clearer picture of the tumor's blood supply, vascular imaging can assist in determining the tumor size and location, which is crucial for developing an effective treatment plan and guiding surgical navigation, allowing for visualization of the tumor and surrounding blood vessels during the procedure [15, 16].

While structural images are the mainstay of planning, functional images can be considered according to necessity, taking into account that each resource has an economic, logistical and temporal impact. Therefore, while any lesion regardless of its nature and location is worthy of a CT scan and MRI, only in selected cases, functional assessment should be considered.

Notably, the collection of these images is crucial not only for the first planning phase but also for the next one, which is neuronavigation.

4.1.2 Neuronavigation

Conceived in 1980, neuronavigation systems have revolutionized the field of neurosurgery by providing real-time guidance during complex procedures [17]. These systems utilize optical or electromagnetic detectors coupled with computerized image-processing modules to track the position of a probe in relation to a fixed reference frame. By localizing anatomical landmarks within the operative field and registering them with identical landmarks on a 3D model constructed using data from preoperative imaging scans, neuronavigation enables the extrapolation of preoperative imaging and plans within the patient's cranium in real time. These image-to-patient techniques increase the chance of performing a safe and functional gross total resection of brain tumors [18, 19]. A further advancement in navigation has been given by the implementation of functional images, such as DTI and BOLD, which allow planning the correct and safe approach and corridor to the lesion, as well as offering a fundamental aid during excision to ensure function preservation [20, 21]. Neuronavigation's main objective is to facilitate extensive lesion resection while minimizing the risk of neurological sequelae and favouring the outcome [22]. This is possible thanks to the aid provided by neuronavigation in planning the surgery, localizing lesions, creating smaller craniotomies, reducing surgery time, and finally decreasing morbidity and mortality.

Concerning the limits, one of the main disadvantages of neuronavigation is the brain shift observed after craniotomy and dura opening as well as the brain deformation occurring during tumor resection which significantly undermines the precision of neuronavigation [23]. Intraoperative MRI could deal with this limit, but as a matter of fact, these facilities are not always available [24]. Another solution is provided by intra-operative ultrasound scans which can be used before dural opening, after dural opening, and during resection to correct brain shift every time needed [25, 26].

In conclusion, neuronavigation has greatly improved the precision, accuracy, and safety of neurosurgical procedures. This technology enables surgeons to navigate the complex anatomy of the brain with greater confidence, resulting in better outcomes for patients. However, there are limitations to consider, such as the biological variability among individuals and brain shift/deformation occurrence. Nevertheless, as technology continues to advance, we can expect to see further improvements.

4.1.3 New Advanced Technologies

The use of augmented reality (AR) and virtual reality (VR) has steadily increased over the last decade, entailing a significant refinement of the technique, making it more precise, accurate, and safe for patients. Their application covers all aspects of neurosurgery, from residents' training, surgical planning, surgical guidance and also to inform patients [27–30].

Intraoperatively, microscope-guided interventions (MAGI) provide preoperative 3D images superimposed on the oculars of the surgical microscope at AR (Fig. 4.1). The advantage of MAGI over the pointer-based navigation system is obvious, as the surgeon does not need to shift focus from the surgical field to the screen. Additionally, MAGI can provide information regarding the location of nearby structures, thus enhancing orientation and precision. Similarly, AR and VR are being used in image-enhanced endoscopy, where real and virtual images are superimposed with multiple layers to provide enhanced surgical exposure [31, 32].

The use of these advanced technology systems, therefore, constitutes a useful tool for neurosurgeons, gradually becoming a must-have to ensure improved surgery and greater patient safety.

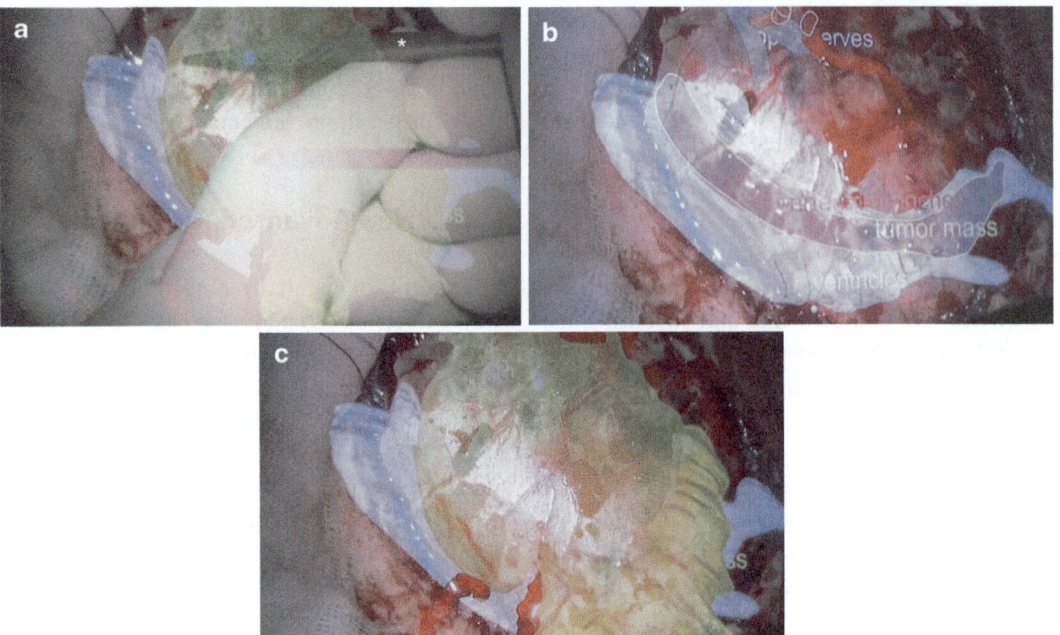

Fig. 4.1 An illustrative case of reality augmentation applied to the neurosurgical context. (**a**) Superimposition of 3D AR images under the microscope during the navigation phase (*navigator; in *green* the tumor; in *light blue* the ventricles); (**b**) in *blue* the ventricles, in *red* the vascular structures, in *blue* the nerves; (**c**) in *green* the tumor; in *light blue* the ventricles; in *blue* the nerves

4.2   Intra-operative Imaging

As new imaging technologies continue to emerge, the potential as surgical tools has led to the adoption of various diagnostic imaging devices in the operating room.

The use of multimodal imaging should be the goal in the long run, and synergy between technologies is the key to this aim.

4.2.1   Structural Intra-operative Imaging: iMRI and IOUS

As far as intra-operative imaging is concerned, the instruments with the greatest potential to date are certainly Intra-operative MRI (iMRI) and Intra-operative ultrasound (IOUS).

One of the most significant advantages of iMRI is its ability to obtain serial intra-operative imaging, which bypasses the effect of brain shift by allowing the operator to orientate himself dur-

ing anatomical changes resulting from surgery and to discern whether there is still pathological residue or not [33]. This is particularly relevant in tumors adjacent to the corticospinal tract, where an intraoperative modification in the tumor to corticospinal tract distance can be observed. As a consequence, as shown in several studies, IMRi ensures a higher extent of resection (EOR) with less morbidity [34]. In addition, Hatiboglu et al. found that, in gliomas, even when the surgeon feels that the goals of surgery have been achieved, iMRI demonstrated unexpected residual tumors resulting in additional resection in 47% of cases [35]. Golub et al. showed in a meta-analysis published in 2020 that iMRI was superior to conventional navigation in achieving GTR and improving patient progression-free survival (PFS) and even overall survival (OS) [36].

Another advantage is the potential of IMRi to decrease surgical complications by enabling visualization beyond the surface that is surgically exposed. Identifying complications intraoperatively can theoretically allow for earlier fixation, ultimately reducing neurological sequelae and the risk of reoperation [37].

However, despite these considerations, iMRI brings several structural limitations that are difficult to overcome. First among them is the increased operative time compared to traditional surgeries. Indeed, iMRI workflow is extremely time-consuming requiring a specific effort to prepare/move the patient to MRI gantry, to acquire the images, and to resume surgery. As a consequence, iMRI can be employed only once or twice during surgery, making it more similar to an off-line technique, rather than on-line. Another aspect to be considered is image quality related to surgically induced artefacts including motion, metallic susceptibility, radiofrequency noise from inadequately shielded electronics in the operating room, the brain-air interface, and blood products. In addition, there are concerns related to repeated contrast-enhanced T1-weighted images due to alterations in the blood-brain barrier caused by surgical manipulation [38]. Last but not the least, the economic efficiency of iMRI must be taken into consideration for the healthcare system as a whole and for a hospital system contemplating its purchase. One of the major hindrances to universal implementation is the high cost of purchasing a system, ranging from $3 to $7 million, not including the cost of renovating the operative suite [36].

Alternatively, ultrasound (US) is an affordable, safe, and repeatable imaging technique that can be easily integrated into surgical workflow allowing live imaging during surgery [39]. One of the major advantages of US is the multiparametric nature of the images it can provide. In fact, in addition to the classic B-mode that differentiates structures on the basis of echogenicity, there are different modalities such as Doppler, contrast-enhanced ultrasound (CEUS), and elastography which can be of help in characterizing and orientating in the surgical field [40]. Color Doppler provides a colour map of blood flow and is useful for the localization of critical vessels in relation to the tumor; power Doppler is more sensitive to smaller and deeper vessels and is useful for detecting low flow and microvessels [41]. The possibility to use contrast (i.e. CEUS) can highlight tumors, define feeding arteries and draining veins, and characterize the tumor's microvasculature and perfusion. CEUS can also help in differentiating glioma grade, with LGGs exhibiting minimal to mildly greater enhancement and HGGs demonstrating avid contrast enhancement with disorganized vascularity. It has also been proven helpful in detecting residual disease following glioma resection, and it has a synergistic role with 5-ALA [42]. Another tool is elastography, such as strain elastography (SE) and shear-wave elastography (SWE). While SE is qualitative and operator-dependent, SWE is quantitative and repeatable. Studies have reported an improved definition of tumor margins and discrimination of disease grade using both SE and SWE (Fig. 4.2) [43].

As with MRI, US can lead to a higher extent of resection, but with the possibility of using it at any time and with less effort. On the other hand, ultrasonographic imaging recognizes a steeper learning curve, although systems have been introduced to facilitate US understanding, such as the possibility of merging MR images with US or the possibility of navigating the probe.

4.2.2 Fluorescence-Guided Surgery

Fluorescence-guided surgery (FGS) has been already established as capable of providing an advantage in terms of extent of resection (EOR), and subsequently, progression-free survival (PFS) and overall survival (OS). The superiority of FGS over white-light surgery has been demonstrated in various studies. The ability to achieve gross-total resection or even supramaximal resection is significantly enhanced. Fluorophores can target areas of blood-brain barrier breakdown, inflammation, or glioma cells, and are administered through various routes. Surgeons should be aware of how the method of fluorophore administration can impact tumor fluorescence [44].

Fluorophores such as Indocyanine Green (ICG) and fluorescein work by passive targeting and can be administered intravenously during surgery within seconds (in the case of ICG as a

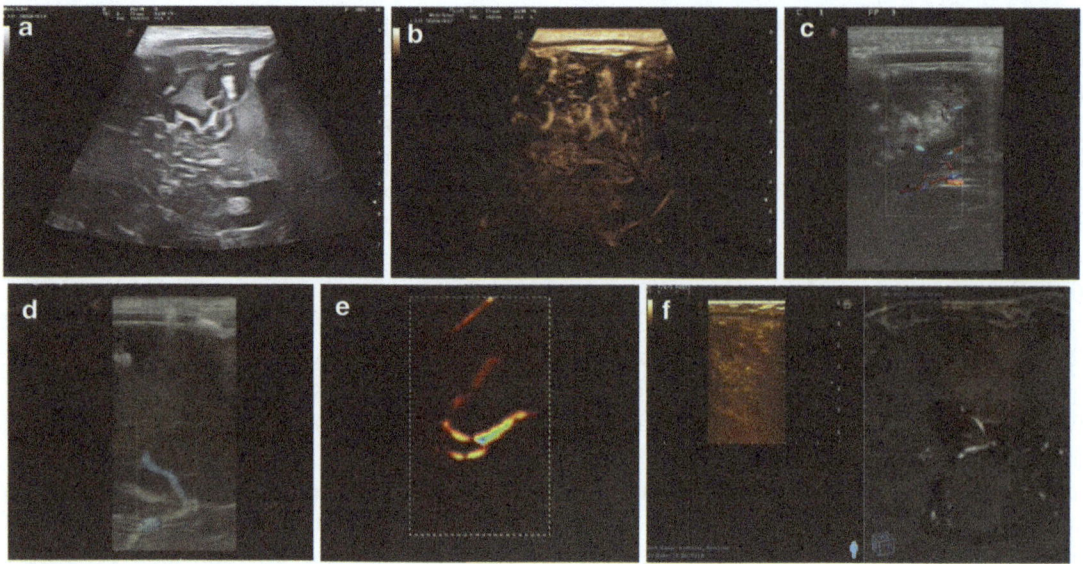

Fig. 4.2 US multimodal scan. (**a**) B-mode; (**b**) CEUS; (**c, d**) color Doppler; (**e**) power Doppler; (**f**) superimposition of CEUS and B-mode

vascular angiography agent) or shortly before surgery (in the case of fluorescein). 5-ALA is an oral agent that is administered several hours before surgery and can persist in the target tissue for longer periods. Newly studied molecular targeting agents, such as BLZ100 and EGF conjugates, are also administered during surgery, but they may last in tumor tissue for up to several days. Understanding the administration and properties of different fluorophores is essential for their effective use as a surgical adjunct in glioma surgery.

Among the fluorophores, 5-aminolevulinic acid (5-ALA) and sodium fluorescein (SF) are the most extensively studied fluorescent dyes. 5-ALA is specifically metabolized by neoplastic cells, making it more selective. On the other hand, SF is not selective for malignant glioma cells, but it can identify blood-brain barrier (BBB) impairment similar to the gadolinium used in contrast-enhanced MRI [44].

5-ALA is a natural biochemical precursor that is metabolized by heme biosynthesis, producing protoporphyrin IX (PpIX) in tumor cells due to the downregulation of ferrochelatase [45]. PpIX shows fluorescent properties and can be used to distinguish between neoplastic and non-neoplastic

tissue during surgery. FGS using 5-ALA has been shown to highlight infiltrating tumor areas in glioblastoma [46]. Administering 5-ALA earlier than the current FDA recommendation (4–5 h before anaesthesia induction) may improve its effectiveness in guiding tumor resection. A systematic review and meta-analysis by Stummer et al. (2014) analysed 16 studies comprising a total of 1392 patients with glioblastoma who underwent surgery with or without 5-ALA. The analysis found that the use of 5-ALA was associated with a higher rate of gross total resection (OR = 2.66, 95% CI: 2.08–3.39, $p < 0.001$) and a longer progression-free survival (HR = 0.65, 95% CI: 0.56–0.76, $p < 0.001$) (Fig. 4.3) [47].

Sodium fluorescein accumulates in areas of BBB disruption and emits fluorescence upon excitation by light [48]. The YELLOW 560 nm filter can be used to highlight pathological tissue from healthy tissue, especially at the tumor's borders. A recent multicentre phase II trial demonstrated the high sensitivity and specificity of SF in detecting glioma cells, resulting in a significant rate of GTR (82.6%) and 6-month PFS (56.6%) [49]. However, the intensity of fluorescence is time-dependent, and SF may diffuse beyond the tumor's boundary due to surgical manipulation [50].

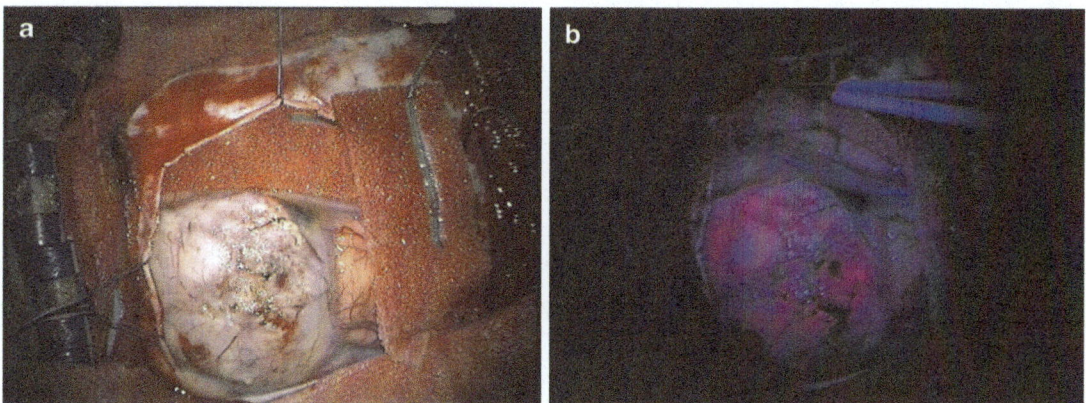

Fig. 4.3 Application of 5-ALA during an operation. Comparison of tumor aspect in white light (**a**) and 5-ALA fluorescence (**b**) of the same lesion

Some studies suggest using both 5-ALA and SF to improve sensitivity and specificity in detecting glioma cells. However, the mechanism of action of SF in non-contrast-enhanced regions of high-grade glioma is still unclear [51].

To compare both, Della Puppa et al. compared the two using the current recommended dosage and timing of administration. Although the sample size was small, analysing the different classes of EOR among subgroups, they found an EOR of more than 90% in 87.5% of patients for 5-ALA, 80% of patients for both, and 77.3% for only SF [52].

Recently, delayed administration of ICG before glioma surgery has been reported. Unlike 5-ALA and fluorescein, ICG is a near-infrared (NIR) fluorophore with unique utility in labelling tumor tissue. NIR imaging provides higher tissue penetration and excellent signal-to-noise ratio (SNR). Both preclinical and clinical studies have reported the use of ICG for glioma surgery within a few minutes after systemic administration, taking advantage of the higher vascular permeability of gliomas compared to normal brain. Haglund et al. used ICG for enhanced optical imaging in human gliomas. Hansen et al. found that ICG injected intravenously into tumor-bearing rats fluoresced intensely at 60–120 mg/kg for at least 1 h after injection. This study showed the ability of ICG to distinguish rat brain tumors from normal parenchyma with adequate tumor-to-normal brain background ratio, with minimal post-

resection residual tumor cells. ICG has a plasma half-life of 3–4 min, with only a small amount of the originally injected volume remaining in the blood after 10 min, as demonstrated in preclinical studies [53].

In addition to the fluorophores mentioned above, there are current studies on fluorophores with more directed mechanisms of action, such as specific receptor targets: BLz-100 [54], Alkyl Phosphocholine Analogs [55], and Epidermal Growth Factor Receptor (EGFR) Targeted Fluorophores [56].

4.3   Intraoperative Functional Mapping and Monitoring to Guide Surgery

Intraoperative neurophysiological monitoring (IONM) is currently employed to localize and evaluate the functional integrity of specific neural structures. The electrical activity of one or more neural pathways in an anaesthetized patient is continuously assessed with a two-fold purpose: firstly, to identify any surgical or physiological disturbances to the nervous system while they are still reversible, and secondly, to minimize any harm caused to these structures during surgical resection.

The electrophysiological techniques used are manifold: somatosensory-evoked potentials (SSEPs), motor-evoked potentials (MEPs), direct electrical stimulation (DES), including transcranial motor-evoked potentials (tcMEPs), brainstem auditory-evoked potentials (BAEPs), electroencephalography (EEG), and electromyography (EMG); knowledge and mastery of the advantages of these techniques ensure greater intraoperative safety.

4.3.1 Motor-Evoked Potentials (MEPs)

To evoke MEPs, either transcranial electric stimulation (TES) or direct cortical stimulation (DCS) can be used. An MEP can be elicited by applying a short train of high-frequency pulses consisting of five pulses with an interstimulus interval of 2–4 ms, corresponding to a pulse frequency of 250–500 Hz within the train. TES provides the advantage of using contralateral unoperated hemisphere MEPs for systemic control. However, in brain tumor surgery, the position of ipsilateral scalp stimulating electrodes may need to be adjusted to accommodate the incision and craniotomy, which may increase the TES intensity needed to obtain MEPs from the operated hemisphere, potentially leading to deep activation and false-negative results for superficial injury. Nevertheless, obtaining MEPs before dura opening and during dura closing when delayed vascular injury might occur extends the monitoring duration. Monitoring at least three contralateral hand and arm, two face, and two leg muscles is recommended, with more muscles added based on the tumor location and preoperative motor status [57, 58].

4.3.2 Somatosensory-Evoked Potentials (SSEP)

Somatosensory-evoked potentials (SSEP) phase reversal serves as one of the valid parameters for central sulcus positioning during tumor resections. Upon opening the dura mater, a strip electrode is inserted as the recording electrode. Stimulating electrodes are placed near the median nerve or posterior tibial nerve on the opposite side of the tumor to obtain a stable SSEP. Next, to determine the structural position based on waveform direction, the electrode of N20 represents the postcentral gyrus position, and that of P22 represents the precentral gyrus position. If the waveform is inverted, the central groove lies between these two locations. Therefore, during brain tumor surgery, median and tibial nerve SEPs are commonly used to detect ischemia affecting the somatosensory cortex or lemniscal pathways. A decline in SEP amplitudes has been shown to be related to critical cortical perfusion of brain parenchyma below 15 mL/100 g/min. Bilateral stimulation and recordings of technical control responses and cortical monitoring responses are recommended, including median nerve N20 and tibial nerve P37. Unaffected hemisphere recordings serve as systemic controls to detect confounding factors unrelated to surgical resection [59, 60].

4.3.3 Direct Electrical Stimulation (DES)

Direct electrical stimulation (DES) involves applying electric current to the cerebral cortex and subcortex to localize functional regions during craniotomy. This technique uses single-pulse or high-frequency multi-pulse electrical stimulation and is commonly used during surgeries involving functional areas of the brain, particularly in the excision of low-grade gliomas. Technically, a 1 mm increase in distance is generally associated with a 1 mA increase in stimulation threshold. DES is effective in preserving neurological function by predicting the edges of corticospinal tracts and is the only way to monitor the function of the language brain region in real time. Intraoperative DES technology uses different protocols under different anaesthesia strategies. During awake craniotomies, the low-frequency (LF) method is commonly used, which elicits a continuum of positive or negative responses depending on the area of the cortex stimulated. MEP monitoring in motor eloquent areas is preferably done using direct cortical stimulation, and a suction stimulation probe is a new technique that combines a suction tip with a stimulation probe, making it easier to use in a continuous dynamic mapping fashion [61, 62].

4.3.4 Visual-Evoked Potentials (VEPs)

Visual-evoked potentials (VEPs) are elicited by stimulation of the retina and transmitted through the optic nerve to the primary visual cortex. During neurosurgical procedures that carry a risk of injury to the optic pathway, intraoperative VEP monitoring has been used to assess the functional integrity of visual function. This type of monitoring can detect reversible damage to the visual pathway during surgery, allowing for precautionary measures to be taken to avoid permanent impairment.

Continuous monitoring of visual function is especially important during surgeries that put the visual pathway at risk, but the use of intraoperative VEP monitoring is not yet widespread. Preservation of VEPs has been shown to predict preserved visual function [63].

During the resection of lesions in the visual cortex, VEP monitoring may not detect new major visual field defects resulting from injury to the posterior visual pathway. However, intraoperative VEPs are sensitive enough to reveal mechanical manipulation of the anterior visual pathway in an early reversible stage [64, 65].

4.3.5 Other Nerve Monitoring

During infratentorial brain tumor surgery, monitoring or mapping of cranial nerves (CNs) or nuclei is crucial. Brainstem auditory evoked potentials (BAEP) are commonly used, which involve delivering acoustic stimuli through earplugs and recording near- and far-field potentials from electrodes at the mastoid process or earlobes [66]. Monitoring changes in the amplitude reduction of waves III and V and interwave latencies is important for interpreting BAEP waves with neuroanatomical consideration. Early attention to changes in wave II or III may allow for earlier intervention to reversible damage.

Other cranial motor nerves can be monitored by free-running EMG or transcranial corticobulbar motor evoked potential (MEP). The vagus nerve can be assessed by recording the MEP of the laryngeal muscles via surface electrodes attached to an endotracheal tube, and the hypoglossal nerve can be assessed via paired needle electrodes inserted into the tongue muscle [67]. Free-running EMG for bulbar muscles is performed using cathode and anode electrodes, while corticobulbar MEP requires extra caution due to the proximity of stimulation electrodes to bulbar muscles. To avoid direct current spread, a pair of stimulations are applied at short intervals, consisting of single-pulse stimulation and multi-pulse stimulation. Cranial nuclei, particularly the facial colliculus, can be mapped in the brainstem during surgery by direct stimulation [68]. Implementing IOM in brainstem surgery can reduce the risk of serious functional deficits such as dysphasia, dysphonia, facial palsy, or hearing loss.

4.3.6 Brain Mapping of Speech and Cognition Functional Area

For brain mapping of the motor functional area, the limbs and face on the opposite side of the stimulus point are fully exposed. Positive reactions of the motor functional area manifest as involuntary movements of contralateral limbs or corresponding parts of the face, accompanied by an electromyography (EMG) response. However, in the awake state, voluntary movements can interfere with EMG and MEP recordings. Therefore, the activity of the muscle opposite to the surgical site is also recorded as control to optimize the interpretation of EMG and MEP of the muscles of interest [69]. Additionally, continuous monitoring of MEP in insular and deep temporal regions, makes it a useful assistive strategy for motor functional mapping. Sensory functional areas are identified by pulsed abnormal sensations, such as burning and numbness in the opposite limb or head, and can also cause body movement.

Monopolar stimulation is preferred for identifying the corticospinal tract because of its more radiant electric field properties compared to the bipolar probe. Monopolar stimulation has been reported to be effective in insular glioma resections. Recently, a triple brain mapping method involving transcranial, monopolar, and bipolar stimulation has been proposed to more accurately locate the motor functional area. As a result, the combined application is considered superior in preserving motor function and enhancing EOR [70, 71].

4.3.7 Electrocorticography (ECoG)

The EEG monitoring allows us to locate the origin of epilepsy, to interpret the meaning of the IONM, and to enhance safety of DES. With advances in IONM equipment and technology, the ECG can simultaneously monitor spontaneous and stimulus-triggered epileptiform waves. If intraoperative seizures occur during electrocorticographic (ECoG) monitoring, electrical stimulation is stopped and anti-epileptic drugs are administered. The current intensity of DES is controlled to avoid false-positive consequences. Circular grid electrodes have recently been developed, enabling 360° monitoring and improving functional outcomes [72].

4.3.8 Electromyography (EMG)

During surgery, free-running EMG is used to monitor peripheral nerves, roots, or cranial motor nerves [73]. Intraoperative EMG signals are activated immediately following damage or irritation to cranial motor nerves, whereas abnormal EMG signals in outpatient clinics typically take days or weeks to develop after nerve injury. The mechanism behind intraoperative EMG is still unclear. The duration, morphology, and persistence of EMG signals may reflect the severity of nerve injury, with a longer EMG train indicating a higher likelihood of neural deficits after surgery. The presence of a high frequency, sinusoidal, and symmetric sequence of EMG discharges may indicate probable neural injury. However, injuries resulting from sharp transection or gradual ischemia may not produce any EMG signals [74].

References

1. Hirsch GV, Bauer CM, Merabet LB. Using structural and functional brain imaging to uncover how the brain adapts to blindness. Ann Neurosci Psychol. 2015;2:2.
2. Keller SS, Roberts N. Measurement of brain volume using MRI: software, techniques, choices and prerequisites. J Anthropol Sci. 2009;87:127–51.
3. Fischl B, Dale AM. Measuring the thickness of the human cerebral cortex from magnetic resonance images. Proc Natl Acad Sci USA. 2000;97(20):11050–5.
4. Belliveau JW, Kennedy DNJ, McKinstry RC, Buchbinder BR, Weisskoff RM, Cohen MS, et al. Functional mapping of the human visual cortex by magnetic resonance imaging. Science. 1991;254(5032):716–9.
5. Kwong KK, Belliveau JW, Chesler DA, Goldberg IE, Weisskoff RM, Poncelet BP, et al. Dynamic magnetic resonance imaging of human brain activity during primary sensory stimulation. Proc Natl Acad Sci USA. 1992;89(12):5675–9.
6. Ambrose J. Computerized transverse axial scanning (tomography). 2. Clinical application. Br J Radiol. 1973;46(552):1023–47.
7. Poggi S, Pallotta S, Russo S, Gallina P, Torresin A, Bucciolini M. Neuronavigation accuracy dependence on CT and MR imaging parameters: a phantom-based study. Phys Med Biol (England). 2003;48:2199–216.
8. Symms M, Jäger HR, Schmierer K, Yousry TA. A review of structural magnetic resonance neuroimaging. J Neurol Neurosurg Psychiatry. 2004;75(9):1235–44.
9. O'Donnell LJ, Westin C-F. An introduction to diffusion tensor image analysis. Neurosurg Clin N Am. 2011;22(2):185–96, viii.
10. Hagmann P, Jonasson L, Maeder P, Thiran J-P, Wedeen VJ, Meuli R. Understanding diffusion MR imaging techniques: from scalar diffusion-weighted imaging to diffusion tensor imaging and beyond. Radiographics. 2006;26(Suppl 1):S205–23.
11. Matthews PM, Jezzard P. Functional magnetic resonance imaging. J Neurol Neurosurg Psychiatry. 2004;75(1):6–12.
12. Uğurbil K, Toth L, Kim DS. How accurate is magnetic resonance imaging of brain function? Trends Neurosci. 2003;26(2):108–14.
13. Stufflebeam SM. Clinical magnetoencephalography for neurosurgery. Neurosurg Clin N Am. 2011;22(2):153–67, vii–viii.
14. Holzgreve A, Albert NL, Galldiks N, Suchorska B. Use of PET imaging in neuro-oncological surgery. Cancers (Basel). 2021;13(9):2093.

15. Culbreth GG, Walker AE, Curry RW. Cerebral angiography in brain tumor suspects. J Neurosurg. 1950;7(2):127–38.

16. Tomura N, Hashimoto M, Sashi R, Hirano H, Kobayashi M, Hirano Y, et al. Superselective angio-CT of brain tumors. AJNR Am J Neuroradiol. 1996;17(6):1073–80.

17. Upadhyay UM, Golby AJ. Role of pre- and intraoperative imaging and neuronavigation in neurosurgery. Expert Rev Med Devices. 2008;5(1):65–73.

18. Eggers G, Mühling J, Marmulla R. Image-to-patient registration techniques in head surgery. Int J Oral Maxillofac Surg. 2006;35(12):1081–95.

19. Slavin KV. Neuronavigation in neurosurgery: current state of affairs. Expert Rev Med Devices (England). 2008;5:1–3.

20. Nimsky C, Ganslandt O, Fahlbusch R. Functional neuronavigation and intraoperative MRI. Adv Tech Stand Neurosurg. 2004;29:229–63.

21. Willems PWA, van der Sprenkel JWB, Tulleken CAF, Viergever MA, Taphoorn MJB. Neuronavigation and surgery of intracerebral tumours. J Neurol. 2006;253(9):1123–36.

22. Willems PWA, Taphoorn MJB, Burger H, Berkelbach van der Sprenkel JW, Tulleken CAF. Effectiveness of neuronavigation in resecting solitary intracerebral contrast-enhancing tumors: a randomized controlled trial. J Neurosurg. 2006;104(3):360–8.

23. Gerard IJ, Kersten-Oertel M, Petrecca K, Sirhan D, Hall JA, Collins DL. Brain shift in neuronavigation of brain tumors: a review. Med Image Anal. 2017;35:403–20.

24. Kuhnt D, Bauer MHA, Nimsky C. Brain shift compensation and neurosurgical image fusion using intraoperative MRI: current status and future challenges. Crit Rev Biomed Eng. 2012;40(3):175–85.

25. Gerard IJ, Kersten-Oertel M, Hall JA, Sirhan D, Collins DL. Brain shift in neuronavigation of brain tumors: an updated review of intra-operative ultrasound applications. Front Oncol. 2020;10:618837.

26. Rasmussen I-AJ, Lindseth F, Rygh OM, Berntsen EM, Selbekk T, Xu J, et al. Functional neuronavigation combined with intra-operative 3D ultrasound: initial experiences during surgical resections close to eloquent brain areas and future directions in automatic brain shift compensation of preoperative data. Acta Neurochir (Wien). 2007;149(4):365–78.

27. Perin A, Galbiati TF, Ayadi R, Gambatesa E, Orena EF, Riker NI, et al. Informed consent through 3D virtual reality: a randomized clinical trial. Acta Neurochir (Wien). 2020;163:301.

28. Alessandro P, Giovanni C, Benedetta RC, Luca R, Claudia F, Francesco GT, et al. The "STARS-CT-MADE" study: advanced rehearsal and intraoperative navigation for skull base tumors. World Neurosurg. 2021;154:e19. Available from: https://www.sciencedirect.com/science/article/pii/S1878875021008895.

29. Perin A, Gambatesa E, Galbiati TF, Fanizzi C, Carone G, Rui CB, et al. The "STARS-CASCADE" study: virtual reality simulation as a new training approach in vascular neurosurgery. World Neurosurg. 2021;154:e130–46.

30. Perin A, Gambatesa E, Rui CB, Carone G, Fanizzi C, Lombardo FM, et al. The "STARS" study: advanced pre-operative rehearsal and intraoperative navigation in neurosurgical oncology. J Neurosurg Sci. 2022;67:671.

31. Mishra R, Narayanan MDK, Umana GE, Montemurro N, Chaurasia B, Deora H. Virtual reality in neurosurgery: beyond neurosurgical planning. Int J Environ Res Public Health. 2022;19(3):1719.

32. Cannizzaro D, Zaed I, Safa A, Jelmoni AJM, Composto A, Bisoglio A, et al. Augmented reality in neurosurgery, state of art and future projections. A systematic review. Front Surg (Switzerland). 2022;9:864792.

33. Jenkinson MD, Barone DG, Bryant A, Vale L, Bulbeck H, Lawrie TA, et al. Intraoperative imaging technology to maximise extent of resection for glioma. Cochrane Database Syst Rev. 2018;1(1):CD012788.

34. Peruzzi P, Puente E, Bergese S, Chiocca EA. Intraoperative MRI (ioMRI) in the setting of awake craniotomies for supratentorial glioma resection. Acta Neurochir Suppl. 2011;109:43–8.

35. Hatiboglu MA, Weinberg JS, Suki D, Rao G, Prabhu SS, Shah K, et al. Impact of intraoperative high-field magnetic resonance imaging guidance on glioma surgery: a prospective volumetric analysis. Neurosurgery. 2009;64(6):1073–81; discussion 1081.

36. Golub D, Hyde J, Dogra S, Nicholson J, Kirkwood KA, Gohel P, et al. Intraoperative MRI versus 5-ALA in high-grade glioma resection: a network meta-analysis. J Neurosurg. 2020;134:484.

37. Schulder M, Carmel PW. Intraoperative magnetic resonance imaging: impact on brain tumor surgery. Cancer Control. 2003;10(2):115–24.

38. Rykkje AM, Li D, Skjøth-Rasmussen J, Larsen VA, Nielsen MB, Hansen AE, et al. Surgically induced contrast enhancements on intraoperative and early postoperative MRI following high-grade glioma surgery: a systematic review. Diagnostics (Basel, Switzerland). 2021;11(8):1344.

39. Dixon L, Lim A, Grech-Sollars M, Nandi D, Camp S. Intraoperative ultrasound in brain tumor surgery: a review and implementation guide. Neurosurg Rev. 2022;45(4):2503–15.

40. Prada F, Ciocca R, Corradino N, Gionso M, Raspagliesi L, Vetrano IG, et al. Multiparametric intraoperative ultrasound in oncological neurosurgery: a pictorial essay. Front Neurosci. 2022;16:881661.

41. Prada F, Del Bene M, Mauri G, Lamperti M, Vailati D, Richetta C, et al. Dynamic assessment of venous anatomy and function in neurosurgery with real-time intraoperative multimodal ultrasound: technical note. Neurosurg Focus. 2018;45(1):E6.

42. Prada F, Perin A, Martegani A, Aiani L, Solbiati L, Lamperti M, et al. Intraoperative contrast-enhanced ultrasound for brain tumor surgery. Neurosurgery. 2014;74(5):542. Available from: https://journals.lww.com/neurosurgery/Fulltext/2014/05000/

Intraoperative_Contrast_Enhanced_Ultrasound_for.9.aspx.

43. Prada F, Del Bene M, Rampini A, Mattei L, Casali C, Vetrano IG, et al. Intraoperative strain elastosonography in brain tumor surgery. Oper Neurosurg (Hagerstown, MD). 2019;17(2):227–36.

44. Schupper AJ, Rao M, Mohammadi N, Baron R, Lee JYK, Acerbi F, et al. Fluorescence-guided surgery: a review on timing and use in brain tumor surgery. Front Neurol. 2021;12:682151.

45. Bottomley SS, Muller-Eberhard U. Pathophysiology of heme synthesis. Semin Hematol. 1988;25(4):282–302.

46. Hadjipanayis CG, Widhalm G, Stummer W. What is the surgical benefit of utilizing 5-aminolevulinic acid for fluorescence-guided surgery of malignant gliomas? Neurosurgery. 2015;77(5):663–73.

47. Stummer W, Pichlmeier U, Meinel T, Wiestler OD, Zanella F, Reulen H-J. Fluorescence-guided surgery with 5-aminolevulinic acid for resection of malignant glioma: a randomised controlled multicentre phase III trial. Lancet Oncol. 2006;7(5):392–401.

48. Acerbi F. Fluorescein assistance in neuro-oncological surgery: a trend of the moment or a real technical adjunct? Clin Neurol Neurosurg (Netherlands). 2016;144:119–20.

49. Acerbi F, Broggi M, Schebesch K-M, Höhne J, Cavallo C, De Laurentis C, et al. Fluorescein-guided surgery for resection of high-grade gliomas: a multicentric prospective phase II study (FLUOGLIO). Clin Cancer Res. 2018;24(1):52–61.

50. Hamamcıo MK, Akc MO, Göker B, Kasımcan MÖ, Kırıs T. The use of the YELLOW 560 nm surgical microscope filter for sodium fluorescein-guided resection of brain tumors: our preliminary results in a series of 28 patients. Clin Neurol Neurosurg. 2016;2022(143):39–45.

51. Zeppa P, De Marco R, Monticelli M, Massara A, Bianconi A, Di Perna G, et al. Fluorescence-guided surgery in glioblastoma: 5-ALA, SF or both? Differences between fluorescent dyes in 99 consecutive cases. Brain Sci. 2022;12(5):555.

52. Della Puppa A, Ciccarino P, Lombardi G, Rolma G, Cecchin D, Rossetto M. 5-Aminolevulinic acid fluorescence in high grade glioma surgery: surgical outcome, intraoperative findings, and fluorescence patterns. Biomed Res Int. 2014;2014:232561.

53. Teng CW, Huang V, Arguelles GR, Zhou C, Cho SS, Harmsen S, et al. Applications of indocyanine green in brain tumor surgery: review of clinical evidence and emerging technologies. Neurosurg Focus. 2021;50(1):E4.

54. Yamada M, Miller DM, Lowe M, Rowe C, Wood D, Soyer HP, et al. A first-in-human study of BLZ-100 (tozuleristide) demonstrates tolerability and safety in skin cancer patients. Contemp Clin Trials Commun. 2021;23:100830.

55. Weichert JP, Clark PA, Kandela IK, Vaccaro AM, Clarke W, Longino MA, et al. Alkylphosphocholine analogs for broad-spectrum cancer imaging and therapy. Sci Transl Med. 2014;6(240):240ra75.

56. Zhou Q, van den Berg NS, Rosenthal EL, Iv M, Zhang M, Vega Leonel JCM, et al. EGFR-targeted intraoperative fluorescence imaging detects high-grade glioma with panitumumab-IRDye800 in a phase 1 clinical trial. Theranostics. 2021;11(15):7130–43.

57. Sala F, Palandri G, Basso E, Lanteri P, Deletis V, Faccioli F, et al. Motor evoked potential monitoring improves outcome after surgery for intramedullary spinal cord tumors: a historical control study. Neurosurgery. 2006;58(6):1129–43.

58. Asimakidou E, Abut PA, Raabe A, Seidel K. Motor evoked potential warning criteria in supratentorial surgery: a scoping review. Cancers (Basel). 2021;13(11):2803.

59. Friedman WA. Somatosensory evoked potentials in neurosurgery. Clin Neurosurg. 1988;34:187–238.

60. Grundy BL. Monitoring of sensory evoked potentials during neurosurgical operations: methods and applications. Neurosurgery. 1982;11(4):556–75.

61. Aaronson DM, Martinez Del Campo E, Boerger TF, Conway B, Cornell S, Tate M, et al. Understanding variable motor responses to direct electrical stimulation of the human motor cortex during brain surgery. Front Surg. 2021;8:730367.

62. Mahon BZ, Miozzo M, Pilcher WH. Direct electrical stimulation mapping of cognitive functions in the human brain. Cogn Neuropsychol (England). 2019;36:97–102.

63. Sasaki T, Itakura T, Suzuki K, Kasuya H, Munakata R, Muramatsu H, et al. Intraoperative monitoring of visual evoked potential: introduction of a clinically useful method. J Neurosurg. 2010;112(2):273–84.

64. Kamio Y, Sakai N, Sameshima T, Takahashi G, Koizumi S, Sugiyama K, et al. Usefulness of intraoperative monitoring of visual evoked potentials in transsphenoidal surgery. Neurol Med Chir (Tokyo). 2014;54(8):606–11.

65. Gutzwiller EM, Cabrilo I, Radovanovic I, Schaller K, Boëx C. Intraoperative monitoring with visual evoked potentials for brain surgeries. J Neurosurg. 2018;130(2):654–60.

66. Aravabhumi S, Izzo KL, Bakst BL. Brainstem auditory evoked potentials: intraoperative monitoring technique in surgery of posterior fossa tumors. Arch Phys Med Rehabil. 1987;68(3):142–6.

67. Matsushima K, Kohno M, Ichimasu N, Tanaka Y, Nakajima N, Yoshino M. Intraoperative continuous vagus nerve monitoring with repetitive direct stimulation in surgery for jugular foramen tumors. J Neurosurg. 2021;135:1036.

68. Berges C, Fraysse B, Yardeni E, Rugiu G. Intraoperative facial nerve monitoring in posterior fossa surgery: prognostic value. Skull Base Surg. 1993;3(4):214–6.

69. Bertani G, Fava E, Casaceli G, Carrabba G, Casarotti A, Papagno C, et al. Intraoperative mapping and monitoring of brain functions for the resection of low-grade gliomas: technical considerations. Neurosurg Focus. 2009;27(4):E4.

70. Zhou T, Yu T, Li Z, Zhou X, Wen J, Li X. Functional mapping of language-related areas from natural, narrative speech during awake craniotomy surgery. Neuroimage. 2021;245:118720.
71. Garrett MC, Pouratian N, Liau LM. Use of language mapping to aid in resection of gliomas in eloquent brain regions. Neurosurg Clin N Am. 2012;23(3):497–506.
72. Hill NJ, Gupta D, Brunner P, Gunduz A, Adamo MA, Ritaccio A, et al. Recording human electrocortico-graphic (ECoG) signals for neuroscientific research and real-time functional cortical mapping. J Vis Exp. 2012;(64):3993.
73. Woods WW, Shea PA. The value of electromyography in neurology and neurosurgery. J Neurosurg. 1951;8(6):595–607.
74. Mills KR. The basics of electromyography. J Neurol Neurosurg Psychiatry. 2005;76(Suppl 2):ii32–5.

Next Frontiers in Surgical Management

5

Beatrice C. Bono, Edoardo M. Barbieri,
Federico Pessina, and Marco Riva

5.1   Background

The surgical management of tumors of the central nervous system has been pursuing new therapeutic and clinical needs upon the push of the recent developments of the molecular era, advanced imaging and radiomics, and immunomodulatory/targeted therapies.

The two most common intracranial malignancies are the metastases and glial lesions. In this context, considerable progress has been made in the field of brain metastases, with the achievement of significant benefits in terms of progression-free (PFS) and overall survival (OS). On the other hand, however, this is not fully achieved for glial lesions, particularly for the high-grade gliomas (HGGs), especially with the wild-type status of the IDH 1/2. Intracranial malignancies are still characterized by a poor prognosis, with limited survival and a profound impact on the patient's life even in the post-Stupp protocol era (i.e., a regimen of adjuvant radiotherapy and temozolomide following surgical resection).

This chapter seeks to introduce the latest updates regarding new techniques, technologies, and functional strategies for the surgical treatment of intracranial malignant tumors, focusing attention on high-grade glial lesions both at the initial diagnosis and at the disease recurrence.

5.2   The Role of Surgical Treatment, the Impact of the Extent of Resection: Toward *Supra-Total* Resection?

Three cornerstones can be considered when it comes to surgical treatment of intracranial malignant lesions: (1) oncological radicality, (2) the full preservation of the neurological functions, and (3) the achievement of a proper histological and molecular diagnosis.

Regarding the first issue, it is now well known that the extent of the resection (EOR) is one of the most impactful factors related to the prognosis, both in terms of overall (OS) and progression-free (PFS) survival. As such, EOR is still considered the primary modifiable factor in the treatment paradigm of HGGs. In fact, oncological brain surgery has been pursuing ever-wider resection margins [1, 2] in the last decade, addressing the tissue beyond the MRI contrast-

B. C. Bono · F. Pessina · M. Riva (✉)
Department of Biomedical Sciences, Humanitas
University, Pieve Emanuele, Milan, Italy

Neurosurgery Department, IRCCS Humanitas
Research Hospital, Rozzano, Milan, Italy
e-mail: marco.riva@hunimed.eu

E. M. Barbieri
Department of Biomedical Sciences, Humanitas
University, Pieve Emanuele, Milan, Italy

enhancing lesion core until reaching eloquent functional limits. This strategy has been termed *supratotal resection*, also as it consists of the removal of brain tissue in and beyond the T2/FLAIR-hyperintense area. This surgical behavior seeks to intercept tumor cells at the invasive edge of a disease, such as HGGs, that is diffusely infiltrative, therefore making a theoretical "complete resection" unfeasible. In addition, current studies are also investigating the cell and tissue composition of the microenvironment of the lesion core, the invasive edge, and the adjacent brain tissue and whether a likely differential composition has a role in the likely timing and site of relapse. The results of these studies could help in optimizing current therapies and finding new therapeutic targets. The surgical management should thus be aware of this cellular and tissue spatial heterogeneity of the HGGs.

There are thus few fundamental issues that can be considered. How to properly identify and characterize the peritumoral area to include within the resection? How to distinguish the FLAIR pathological "periphery" from edema? How to describe the actual disease extent? How to balance the need for more extensive resection with likely increasing risks of injuring normal tissues with eventual neurological deficits?

This issue is pivotal in the current surgical treatment as the *supratotal resection* in high-grade gliomas, when feasible, leads to a significant prognostic benefit, both in terms of PFS and OS [2–4]. The complete resection of the FLAIR tumor area also referred to as FLAIRectomy, increases the median survival by about 5–13 months, compared to what has been observed when only the contrast-enhanced tumor is resected [2, 3, 5–7].

However, high-level scientific evidence is still lacking and a common consensus on "what should be done" has not been agreed yet. The inconsistent definition of supramaximal resection, as either the 1 cm beyond the T1-contrast enhanced area or the surrounding FLAIR abnormal tissue, is a further limitation [8].

New technologies can help us to better understand the extent of the problem, guiding the neurosurgeon toward a safer surgical technique tailored to the specific patient.

5.3 Information-Guided Brain Surgery

Conventional MR imaging historically considered contrast-enhanced magnetic resonance (ceMRI) as the gold standard for the preoperative evaluation of a neuro-oncological patient. Over the last few years, however, with the growing diffusion of intraoperative neuronavigation systems, new techniques have been introduced with the aim of better characterizing the tumor, its metabolic activity, and its biological behavior.

As elsewhere mentioned, advanced MRI techniques, such as diffusion, perfusion analyses, and spectroscopy maps allow to obtain both qualitative and quantitative data about the tumor's intrinsic features [9–17].

In addition to advanced MRI, amino acid Positron Emission Tomography (PET) is increasingly being used in recent years also for the preoperative assessment of the lesional heterogeneity through the identification of the tumor areas that show higher metabolic activity and can thus be separately reached and surgically sampled. Recent studies have demonstrated how amino acid PET is not only capable of predicting the histological grade of the tumor but also of visualizing hypermetabolic areas outside the area that is conventionally considered positive in FLAIR sequences [18, 19], therefore playing a pivotal role in prognostication and in surgical guidance. These aspects are particularly useful in those tumors that are poorly (or not at all) enhancing, to guide and define the resection margins, and to avoid any downgrading of the tumor on definitive histo-molecular examination.

5.4 Maximizing the Extent of Resection and Enhancing the Detection of the Glioma Edge: The Role of Intraoperative Tools

Recent innovations have focused on improving our ability to detect and delineate tumor tissue from the surrounding brain in the operating room. Intraoperative technologies such as neuronavigation, intraoperative MRI, and intraoperative ultrasound have aided surgeons in localizing and resecting the bulk tumor tissue. However, enhanced real-time information is required to better guide resection of HGGs at the infiltrative margin, with direct visualization of the leading edge of tumors to pursue a maximial resection. These technologies are also essential to support surgical decision-making weighing both the need to maximize tumor resections and functional preservation of the patients, i.e., safety.

5.4.1 Intraoperative Ultrasound (ioUS) and Intraoperative MRI (iMRI)

The major disadvantage of most preoperative image-based neuronavigation techniques is the well-known brain-shift issue. It is well known that during surgery, and even since its earliest stages, the accuracy of neuronavigation decreases. This inevitably influences the subsequent stages of resection, if this is merely based on preoperative image guidance. Given these premises, it seems intuitive that the use of intraoperative imaging techniques that allow for real-time navigation made a significant contribution to maximizing the EOR, in the context of a high-precision surgery.

Intraoperative imaging has the fundamental purpose of correcting the error caused by the brain shift in *real time*. IoUS is simple (although operator-dependent), repeatable, and cost-effective. With the development of new high-definition ultrasound systems, it is also possible to dispose of extremely detailed images, which can be merged in real time with the preoperative MRI dataset to update the spatial distribution of dataset [20]. An analogous, but conceptually different, argument can also be made for iMRI. According to a recent systematic review, iMRI has demonstrated its efficacy in increasing the extent of resection with a significant impact in terms of patient survival [21]. However, it is a time-consuming technology with fairly high costs.

5.4.2 Fluorescence

Recently, the idea of fluorescence-guided surgery has experienced increasing popularity. 5-Aminolevulinic acid (5-ALA), a precursor molecule in the heme biosynthetic pathway, that, when exogenously administered, accumulates intracellularly in high-grade gliomas as protoporphyrinogen IX (PpIX) [22, 23]. The latter is a fluorophore that fluoresces when excited by violet-blue light (370–440 nm), thus helping in the identification of tumor tissue in the surgical field. Interestingly, this does not seem to hold true for low-grade gliomas, for which 5-ALA seems to have a very low sensitivity [23].

A phase III multicentre trial evaluating 5-ALA fluorescence-guided resection as opposed to white light resection identified higher rates of complete resection and significantly improved progression-free survival (PFS) while failing to find significant improvements in overall survival (OS) [24]. Nonetheless, the study was deemed to be underpowered to detect a significant difference in OS [25] and since then 5-ALA has been extensively used as a tool in HGG surgery.

Recently, fluorescein sodium salt has shown promising results as an intraoperative "contrast enhancer" [26] highlighting areas of blood-brain barrier disruption, but further data are needed to support its widespread employment in HGG surgery [27]. The feasibility of miniatured confocal laser microscopy combined with fluorescein sodium as a method for intraoperative high-resolution cellular visualization is also currently being studied [28].

5.4.3 Raman Spectroscopy, Stimulated Raman Scattering (SRS), and Stimulated Raman Histology (SRH)

Raman spectroscopy (RS) is a label-free image tool that allows for the intraoperative characterization of the resected tissue through the analysis of the biochemical–spectral differences between the tumor and the healthy brain [29–33].

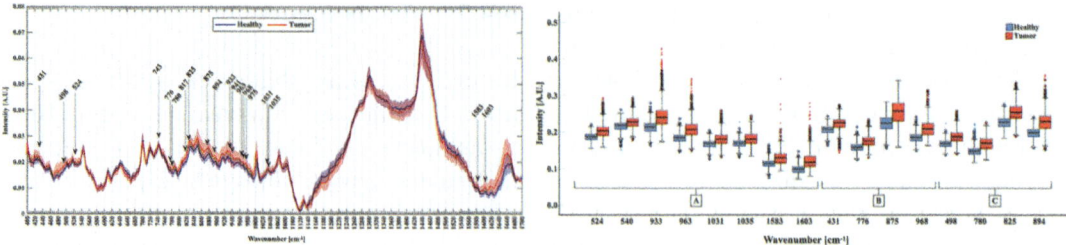

Fig. 5.1 Images showing the normalized Raman spectra for healthy and tumor patients (on the left), and their band intensities comparison grouped for biological significance (on the right). (Courtesy of Riva et al., 2021)

The so-called Raman shift, which can be observed with the aid of spectroscopy, is the physical process through which a molecule absorbs or decreases its energy by modifying its scattered photonic frequency. This method can be used to identify molecules based on Raman-active chemical bonds, giving interesting insights into the biomolecular composition of surgical specimens. The use of Raman spectroscopy applied to neurosciences dates to the early 1990s [34]. Since then, many studies have been conducted on both frozen and fresh ex vivo brain tissue employing the RS for the characterization of glioma infiltration.

When the RS is used for ex vivo sampling, tumor specimens are collected during the resection under image guidance and provided to the Raman specialist. The Raman spectra are then extracted, and, with the aid of machine learning techniques, categorized to obtain a detailed biochemical composition of the sample. An intraoperative diagnosis is therefore possible with satisfactory results in terms of accuracy, sensibility, and specificity [31] (Fig. 5.1).

A conceptually similar technology is represented by stimulated Raman scattering (SRS) microscopy. SRS is a visualization tool that uses molecular vibrational properties to produce label-free contrast-enhanced histologic images (stimulated Raman histology, SRH), which are similar in appearance to that observed in standard microscopic staining [35–38]. Compared to the RS (and to other optical technologies), the SRH is characterized by sub-cellular image resolution with diagnostic accuracy rates that are compara-

ble to the ones and are reported with standard histologic analyses. Moreover, this technology offers the possibility to obtain true real-time histologic information on the tumor tissue, potentially guiding the surgeon during the intraoperative decision-making process and, ultimately, allowing for wider resections.

5.5 Surgery for Recurrent HGGs

The role of surgical treatment in glioblastoma recurrences is still unclear, and a consensus has not yet been reached about the correct management of such cases. However, emerging evidence has recently shown how the surgery of HGG recurrences can significantly prolong overall survival, giving the patient a benefit that is almost comparable to that conferred upon the first diagnosis, therefore justifying the rationale for reoperation in these patients [33, 39–43].

5.6 Novel Therapeutic Approaches

In spite of recent advances in the field of neuro-oncology, a definitive cure for glioblastoma still seems to be an unreachable goal: even when supramaximally resected and treated with adjuvant radio-chemotherapy, it will almost invariably recur [44]. Moreover, glioblastoma recurrences are less likely to be surgically resectable and show greater heterogeneity in terms of molecular expression, thus posing the need for alternative therapies [45, 46]. Several strategies for tackling glioblastoma recurrences not amenable for re-intervention are currently being studied, mostly in phase I and II studies, but the ones in which neurosurgeons are mostly involved include immunotherapy, tumor-treating fields (TTF), focused ultrasound (FUS), localized thermal therapy and local chemotherapy delivery [46], magnetic hyperthermia therapy, and photodynamic therapy.

Immunotherapy, including immune checkpoint blockade, chimeric antigen receptor T (CAR-T) cell therapy, oncolytic virotherapy, and vaccine therapy, has shown very promising preclinical results [46–48]. Nevertheless, most of the hopes were disregarded in phase I and II clinical trials, with only one phase II trial reporting a survival advantage with neo-adjuvant and adjuvant Pembrolizumab (anti-PD-1) with respect to adjuvant Pembrolizumab alone in 35 patients with recurrent, surgically resectable GBM [49, 50]. Similarly, only one phase II trial was able to show a survival advantage in treating GBM recurrences with Rindopepimut, a peptide vaccine targeting EGFRvIII, plus bevacizumab versus bevacizumab alone [51]. The lack of success of these approaches can be partially explained by recent evidence highlighting the role of immune synergism when immunotherapy is administered together with other therapies, which may hamper the ability of the immune system to mount an appropriate inflammatory response against the tumor [52].

TTFs are low-intensity, intermediate frequency, alternating electric fields that have antiproliferative properties and that have shown to be a promising option in both primary and recurrent GBM [53]. Despite evidence of beneficial effects on quality of life in patients with recurrent GBM [54, 55], additional trials are still needed to demonstrate a significant effect on survival.

Focused ultrasound (FUS) may help overcome one of the main limitations in the treatment of glioblastoma: the blood-brain barrier (BBB). Indeed, a single-center trial demonstrated in 2016 the feasibility of repeated pulsed ultrasound in recurrent GBM [56], with the aim of transiently disrupting the BBB and favoring drug delivery to the tumor. Trials evaluating whether FUS can effectively increase the efficacy of systemic chemotherapy are currently ongoing [57].

Localized thermal therapy exploits heat to induce intratumoral apoptosis and necrosis. The most employed techniques are Laser Interstitial Thermal Therapy (LITT), where an optical fiber is stereotactically inserted into the tumor through a burr hole and heats the tissue through laser light, and magnetic hyperthermia, in which magnetic nanoparticles inserted within the tumor are stimulated by an external alternating magnetic field producing heat. LITT has been also shown to induce transient blood–brain barrier disruption at the margin and peritumoral region up to 6 weeks following treatment, providing an opportunity for delivering an antitumor drug agent [58]. In fact, the BBB is essentially intact, thus limiting the penetration of therapeutic agents. Although both techniques have been shown to be feasible options to treat recurrent GBMs [59], they are still in their infancy, and trials unequivocally proving their efficacy are still needed. Furthermore, concerns about the possible side effects of these techniques on healthy brain tissue, such as thermal-induced necrosis requiring surgery or high-dose steroid treatment, have been raised.

An additional method to overcome the obstacles posed by the BBB is represented by convection-enhanced delivery (CED). Initially developed as an improvement of the much more limited diffusion-mediated intracavitary drug delivery [60], CED allows local conveyance of both conventional chemotherapeutics and newer drugs, including targeted fusion toxins and chimeric monoclonal antibodies. The formers were tested in a phase III trial (PRECISE trial) evaluating the survival benefit of convection-enhanced delivery of a chimeric pseudomonas exotoxin fused with recombinant human IL-13 [61]. Despite being unable to identify a statistically significant survival benefit in the CED arm, this trial's power has been questioned because of a flawed statistical design and poor adherence to protocol specifications. The disclosure of CED's full therapeutic potential is supposedly also restrained by its numerous technical hurdles, including appropriate infusion rate, physical and chemical properties of the infusate, both tumor and surrounding tissue properties, and appropriate catheter placement [62]. To overcome this latter challenge, a modular robotic system designed to perform neurosurgical procedures has been tested in the first in vivo trial [63]. The trial confirmed that this method of catheter placement is functional and safely feasible and further in vivo studies are underway. Taken together, these studies establish CED as a promising therapeutic modality whose efficacy may improve in parallel with technological advancements.

5.7 Functional Preservation: Relevance for the Quality of Life and Survival

In an era of re-definition of the EOR, seeking wider resections, it is essential to be aware that too much aggressiveness can be detrimental as postoperative deficits, especially in strength, diminish the survival benefit conveyed by surgery [64] and can hamper the access to established adjuvant treatments and to investigational approaches.

As resections are pushed to the edge and even further, some patients can experience postoperative deficits. It is thus of paramount relevance to avoid the occurrence of postoperative deficits and, when these nonetheless occur, explore interventions to accelerate patient recovery.

Intraoperative neurophysiological techniques [65–69] provide the neurological surgeon with essential monitoring and mapping tools that proved effective in reducing postoperative morbidity, thus having an established role in supporting wider safe resections [70].

However, some patients do experience postoperative deficits, especially due to ischemic injury often detected in early postoperative DWI scans. Along with rehabilitation therapy, techniques that increase the speed and rate of recovery have been explored recently. It is in fact essential that patients recover from their deficits at best and quickly to avoid starting the recommended adjuvant therapies in the due time. In this regard, initial studies investigated the role of transcranial magnetic stimulation (TMS). TMS is a noninvasive electrophysiological technique for the stimulation of the human motor cortex and motor tracts, with the repetitive controlled application of TMS known to induce neuroplasticity. In a recent study prolonged repetitive TMS has been shown to improve motor recovery resulting from ischemic injury patients who underwent the surgical resection of a glioma [71].

5.8 Final Remarks

Current advancements in the surgical treatments of the HGGs are thus aiming at increasing and improving the detection and treatment of the infiltrative edge while preserving the safety of the procedure. As a result, the development and refinement of technologies capable of delineating tumors from the surrounding brain may permit more effective and safer treatment of the invasive margin that is responsible for tumor recurrence, treatment resistance, and ultimately, the demise of most patients.

Addressing this peritumoral environment could also shed further light on the constituting cellular populations, with a potential knowledge essential to drive oncological treatments, in the multimodal context that characterized the management of this disease. Recurrence primarily occurs at the leading tumor margin, where there is a unique immune biological footprint relative to the tumor core, with also differential sensitivity to antitumor drug agents and with different BBB permeability.

While increasing the EOR and protecting the neurological status of the patient, further effort should also be pursued in boosting the recovery after surgery, regardless of the cause, either iatrogenic or due to the disease itself.

Promising effective strategies are both available and under investigation, with further work needed to provide results with a proper level of evidence and to finally increase the armamentarium the brain surgeon is endowed with to effectively contribute to the multidisciplinary treatment of patients with high-grade gliomas.

References

1. Giambra M, et al. The peritumoral brain zone in glioblastoma: where we are and where we are going. J Neurosci Res. 2023;101:199–216.
2. Pessina F, et al. Maximize surgical resection beyond contrast-enhancing boundaries in newly diagnosed glioblastoma multiforme: is it useful and safe? A single institution retrospective experience. J Neurooncol. 2017;135:129–39.
3. Li YM, Suki D, Hess K, Sawaya R. The influence of maximum safe resection of glioblastoma on survival in 1229 patients: can we do better than gross-total resection? J Neurosurg. 2016;124:977–88.
4. Pessina F, et al. Value of surgical resection in patients with newly diagnosed grade III glioma treated in a multimodal approach: surgery, chemotherapy and radiotherapy. Ann Surg Oncol. 2016;23:3040–6.
5. Jain R, et al. Outcome prediction in patients with glioblastoma by using imaging, clinical, and genomic biomarkers: focus on the nonenhancing component of the tumor. Radiology. 2014;272:484–93.
6. Beiko J, et al. IDH1 mutant malignant astrocytomas are more amenable to surgical resection and have a survival benefit associated with maximal surgical resection. Neuro Oncol. 2014;16:81–91.
7. Molinaro AM, et al. Association of maximal extent of resection of contrast-enhanced and non-contrast-enhanced tumor with survival within molecular subgroups of patients with newly diagnosed glioblastoma. JAMA Oncol. 2020;6:495.
8. Karschnia P, et al. Prognostic validation of a new classification system for extent of resection in glioblastoma: a report of the RANO *resect* group. Neuro Oncol. 2023;25:940–54.
9. Fathi Kazerooni A, Bakas S, Saligheh Rad H, Davatzikos C. Imaging signatures of glioblastoma molecular characteristics: a radiogenomics review. J Magn Reson Imaging. 2020;52:54–69.
10. Hygino da Cruz LC, Vieira IG, Domingues RC. Diffusion MR imaging: an important tool in the assessment of brain tumors. Neuroimaging Clin N Am. 2011;21:27–49.
11. Romano A, et al. Apparent diffusion coefficient obtained by magnetic resonance imaging as a prognostic marker in glioblastomas: correlation with MGMT promoter methylation status. Eur Radiol. 2013;23:513–20.
12. Choi HJ, et al. MGMT promoter methylation status in initial and recurrent glioblastoma: correlation study with DWI and DSC PWI features. Am J Neuroradiol. 2021;42:853–60.
13. Sunwoo L, et al. Correlation of apparent diffusion coefficient values measured by diffusion MRI and MGMT promoter methylation semiquantitatively analyzed with MS-MLPA in patients with glioblastoma multiforme. J Magn Reson Imaging. 2013;37:351–8.
14. Moon W-J, Choi JW, Roh HG, Lim SD, Koh Y-C. Imaging parameters of high grade gliomas in relation to the MGMT promoter methylation status: the CT, diffusion tensor imaging, and perfusion MR imaging. Neuroradiology. 2012;54:555–63.
15. Sternberg EJ, Lipton ML, Burns J. Utility of diffusion tensor imaging in evaluation of the peritumoral region in patients with primary and metastatic brain tumors. Am J Neuroradiol. 2014;35:439–44.
16. Shiroishi MS, Boxerman JL, Pope WB. Physiologic MRI for assessment of response to therapy and prognosis in glioblastoma. Neuro Oncol. 2016;18:467–78.
17. Anzalone N, et al. Brain gliomas: multicenter standardized assessment of dynamic contrast-enhanced and dynamic susceptibility contrast MR images. Radiology. 2018;287:933–43.
18. Ninatti G, et al. Preoperative [11C]methionine PET to personalize treatment decisions in patients with lower-grade gliomas. Neuro Oncol. 2022;24:1546–56.
19. Pessina F, et al. Role of 11C methionine positron emission tomography (11CMETPET) for surgery and radiation therapy planning in newly diagnosed glioblastoma patients enrolled into a phase II clinical study. J Clin Med. 2021;10:2313.
20. Riva M, et al. 3D intra-operative ultrasound and MR image guidance: pursuing an ultrasound-based management of brainshift to enhance neuronavigation. Int J Comput Assist Radiol Surg. 2017;12:1711–25.
21. Kubben PL, et al. Intraoperative MRI-guided resection of glioblastoma multiforme: a systematic review. Lancet Oncol. 2011;12:1062–70.
22. Traylor JI, Pernik MN, Sternisha AC, McBrayer SK, Abdullah KG. Molecular and metabolic mechanisms underlying selective 5-aminolevulinic acid-induced fluorescence in gliomas. Cancers (Basel). 2021;13:580.
23. Ferraro N, et al. The role of 5-aminolevulinic acid in brain tumor surgery: a systematic review. Neurosurg Rev. 2016;39:545–55.
24. Stummer W, et al. Fluorescence-guided surgery with 5-aminolevulinic acid for resection of malignant glioma: a randomised controlled multicentre phase III trial. Lancet Oncol. 2006;7:392–401.
25. Stummer W, et al. Counterbalancing risks and gains from extended resections in malignant glioma surgery: a supplemental analysis from the randomized 5-aminolevulinic acid glioma resection study. J Neurosurg. 2011;114:613–23.
26. Catapano G, et al. Fluorescein-guided surgery for high-grade glioma resection: an intraoperative "contrast-enhancer". World Neurosurg. 2017;104:239–47.
27. Acerbi F, et al. Fluorescein-guided surgery for resection of high-grade gliomas: a multicentric prospective phase II study (FLUOGLIO). Clin Cancer Res. 2018;24:52–61.
28. Acerbi F, et al. Ex vivo fluorescein-assisted confocal laser endomicroscopy (CONVIVO® system) in patients with glioblastoma: results from a prospective study. Front Oncol. 2020;10:606574.
29. Cameron JM, et al. Interrogation of IDH1 status in gliomas by Fourier transform infrared spectroscopy. Cancers (Basel). 2020;12:3682.

30. Gajjar K, et al. Diagnostic segregation of human brain tumours using Fourier-transform infrared and/or Raman spectroscopy coupled with discriminant analysis. Anal Methods. 2013;5:89–102.

31. Riva M, et al. Glioma biopsies classification using Raman spectroscopy and machine learning models on fresh tissue samples. Cancers (Basel). 2021;13:1073.

32. Sciortino T, et al. Raman spectroscopy and machine learning for IDH genotyping of unprocessed glioma biopsies. Cancers (Basel). 2021;13:4196.

33. Ma R, Taphoorn MJB, Plaha P. Advances in the management of glioblastoma. J Neurol Neurosurg Psychiatry. 2021;92:1103–11.

34. Mizuno A, Tsuji M, Fujii K, Kawauchi K, Ozaki Y. Near-infrared Fourier transform Raman spectroscopic study of cornea and sclera. Jpn J Ophthalmol. 1994;38:44–8.

35. Freudiger CW, et al. Label-free biomedical imaging with high sensitivity by stimulated Raman scattering microscopy. Science. 2008;1979(322):1857–61.

36. Lu F-K, et al. Label-free DNA imaging in vivo with stimulated Raman scattering microscopy. Proc Natl Acad Sci. 2015;112:11624–9.

37. Saar BG, et al. Video-rate molecular imaging in vivo with stimulated Raman scattering. Science. 2010;1979(330):1368–70.

38. Orillac C, Hollon T, Orringer DA. Clinical translation of stimulated Raman histology. Methods Mol Biol. 2022;2393:225–36. https://doi.org/10.1007/978-1-0716-1803-5_12.

39. Montemurro N, Perrini P, Blanco MO, Vannozzi R. Second surgery for recurrent glioblastoma: a concise overview of the current literature. Clin Neurol Neurosurg. 2016;142:60–4.

40. Sughrue ME, Sheean T, Bonney PA, Maurer AJ, Teo C. Aggressive repeat surgery for focally recurrent primary glioblastoma: outcomes and theoretical framework. Neurosurg Focus. 2015;38:E11.

41. Wann A, et al. Outcomes after second surgery for recurrent glioblastoma: a retrospective case–control study. J Neurooncol. 2018;137:409–15.

42. Voisin MR, Zuccato JA, Wang JZ, Zadeh G. Surgery for recurrent glioblastoma multiforme: a retrospective case control study. World Neurosurg. 2022;166:e624–31.

43. Perrini P, et al. Survival outcomes following repeat surgery for recurrent glioblastoma: a single-center retrospective analysis. J Neurooncol. 2017;131:585–91.

44. van Solinge TS, Nieland L, Chiocca EA, Broekman MLD. Advances in local therapy for glioblastoma—taking the fight to the tumour. Nat Rev Neurol. 2022;18:221–36.

45. Campos B, Olsen LR, Urup T, Poulsen HS. A comprehensive profile of recurrent glioblastoma. Oncogene. 2016;35:5819–25.

46. Weller M, Cloughesy T, Perry JR, Wick W. Standards of care for treatment of recurrent glioblastoma—are we there yet? Neuro Oncol. 2013;15:4–27.

47. Weller M. Novel diagnostic and therapeutic approaches to malignant glioma. Swiss Med Wkly. 2011; https://doi.org/10.4414/smw.2011.13210.

48. Weller M, Le Rhun E, Preusser M, Tonn J-C, Roth P. How we treat glioblastoma. ESMO Open. 2019;4:e000520.

49. Medikonda R, Dunn G, Rahman M, Fecci P, Lim M. A review of glioblastoma immunotherapy. J Neurooncol. 2021;151:41–53.

50. Cloughesy TF, et al. Neoadjuvant anti-PD-1 immunotherapy promotes a survival benefit with intratumoral and systemic immune responses in recurrent glioblastoma. Nat Med. 2019;25:477–86.

51. Reardon DA, et al. Rindopepimut with bevacizumab for patients with relapsed EGFRvIII-expressing glioblastoma (ReACT): results of a double-blind randomized phase II trial. Clin Cancer Res. 2020;26:1586–94.

52. Riva M, et al. Radiotherapy, temozolomide, and anti-programmed cell death protein 1 treatments modulate the immune microenvironment in experimental high-grade glioma. Neurosurgery. 2021;88:E205–15.

53. Mittal S, et al. Alternating electric tumor treating fields for treatment of glioblastoma: rationale, preclinical, and clinical studies. J Neurosurg. 2018;128:414–21.

54. Stupp R, et al. NovoTTF-100A versus physician's choice chemotherapy in recurrent glioblastoma: a randomised phase III trial of a novel treatment modality. Eur J Cancer. 2012;48:2192–202.

55. Stupp R, et al. Maintenance therapy with tumor-treating fields plus temozolomide vs temozolomide alone for glioblastoma. JAMA. 2015;314:2535.

56. Carpentier A, et al. Clinical trial of blood-brain barrier disruption by pulsed ultrasound. Sci Transl Med. 2016;8:343re2.

57. Bunevicius A, McDannold NJ, Golby AJ. Focused ultrasound strategies for brain tumor therapy. Oper Neurosurg. 2020;19:9–18.

58. Salehi A, et al. Therapeutic enhancement of blood–brain and blood–tumor barriers permeability by laser interstitial thermal therapy. Neurooncol Adv. 2020;2:vdaa071.

59. Maier-Hauff K, et al. Efficacy and safety of intratumoral thermotherapy using magnetic iron-oxide nanoparticles combined with external beam radiotherapy on patients with recurrent glioblastoma multiforme. J Neurooncol. 2011;103:317–24.

60. Brem H, et al. Placebo-controlled trial of safety and efficacy of intraoperative controlled delivery by biodegradable polymers of chemotherapy for recurrent gliomas. Lancet. 1995;345:1008–12.

61. Kunwar S, et al. Phase III randomized trial of CED of IL13-PE38QQR vs Gliadel wafers for recurrent glioblastoma. Neuro Oncol. 2010;12:871–81.

62. Vogelbaum M, Healy A. Convection-enhanced drug delivery for gliomas. Surg Neurol Int. 2015;6:59.

63. Secoli R, et al. Modular robotic platform for precision neurosurgery with a bio-inspired needle: system overview and first in-vivo deployment. PLoS One. 2022;17:e0275686.

64. Aabedi AA, et al. Association of neurological impairment on the relative benefit of maximal extent of resection in chemoradiation-treated newly diagnosed isocitrate dehydrogenase wild-type glioblastoma. Neurosurgery. 2022;90:124–30.

65. Bello L, et al. Functional approach to brain tumor surgery: awake setting. In: Deletis V, Shils J, Sala F, Seidel K, editors. Intraoperative neurophysiology. Academic Press; 2020.

66. Bello L, et al. Neurophysiology of language and cognitive mapping. In: Deletis V, Shils J, Sala F, Seidel K, editors. Intraoperative neurophysiology. Academic Press; 2020.

67. Bello L, et al. Tailoring neurophysiological strategies with clinical context enhances resection and safety and expands indications in gliomas involving motor pathways. Neuro Oncol. 2014;16:1110–28.

68. Riva M, et al. Monopolar high-frequency language mapping: can it help in the surgical management of gliomas? A comparative clinical study. J Neurosurg. 2016;124:1479–89.

69. De Witt Hamer PC, Robles SG, Zwinderman AH, Duffau H, Berger MS. Impact of intraoperative stimulation brain mapping on glioma surgery outcome: a meta-analysis. J Clin Oncol. 2012;30:2559–65.

70. Weller M, et al. EANO guidelines on the diagnosis and treatment of diffuse gliomas of adulthood. Nat Rev Clin Oncol. 2021;18:170–86.

71. Ille S, et al. Navigated repetitive transcranial magnetic stimulation improves the outcome of postsurgical paresis in glioma patients—a randomized, double-blinded trial. Brain Stimul. 2021;14:780–7.

Current and Future Drugs for Brain Tumors Treatment

6

Francesco Bruno, Alessia Pellerino, Elena Maria Marchesani, and Roberta Rudà

6.1 Drugs for *IDH*-Wildtype Glioblastoma, Grade 4 WHO 2021: First-Line Treatments

Glioblastoma (GBM) is the most common malignant brain tumor [1, 2].

Even if knowledge of cellular mechanisms fostering tumor growth has increased in the last decades and strenuous efforts have been made to improve surgical techniques and treatment modalities, to date the prognosis of patients with glioblastoma still remains poor [3, 4]. Standard treatment consists of concomitant radiochemotherapy followed by adjuvant chemotherapy (CT). Temozolomide (TMZ), a DNA alkylating agent, is used both in association with radiotherapy (RT) and, after the completion of RT, as a single-agent adjuvant CT, thus representing the gold standard for first-line treatment in GBM [5]. TMZ causes guanine methylation at O6 and N7 positions of DNA, which results in mismatch with thymine and provokes DNA breaks. Consequently, the cell cycle is blocked at the progression of G2/M phase, which induces cell death [6]. A high activity of the enzyme O6-methylguanine-methyl-transferase (*MGMT*) is associated with resistance to TMZ and other alkylating agents. Therefore, a down-regulation of the *MGMT* activity based on gene promoter methylation correlates with an improved response to TMZ.

Concurrent temozolomide (TMZ) is given with a dose of 75 mg/m^2/daily during the entire RT period (which usually consists of a 60 Gy radiation schedule distributed over 30 days). Then, TMZ should be resumed 4 weeks after completion of RT, with a dose of 150–200 mg/m^2/daily day 1–5 every 28 days for 6–12 monthly cycles [3, 5]. This treatment modality was introduced in the clinical practice as a standard of care based on the results of a seminal trial on 573 participants, where concurrent RT/TMZ followed by adjuvant TMZ was compared to RT alone. In this study, the median overall survival (mOS) was longer for patients in the arm of concurrent RT/TMZ treatment (14.6 vs 12.1 months; hazard ratio [HR], 0.63 [95% CI, 0.52–0.75]; $p < 0.001$) [3]. The presence of *MGMT*p methylation provided an additional benefit in terms of OS among patients treated with concurrent and adjuvant TMZ as compared to RT alone (21.7 months [95% CI, 17.4–30.4] vs 15.3 months [95% CI, 13.0–20.9], $p = 0.010$) [7]. Also, patients undergoing concurrent and adjuvant TMZ had a similar quality of life to those undergoing RT alone [8].

Noteworthy, a reduced concomitant schedule of RT (42 Gy over 15 days) with concurrent TMZ followed by adjuvant TMZ was proven to be more effective than RT alone in a clinical trial on

F. Bruno · A. Pellerino · E. M. Marchesani
R. Rudà (✉)
Division of Neuro-Oncology, Department of Neuroscience "Rita Levi Montalcini", University of Turin, Turin, Italy

562 patients aged 65 years or older (mOS being 9.3 vs 7.6 months; HR: 0.67 [95% CI, 0.56–0.80]; $p < 0.001$) [9]. For this reason, a short-course RT/TMZ modality is now recommended in the elderly population, and may also be an effective and safer option in patients with large tumor volumes and/or displaying poorer performance status [5, 9]. Moreover, for frail patients unlikely to tolerate the combination of chemotherapy and radiation, treatment with either RT alone (if *MGMT*-unmethylated) or TMZ alone (if *MGMT*-methylated) may be an option [5, 10, 11].

The association of maintenance TMZ with tumor-treating fields (TTFs), alternating low-intensity electric fields delivered on the scalp by a portable device, has also been explored and proved to be effective in a clinical trial as compared to maintenance TMZ alone (mOS 20.9 vs 16.0 months; HR 0.63 [95% CI, 0.53–0.76], $p < 0.001$) [4].

The 2021 WHO Classification has expanded the diagnosis of GBM to diffuse astrocytic gliomas isocitrate dehydrogenase-wildtype (*IDH*-wildtype) with characteristic molecular alterations (i.e. *EGFR* amplification, *pTERT* mutation, or chromosome 7 gain/chromosome 10 loss), even if typical histological findings of GBM (i.e. necrosis or endothelial proliferation), or typical MRI findings are not present [1, 12]. Before the 2021 Classification, the inclusion of those rare tumors in clinical trials on GBM patients was not possible, as in previous classifications the diagnosis of GBM always required traditional histopathological criteria. Therefore, which is the best treatment modality for patients with "molecularly defined" GBM remains an open issue. Interestingly, in a post hoc analysis of the CATNON trial (in which patients with grade 3 1p19q-intact gliomas based on the 2007 Classification were randomised to receive RT alone, RT followed by TMZ, concurrent RT and TMZ, or concurrent RT and TMZ followed by maintenance TMZ) [13], TMZ did not add benefit beyond that provided by RT, regardless of *MGMT*p status, in patients with *IDH*-wildtype tumors with molecular features of GBM, as defined by the 2021 Classification [14].

6.2 Drugs for *IDH*-Wildtype Glioblastoma, Grade 4 WHO 2021: Nitrosoureas and Bevacizumab in the Setting of Recurrence

Disease progression occurs in almost all GBM patients after first-line treatment [15]. Thus far, no highly effective treatment has been found for disease recurrence, and the choice of the best second-line therapy remains an open issue [16].

To date, the most common medical treatments at recurrence consist of nitrosourea-based regimens and/or antiangiogenic therapy.

6.2.1 Nitrosoureas

Nitrosoureas, damage DNA by alkylation, leading to cell death. They generate reactive compounds, like chloroethyldiazohydroxide and isocyanates, that form DNA cross-links and hinder repair processes. Metabolized in the liver, their lipophilicity enables them to cross the blood-brain barrier, achieving therapeutic levels in the brain.

- Carmustine (BCNU) is administered intravenously with two schedules of administration: 80 mg/mq on days 1–3 every 6 weeks or 240 mg/mq on day 1 every 6 weeks. Two phase 2 clinical trials and one retrospective study assessed the use of BCNU monotherapy for recurrent or progressive GBM [17–19]. Overall, response rates were modest, and complete remission was never observed. Moreover, BCNU treatment was associated with frequent hematologic toxicity and prolonged hepatic and pulmonary (fibrosis) side effects. For this reason, the clinical use of BCNU is limited.
- Lomustine (CCNU, chloroethyl-cyclohexyl-nitrosourea) is an oral nitrosourea agent which alkylates DNA and RNA, thus acting both with a cell cycle-dependent and independent mechanism. It is administered once from 6 to 8 week intervals at the dose of 110 mg/m^2. Myelosuppression is the most relevant side effect, with nadirs at 4–5 weeks after adminis-

tration. CCNU has been used as control in several phase 2 and 3 trials [20–27], thus achieving the role of the standard of care drug in the recurrence setting in Europe. Of note, the most compelling evidence of CCNU efficacy in diffuse gliomas derives from studies that associated this drug with procarbazine and vincristine, a schedule commonly known as "PCV" [28, 29]. However, while this association has proven to be effective in lower-grade grade 2 and 3 gliomas [28–32], the objective response rate with CCNU schedules in GBM is quite low (around 10%), and almost exclusively limited to patients with *MGMT*p methylation [22, 24, 26].

- Fotemustine has gained prominence in the treatment of recurrent GBM, particularly in some European countries. Efficacy data come from phase 2 studies using different administration schedules [33, 34]. In a prospective phase 2 study, fotemustine was assessed in 43 recurrent GBM patients after standard radiation therapy and temozolomide [33]. The regimen involved induction with 75 mg/m^2 on days 1–8–15 and maintenance with 100 mg/m^2 every 3 weeks. Results showed a 20.9% 6-month PFS, a 7% response rate, and a median OS of 6 months. Disease control was higher in patients with *MGMT*p methylation. In a retrospective study, an induction schedule of 80 mg/m^2 on days 1, 15, 30, 45, and 60, followed by maintenance with 80 mg/m^2 every 4 weeks, yielded a 6-month PFS of 61%, a median PFS of 6.7 months, and an OS of 11.1 months [34]. In a phase 2 trial of combined fotemustine and bevacizumab for GBM at first recurrence after radiochemotherapy with TMZ, the 6-month PFS rate was 42.6%, the median PFS 5.2 months, and the median OS 9.1 months (results that were not significantly superior to those of historical cohorts of fotemustine or bevacizumab alone) [35].

6.2.2 Antiangiogenetic Drugs

Antiangiogenic drugs have been investigated in clinical trials showing some activity in terms of PFS, but disappointing results regarding OS. Bevacizumab (Bev), a human monoclonal antibody which binds circulating VEGF-A, conferred an advantage in 6-months PFS when associated with irinotecan (50%) as compared with Bev alone (42%) in the BRAIN trial [36], leading to the approval by FDA for the use at first recurrence. Likelihood, in Europe, the BELOB trial has shown encouraging results for the combination of Bev and lomustine vs either agent alone [22]. However, the phase 3 trial investigating the combination of Bev plus lomustine in comparison with lomustine alone failed to demonstrate an improvement of OS (median OS 9.1 vs 8.6 months), despite an increase of PFS from 1.5 to 4.2 months [24]. Other phase 2 trials have investigated Bev in association with several drugs, including temozolomide, fotemustine, irinotecan, temsirolimus and erlotinib, but none have displayed a significant impact in OS [35, 37–39]. Bev in GBM patients, in general, is well tolerated and serious adverse events, such as gastrointestinal perforation, thromboembolic events, renal injury, impairment of wound healing process, Posterior Reversible Encephalopathy, congestive heart failure, and uncontrolled hypertension are rare. A post hoc analysis of the ARTE trial has shown a survival benefit from the addition of Bev to radiotherapy in comparison with Bev alone in elderly patients with newly diagnosed GBM that depends on the presence of large contrast-enhancing tumor lesions, while the detection of non-contrast-enhancing tumor on amino acid PET scans indicated inferior survival. These findings suggest that Bev may work as a radiosensitizer in presence of dysfunctional vasculature in GBM [40, 41]. Some preclinical and translational studies have displayed that the effect of VEGF-targeted therapy is transient and dose-dependent on tumor barrier permeability [42, 43]. Notably, lower doses (<10 mg/kg) of Bev may induce reduction of leakiness, improve oxygenation without inducing vessel destruction, and favour the upregulation of angiopoietin-2 (Ang-2), a potent driver of vessel leakiness.

Aflibercept is a recombinant human fusion protein that acts as a soluble decoy receptor for VEGF-A, VEGF-B and placental growth factor, depleting circulating levels of these growth factors. A phase 1 trial suggested that Aflibercept in combination with temozolomide conferred moderate toxicities, including fatigue, hypertension, lymphopenia, ischaemic stroke, and systemic haemorrhage. All patients stopped the treatment: 28 (47%) for disease progression, 21 (36%) for toxicities, 8 (14%) for other reasons, and 2 (3%) patients completed the full treatment course [44]. The phase 2 trial reported limited efficacy of Aflibercept in both grade 3 astrocytomas (radiological response in 44%, 6-month PFS of 25%, median PFS of 24 weeks) and GBM (radiological response in 18%, 6-month PFS of 7.7%, median PFS of 12 weeks) [45].

Tanibirumab is a fully human monoclonal antibody targeting soluble vascular endothelial growth factor receptors-2 (VEGFR-2) that was investigated in a phase 2 trial in 12 patients with recurrent GBM. The best radiological response was a stable disease in 3/12 patients of whom two patients had a long-lasting response till weeks 60 and 40, respectively, and was correlated with the highest expression of VEGFR2 using immunohistochemistry on archival tumor and blood vessels [46].

As VEGF-targeted mAb fail to control disease, we may argue that vascular normalization alone is not the sole factor to overcome treatment resistance of GBM, and other mechanisms may co-exist or even prevail upon targeting of neo angiogenesis.

6.3 Drugs for *IDH*-Mutant Lower Grade Gliomas

IDH-mutant gliomas include astrocytomas grade 2, 3, and 4, and oligodendrogliomas grade 2 and 3. The 2021 WHO Classification provides integrated histomolecular criteria for diagnosis: astrocytomas typically show *ATRX* loss, while 1p/19q codeletion is a molecular hallmark of oligodendrogliomas.

The majority of clinical trials on lower-grade gliomas have been carried out in the past two decades, when molecular information was largely lacking and inclusion criteria were based on morphological diagnosis: for this reason, the impact of different treatment strategies across the new molecular subgroups have been analyzed only by post hoc analyses.

6.3.1 IDH-Mutant Grade 2 Astrocytomas and Oligodendrogliomas

Traditionally, the indication to adjuvant treatments for low-grade astrocytomas or oligodendrogliomas was mainly restricted to patients with a high risk of disease progression after surgery. According to the classic prognostic criteria (commonly referred to as the "Pignatti score"), "high-risk" patients were defined by the presence of at least three out of five of the following factors: age >40 years, astrocytic tumors (histologically defined), presence of neurological deficits after surgery, large tumor diameter, tumor crossing the midline [47]. These criteria were largely used to stratify the risk of low-grade glioma patients in clinical trials in pre-molecular era, and allowed to clarify the role of adjuvant treatments across different subgroups [48]. The EORTC trial 22,845 (which was activated from the late '80s to late '90s) was one of the first studies that compared early versus delayed RT after surgery in low-grade glioma patients, and did not find a negative impact on overall survival for patients with low risk factors who were observed with MRI, thus suggesting that delaying radiation therapy at progression was feasible and safe [49].

Conversely, which was the best treatment strategy for high-risk low-grade glioma patients, and what specific role could have chemotherapy, was investigated by different clinical trials in the pre-molecular era. RTOG 9802 phase 3 trial showed that the addition of PCV to adjuvant RT provided longer PFS and OS as compared to RT alone in high-risk histologically-defined low-grade glioma patients (mPFS 10.4 vs 4.0 years, $p < 0.001$; mOS 13.3 vs 7.8 years, $p = 0.003$) [32]. In this trial, "high-risk" patients were defined based on their age (>40 years) or extent of resection, whereas molecular factors (including *IDH* mutation) were not considered for risk stratification. Interestingly, an exploratory analysis showed that the benefit of the addition of PCV in terms of PFS and OS was maintained among patients with IDH-mutant 1p/19q codeleted oligodendrogliomas and in those with *IDH*-mutant non 1p/19q codeleted astrocytomas, whereas it was not significant in patients with IDH wild type astrocytic tumors: these findings corroborated the evidence that CT with alkylating agents could be useful especially among oligodendroglioma patients, a correlation that had already been reported in older studies [50].

The efficacy of upfront CT with alkylating agents versus first-line RT in high-risk low-grade glioma patients was also investigated in clinical trials. The rationale of such a strategy would be to delay RT to avoid the long-term cognitive effects of patients with a significantly long survival [48, 51]. The EORTC 22033-26033 phase 3 trial evaluated the efficacy of either upfront TMZ or RT as adjuvant strategies in high-risk low-grade glioma patients with PFS as primary outcome [52]. In this trial, high-risk patients were defined based on the presence of at least one of the five Pignatti criteria. The long-term results showed that patients treated with either RT or TMZ had similar PFS (mPFS being 39 and 46 months, $p = 0.220$, for TMZ and RT, respectively). However, when stratified according to tumor subtype, patients with 1p19q codeletion only had a similar benefit from TMZ or RT, whereas non-codeleted patients had a significantly longer PFS with RT.

Similarly, a phase 2 trial investigated the role of upfront TMZ in high-risk low-grade gliomas after incomplete surgery or biopsy [53]. Patients receiving upfront TMZ showed similar outcomes as compared to the historical arm of patients treated with RT of the 9802 trial (mPFS 3.8 vs 4.0 years; mOS 9.7 vs 7.8 years). Moreover, factors associated with a better outcome with TMZ were the presence of 1p19q codeletion, as well as larger resections and tumor volume <68 cm^3 at baseline. Similar results were obtained in a multicentre phase 2 trial employing an intensified schedule of initial TMZ after surgery in low-grade glioma patients [54]: in this study, response rate (according to RANO criteria) among IDH-mutant 1p19q-codeleted oligodendrogliomas (76%) was significantly higher than that among astrocytomas either IDH-mutant (55%) or wild-type (36%). In particular, in this study 67% of patients with IDH-mutant 1p19q-codeleted oligodendroglioma did not recur with a median fol-

low-up of 9.3 years, while 59% did not receive radiotherapy at recurrence with a median follow-up of 8.2 years.

In summary: for patients with high-risk IDH-mutant grade 2 astrocytoma, RT followed by PCV is the current standard of care. In patients with high-risk IDH-mutant 1p19q-codeleted grade 2 oligodendroglioma, RT followed by PCV has also demonstrated to prolong both PFS and OS; however, in these patients, especially in case of large tumor volume, upfront TMZ may be an option with similar efficacy and lesser risk of long-term negative effects on neurocognition. Overall, the employ of TMZ instead of PCV is a common strategy in low-grade glioma patients, owning to its better toxicity profile and ease of administration. However, there are no conclusive data assessing the superiority of TMZ over PCV on tumor control as randomized clinical trials are lacking [5, 55, 56].

6.3.2   IDH-Mutant Grade 3 Astrocytomas and Oligodendrogliomas

The standard adjuvant treatment for IDH-mutant grade 3 astrocytomas is RT followed by TMZ [5]. This strategy has proven to be superior in a the phase 3 open-label "CATNON" trial, which enrolled non-1p19q-codeleted patients with grade 3 histology (regardless of IDH mutation status) and compared four arms of treatments (RT alone, RT followed by adjuvant TMZ, RT with concurrent TMZ, and RT with concurrent TMZ followed by adjuvant TMZ) [13]. Patients receiving adjuvant TMZ after RT had longer PFS and OS compared to those who did not (mPFS 42.8 vs 19.1 months, $p < 0.0001$; mOS 82.3 vs 46.9 months, $p < 0.0001$), whereas the addition of concurrent TMZ did not significantly affect the outcome. Of note, only patients with IDH-mutant tumors benefited from adjuvant TMZ, whereas those with IDH-wildtype tumors had a similar outcome with or without adjuvant TMZ following RT [13, 14]. Based on the CATNON results, RT followed by TMZ also represents the recommended treatment for patients with IDH-mutant grade 4 astrocytomas (a new entity of the 2021 WHO Classification, formerly known as "GBM *IDH*-mutant", or "secondary GBM") according to the guidelines of the European Association on Neuro-Oncology [5].

Similarly, for *IDH*-mutant 1p19q-codeleted grade 3 oligodendrogliomas the current standard treatment is RT followed by CT (in this case, PCV). The combination of RT followed by PCV was superior to RT alone in the phase 3 trials RTOG 9402 and EORTC 26951, which compared the two strategies in patients with anaplastic oligodendrogliomas (as defined per histology) [30, 31, 57]. A post hoc analysis within molecular subgroups of patients with *IDH*-mutant 1p19q-codeleted tumors (thus, molecular oligodendrogliomas according to the current nomenclature) confirmed that RT/PCV vs RT alone correlated to a significantly longer survival in the RTOG 9402 trial (mOS 13.2 vs 7.3 years, $p = 0.020$) and to a trend for a longer survival in the EORTC 26951 trial (mOS 14.2 vs 9.3 years, $p = 0.063$).

Whether upfront CT may be an option for patients with oligodendroglioma *IDH*-mutant 1p19q-codeleted grade 3 (as well as for grade 2) was largely debated, and evaluated in retrospective or observational studies with inconclusive results [58, 59]. According to its original study design, the phase 3 CODEL trial randomised patients with 1p19q-codeleted gliomas grade 3 in three arms of treatments: RT alone; RT and concurrent TMZ followed by adjuvant TMZ; TMZ alone. The arm of TMZ alone showed a significantly shorter PFS as compared to the pooled RT arms (HR 3.12, 1.26–7.69 95% CI, $p = 0.014$), and death from disease progression occurred in 3/12 (25%) of TMZ-alone patients and 4/24 (16.7%) on the RT arms [60]. For this reason, the study design was changed, and two arms of RT + PCV vs RT + TMZ were established (the study, after being reshaped, is currently ongoing). However, the small cohort of patients in the TMZ alone arm ($n = 12$), and the unexpected presence of three *IDH*-wildtype patients (representing a potential sample bias) might have influenced the negative result of alone TMZ-arm in this trial [61]. For instance, the NOA-04 trial suggested that prior CT (PCV or TMZ) followed by RT at treatment failure (defined as disease progression

and/or unacceptable tolerability) may not be inferior to prior RT followed by CT in grade 3 gliomas [62]. Interestingly, a post hoc analysis within molecular subgroups revealed that PCV was superior to TMZ as first option in *IDH*-mutant 1p19q-codeleted grade 3 oligodendrogliomas in terms of PFS (but not OS) [63]. However, the level of evidence is still too low to generate solid conclusions on the superiority of PCV over TMZ in oligodendroglioma patients.

6.3.3 IDH Inhibitors for IDH-Mutant Gliomas

One of the major advancements in the treatment of *IDH*-mutant gliomas is the possibility of inhibiting the *IDH* mutation. In fact, *IDH* mutations are responsible for the production of the oncometabolite D2-hydroxygluterate (D2HG), which has a critical role in tumorigenesis [64, 65].

Two inhibitors, ivosidenib and vorasidenib, have proven to be effective in phase 1 trials against non-enhancing *IDH*-mutant gliomas [66–68]. The two agents were compared in a subsequent perioperative study [69]. Patients with recurrent gliomas carrying *IDH* mutations, predominantly grade 2, who were candidates for re-surgery, were randomised to receive either ivosidenib or vorasidenib at different doses, or no treatment during the 28 days leading up to surgery. D2HG levels in surgical specimens were significantly reduced in patients treated with ivosidenib or vorasidenib in a dose-dependent manner, with reductions of up to 93%. Translational analyses of the data revealed that the reduction in D2HG levels correlated with decreased cell proliferation markers, diminished proneural and stem cell gene expression signatures, upregulated inflammatory pathways, and increased infiltration of CD3+ and CD8+ T cells. Notably, Vorasidenib demonstrated greater intratumor diffusion, more consistent D2HG suppression, and moderately superior clinical activity compared to Ivosidenib, leading to its selection for a phase 3 trial [69].

The pivotal INDIGO phase 3 trial aimed to assess the efficacy of vorasidenib vs placebo in patients with RT/CT-naïve, non-enhancing *IDH*-mutant grade 2 gliomas without immediate need for treatment [70]. The primary endpoint was PFS, while the key secondary endpoint was time-to-next-intervention. The second interim analysis provided compelling results [71]. After a median follow-up of 14 months, the vorasidenib arm showed a significant increase in both PFS (median PFS of 28 vs 11 months, $p < 0.001$) and time-to-next-intervention (HR 0.26, $p < 0.001$) compared to the placebo group. At a 24-month evaluation, 83% of vorasidenib-treated patients did not require a second antitumor treatment, in contrast to only 27% of those on placebo. Importantly, the treatment was well tolerated, with a modest increase of hepatic enzymes as the primary reported adverse event [71].

Lastly, there is strong evidence of the role of *IDH* mutations in determining a higher risk of seizures in *IDH*-mutant [72–75]. For this reason, whether *IDH* inhibitors may be effective on seizure control as well as tumor growth is acquiring increasing interest, with initial evidence supporting this possible indication [76, 77].

This trial serves as a benchmark for the evolution of targeted therapy in gliomas and underscores the potentiality of *IDH* inhibition, especially in the earliest phases of the disease when tumor development is expected to be highly dependent on *IDH* function [78, 79].

6.4 Targeted Therapies in Brain Tumors

The purpose of this section is to provide an overview of the recent advances in the field of precision medicine for brain tumors. We will explore strategies such as targeting the epidermal growth factor receptor (*EGFR*), the fibroblast growth factors receptor (*FGFR*), and multikinases in glioblastoma, as well as *BRAF* mutations in diffuse and circumscribed gliomas. We will also briefly discuss the role of targeted therapies in rarer brain tumors, such as the inhibition of rapamycin (mTOR) pathway in subependymal giant cell astrocytomas (SEGAs) associated with tuberous sclerosis, or of fusions of the neurotrophic tyrosine receptor kinase (NTRK).

6.4.1 Inhibition of the Epidermal Growth Factor Receptor (EGFR)

EGFR signalling is a driver of tumor development, influencing cell growth, survival, invasion, angiogenesis, and tumor metabolism [80]. *EGFR* is a clinical target, and in over 50% of GBM cases, it is either amplified or mutated [81]. Extensive research has been focused on *EGFR* and its mutant form, EGFRvIII, with several strategies proposed for receptor inhibition, including monoclonal antibodies, tyrosine kinase inhibitors (TKIs), and anti-tumor vaccines.

Monoclonal Antibodies
- Cetuximab, the pioneering chimeric antibody targeting *EGFR*, showed no therapeutic benefit in recurrent GBM patients in phase 2 trials, either alone [82] or in combination with bevacizumab and irinotecan [83].
- Panitumumab, a fully human monoclonal anti-*EGFR* antibody, did not prove beneficial for GBM patients in a phase 2 trial with irinotecan (NCT01017653).
- Nimotuzumab, a humanised anti-*EGFR* antibody, did not improve OS or PFS in newly diagnosed patients following the Stupp protocol (phase 3) (NCT00753246) [84]. However, nimotuzumab remains an intriguing therapy, as recent observations indicate enhanced cytotoxicity when combined with TMZ in vivo [85].
- Depatuxizumab-mafodotin (ABT-414) is an antibody-drug conjugate (ADC) composed of an anti-*EGFR* IgG linked to the tubulin inhibitor monomethyl auristatin F [86]. It presented potential efficacy when used in combination with TMZ in recurrent GBM with *EGFR* amplification [27] but this advantage has not been confirmed in newly diagnosed GBM.

Tyrosine Kinase Activity Inhibitors
- Erlotinib, a reversible *EGFR* tyrosine kinase inhibitor, failed to demonstrate improved OS when combined with bevacizumab and TMZ in newly diagnosed patients in two phase 2 studies [37, 87]. Similar outcomes were

observed in a phase 2 study evaluating erlotinib in combination with sorafenib [88].

- Gefitinib, a reversible and specific EGFR tyrosine kinase inhibitor, did not improve OS when combined with RT in newly diagnosed patients [89], nor as adjuvant therapy after RT [90].
- Afatinib, an irreversible pan-inhibitor of the ErbB family (including *EGFR* and EGFRvIII), did not outperform TMZ in a phase 2 study (NCT00727506). However, it showed increased PFS in patients with tumors expressing EGFRvIII or *EGFR* amplification [91].
- Dacomitinib, a pan-HER family inhibitor approved for *EGFR*-mutant NSCLC, provided minimal benefits in GBM when tested as monotherapy in tumors with *EGFR* amplification or the common *EGFR* mutation EGFRvIII [92].

Overall, none of the trials employing *EGFR*-targeted agents showed promising results in GBM patients. Resistance to therapies in GBM has been demonstrated to be a combination of acquired and inherent factors. This resistance appears to be affected by a multitude of factors, including ineffective penetration of the blood-brain barrier, genetic mutations, tumor heterogeneity, and the activation of compensatory signalling pathways. Notably, recent research has revealed that EGFR has pro-survival functions in cancer cells that are independent of its kinase activity. Therefore, it is crucial to achieve a deeper understanding of the functioning of *EGFR* signalling pathways and their interactions with other cellular pathways.

6.4.2 Inhibition of the Fibroblast Growth Factor Receptor (FGFR)

Even if mutations in the fibroblast growth factor receptor (*FGFR*) are uncommon in GBM, the signalling mediated by *FGFR* plays a significant role in influencing GBM progression and patients survival [93]. For example, the fusion between *FGFR* and *TACC* (transforming acidic coiled-coil-containing proteins) amplifies both tumor growth and aneuploidy events [94]. An open-label, phase 2, monotherapy study of pemigatinib, FIGHT-209 (NCT05267106), in patients with previously treated recurrent GBM or other primary CNS tumors with an activating FGFR1-3 mutation or fusion/rearrangement, is ongoing.

6.4.3 Multikinase Inhibitors in GBM

Several multikinase inhibitors have been tested in GBM. These inhibitors block various receptor tyrosine kinases (RTKs) or non-receptor kinases due to common structural features in their ATP/ADP binding sites. Many of these inhibitors have demonstrated the ability to target well-known GBM targets such as *EGFR*, *PDGFR*, and vascular endothelial growth factor receptors (*VEGFR*), and the simultaneous inhibition of multiple kinases may help mitigate drug resistance and compensatory pathways.

Among multikinase inhibitors, regorafenib is probably the one that acquired the greater interest in recent times. Regorafenib is an oral inhibitor of several kinases involved in tumor angiogenesis (VEGFR1-3 and TIE2), oncogenesis (KIT, RET, RAF1, and BRAF), and in the interaction between tumor and microenvironment (platelet-derived growth factor receptor [PDGFR] and fibroblast growth factor receptor [FGFR]), and tumor immunity (colony-stimulating factor 1 receptor [CSF1R]) [95–98]. Regorafenib was initially approved for metastatic colorectal cancer, advanced gastrointestinal stromal tumor (GIST), and advanced hepatocellular carcinoma (HCC) [99–101]. Following the demonstration of an antiangiogenic effect in a rat GS9L glioblastoma model [97], regorafenib was investigated in this setting as well. In the randomised, open-label, phase 2 REGOMA trial, GBM patients at first recurrence were treated with either regorafenib (160 mg daily 21/28 days) or lomustine [26]. Regorafenib improved OS (median OS: 7.4 vs 5.6 months, $p = 0.0009$) and PFS (6-month PFS: 16.9% vs 8.3%, $p = 0.022$) as compared with lomustine. Therefore, regorafenib was approved by different regulatory authorities as a second-line treatment for GBM patients. Recently, some real-life trials showed similar impact on survival but a higher rate of adverse events than in REGOMA, thus raising concerns over tolerability [102–107]. However, the possibility of using a dose escalation protocol to improve tolerability while maintaining a similar efficacy of the standard schedule has been suggested [108]. However, more data are needed to confirm this finding. The ongoing AGILE trial (NCT03970447) will address many open issues in a larger prospective cohort of patients.

6.4.4   BRAF/MEK Inhibitors in BRAF-Mutant Brain Tumors

BRAF, a member of the RAF serine/threonine kinase family, is a key component of the mitogen-activated kinase (MAPK) pathway, which regulates cell responses to growth signals. Dysregulation of this pathway, due to *BRAF* gain-of-function mutations or loss of regulatory proteins, is implicated in tumorigenesis [109]. Notably, *BRAF* alterations are prevalent in various cancers, including gliomas, metastatic melanoma, papillary thyroid cancer, colon carcinomas, and hairy cell leukaemia [110].

In primary brain tumors, *BRAF* V600E mutation is observed in 17% of paediatric low-grade gliomas (PLGGs) and correlates with poor outcomes [111]. Pilocytic astrocytomas often harbour *KIAA1549:BRAF* fusions (50–85%) or *BRAF* V600E mutations (9–15%), which are mutually exclusive [64, 112]. Pleomorphic xanthoastrocytomas exhibit *BRAF* single nucleotide mutations in up to 70% of cases, as well as in diffuse lower-grade gliomas (up to 15% in grade 2 and 3 astrocytomas), glioblastomas, and *glioneuronal* tumors [109].

Combined *BRAF* and *MEK* inhibition has shown promise in improving the outcome of *BRAF* V600E-mutant gliomas. In particular, the phase 2 trial "ROAR", which explored the use of *BRAF/MEK* inhibitors (dabrafenib/trametinib) in patients with *BRAF* V600E-mutant gliomas, provided encouraging results, with 33% and 69% MRI objective response rate among high-grade and low-grade gliomas cohorts, respectively [113]. Also, there are scattered data from small clinical studies with small cohorts of patients which support the use of *BRAF/MEK* inhibitors in rarer tumor subtypes, such as pleomorphic astrocytoma and ganglioglioma [114, 115].

The efficacy of treatments with MAPK-inhibitors are limited by the occurrence of drug-resistance over time, as previously seen in melanoma and other solid cancers [116]. Drug-resistance usually derives from upregulation of other pathways, increased activation or expression of surface receptor tyrosine kinases (RTKs), such as *EGFR*, or loss of feedback inhibition by *ERK*, that can lead to activation of *RAF* signalling, and possibly many other mechanisms [115]. Similarly, resistance to *MAPK*-inhibitors may occur in gliomas treated with targeted therapies. It is still unclear whether the pathophysiology underlying the onset of drug-resistance in gliomas is the same of that seen in other cancers.

Finally, emerging evidence suggesting a potential role of BRAF activation in brain tumor-related epilepsy (BTRE) is acquiring increasing interest. In a meta-analysis on 509 patients with BTRE, 193 had the *BRAF* V600E mutation (34.1%). As expected, *BRAF* mutation prevailed in patients with gangliogliomas; furthermore, it was significantly associated with age at seizure onset [117]. To date, there are no available data investigating whether *MAPK*-inhibitors may affect seizure control in *BRAF*-activated brain tumors with BTRE.

6.4.5   Rapamycin (mTOR) Inhibitors in the Tuberous Sclerosis Complex

Tuberous sclerosis complex (TSC) is a rare genetic disorder characterised by an elevated risk of developing benign tumors and hamartomas in various organs, including the brain, skin, kidneys, heart, lungs, and eyes. Brain abnormalities in TSC patients typically include cortical tubers and subependymal giant cell astrocytomas (SEGAs), which, though slow-growing, can obstruct cerebrospinal fluid pathways, leading to hydrocephalus and intracranial hypertension [1].

The underlying cause of TSC is the loss of function in either the *TSC1* or *TSC2* gene, encoding hamartin and tuberin, respectively. These proteins inhibit Rheb, an activator of the mTORC1 protein complex, which plays a critical role in cellular proliferation and the development of tubers and SEGAs [118, 119]. Dysregulation of the mTOR pathway also contributes to TSC-related epilepsy, making mTOR inhibitors effective against both tumor growth and seizure control [120–122].

Everolimus, an mTOR inhibitor known for its higher affinity for the mTORC1 protein complex compared to rapamycin, serves as an effective treatment option for various conditions associated with tuberous sclerosis complex (TSC) [123, 124]. These conditions include SEGAs, angiomyolipomas, epilepsy [120, 125–127], and neuropsychiatric disorders [120, 128].

The pivotal EXIST-1 trial, a double-blind, placebo-controlled phase 3 study, explored the role of everolimus in TSC-related SEGA [122, 123]. In the initial analysis of the double-blind core phase, everolimus achieved a significant 50% reduction in SEGA volume in 27 patients (35%), while no radiological or clinical responses were seen in the placebo group ($p < 0.0001$). Adverse events associated with everolimus were primarily mild (grade 1 or 2) and did not necessitate treatment discontinuation. Common adverse events (AEs) in the everolimus group included mouth ulceration (32%), stomatitis (31%), convulsions (23%), and pyrexia (22%). Encouraged by these findings, the study extended to a long-term, open-label phase, with similar results [124]. Also, the EFFECTS phase 3 trial yielded similar results, with partial responses seen in 81 patients (67.5%), stable disease in 35 patients (29.2%), and progressive disease in 1 patient (0.8%) [129]. Lastly, the EMINENTS trial investigated the efficacy and safety of a reduced everolimus dose, with comparable results [130].

6.4.6 Neurotrophic Tyrosine Receptor Kinase (NTRK) Inhibitors in NTRK-Activated Gliomas

Neurotrophic tyrosine receptor kinases (NTRKs) are a group of high-affinity receptors consisting of three families (NTRK1-2-3) with similar structures and intracellular signalling pathways. They are known to be involved in several cellular functions such as growth, differentiation, and apoptosis. When hyperactivated (usually due to aberrant fusions with other genes), *NTRK* fusions may play a role as oncogenic primers in several cancer settings [131]. Both paediatric and adult brain tumors may present *NTRK* fusions, which represent interesting targets. *NTRK* fusion prevail in a particular subset of non-brainstem high-grade gliomas in very young children (less than 3 years), where they may be found in up to 40% of cases (particularly *TPM3-NTRK1* and *ETV6-NTRK3* fusions) [132]. A significant prevalence of *NTRK* fusions has also been observed in pilocytic astrocytomas (about 15%) [133]; conversely, in diffuse lower-grade gliomas, as well as in glioblastoma and diffuse intrinsic pontine gliomas, *NTRK* fusions are usually found in less than 2% of cases, while they were not observed in ependymomas or medulloblastomas [131].

Entrectinib (RXDX-101) is the first developed anti-NTRK fusions agent, which displays a secondary effect against *ALK* and *ROS1* fusion, and is proven to penetrate the blood-brain barrier [134]. The efficacy in primary and secondary brain tumors has been assessed in phase-1 and 2 trials (ALKA-372-001, STARTRK-1 [135], STARTRK-2, and STARTRK-NG), with promising results. Furthermore, in a series of paediatric high-grade gliomas reported at ASCO 2019, all 4 patients achieved a radiological response, including a complete response [90].

Larotrectinib (LOXO-101) is highly specific for *NTRK* fusions [136], and has been investigated in several clinical trials on solid tumors of paediatric patients, including primary and secondary brain tumors (NCT02637687, NCT02122913, NCT02637687, and NCT02576431). In particular, 9 patients with primary brain tumors were identified from NCT02637687 and NCT02576431 trials: disease control was achieved in all patients. The best objective response to therapy was partial response in 1 patients (11%), whereas the other patients showed stable disease [137].

A second-generation of *NTRK* inhibitors includes repotrectinib-TPX-0005 and LOXO-195-BAY2731954, that are being explored in clinical trials in order to compare their efficacy with first-generation drugs and, more importantly, to tackle tumor resistance to first-line compounds [138, 139].

References

1. Louis DN, Perry A, Wesseling P, et al. The 2021 WHO classification of tumors of the central nervous system: a summary. Neuro Oncol. 2021;23(8):1231–51. https://doi.org/10.1093/neuonc/noab106.

2. Ostrom QT, Cioffi G, Waite K, Kruchko C, Barnholtz-Sloan JS. CBTRUS statistical report: primary brain and other central nervous system tumors diagnosed in the United States in 2014–2018. Neuro Oncol. 2021;23(Suppl_3):iii1–iii105. https://doi.org/10.1093/neuonc/noab200.

3. Stupp R, Mason WP, van den Bent MJ, et al. Radiotherapy plus concomitant and adjuvant temozolomide for glioblastoma. N Engl J Med. 2005;352(10):987–96. https://doi.org/10.1056/NEJMoa043330.

4. Stupp R, Taillibert S, Kanner A, et al. Effect of tumor-treating fields plus maintenance temozolomide vs maintenance temozolomide alone on survival in patients with glioblastoma: a randomized clinical trial. JAMA. 2017;318(23):2306–16. https://doi.org/10.1001/jama.2017.18718.

5. Weller M, van den Bent M, Preusser M, et al. EANO guidelines on the diagnosis and treatment of diffuse gliomas of adulthood. Nat Rev Clin Oncol. 2021;18(3):170–86. https://doi.org/10.1038/s41571-020-00447-z.

6. Koukourakis GV, Kouloulias V, Zacharias G, et al. Temozolomide with radiation therapy in high grade brain gliomas: pharmaceuticals considerations and efficacy; a review article. Molecules. 2009;14(4):1561–77. https://doi.org/10.3390/molecules14041561.

7. Hegi ME, Diserens AC, Gorlia T, et al. MGMT gene silencing and benefit from temozolomide in glioblastoma. N Engl J Med. 2005;352(10):997–1003. https://doi.org/10.1056/NEJMoa043331.

8. Taphoorn MJ, Stupp R, Coens C, et al. Health-related quality of life in patients with glioblastoma: a randomised controlled trial. Lancet Oncol. 2005;6(12):937–44. https://doi.org/10.1016/S1470-2045(05)70432-0.

9. Perry JR, Laperriere N, O'Callaghan CJ, et al. Short-course radiation plus temozolomide in elderly patients with glioblastoma. N Engl J Med. 2017;376(11):1027–37. https://doi.org/10.1056/NEJMoa1611977.

10. Roa W, Brasher PMA, Bauman G, et al. Abbreviated course of radiation therapy in older patients with glioblastoma multiforme: a prospective randomized clinical trial. J Clin Oncol. 2004;22(9):1583–8. https://doi.org/10.1200/JCO.2004.06.082.

11. Malmström A, Grønberg BH, Marosi C, et al. Temozolomide versus standard 6-week radiotherapy versus hypofractionated radiotherapy in patients older than 60 years with glioblastoma: the Nordic randomised, phase 3 trial. Lancet Oncol. 2012;13(9):916–26. https://doi.org/10.1016/S1470-2045(12)70265-6.

12. Brat DJ, Aldape K, Colman H, et al. cIMPACT-NOW update 3: recommended diagnostic criteria for "Diffuse astrocytic glioma, IDH-wildtype, with molecular features of glioblastoma, WHO grade IV". Acta Neuropathol. 2018;136(5):805–10. https://doi.org/10.1007/s00401-018-1913-0.

13. van den Bent MJ, Tesileanu CMS, Wick W, et al. Adjuvant and concurrent temozolomide for 1p/19q non-co-deleted anaplastic glioma (CATNON; EORTC study 26053-22054): second interim analysis of a randomised, open-label, phase 3 study. Lancet Oncol. 2021;22(6):813–23. https://doi.org/10.1016/S1470-2045(21)00090-5.

14. Tesileanu CMS, Sanson M, Wick W, et al. Temozolomide and radiotherapy versus radiotherapy alone in patients with glioblastoma, IDH-wildtype: post hoc analysis of the EORTC randomized phase III CATNON trial. Clin Cancer Res. 2022;28(12):2527–35. https://doi.org/10.1158/1078-0432.CCR-21-4283.

15. Delgado-López PD, Corrales-García EM. Survival in glioblastoma: a review on the impact of treatment modalities. Clin Transl Oncol. 2016;18(11):1062–71. https://doi.org/10.1007/s12094-016-1497-x.

16. Fazzari FGT, Rose F, Pauls M, et al. The current landscape of systemic therapy for recurrent glioblastoma: a systematic review of randomized-controlled trials. Crit Rev Oncol Hematol. 2022;169:103540. https://doi.org/10.1016/j.critrevonc.2021.103540.

17. van den Bent MJ, Brandes AA, Rampling R, et al. Randomized phase II trial of erlotinib versus temozolomide or carmustine in recurrent glioblastoma: EORTC brain tumor group study 26034. J Clin Oncol. 2009;27(8):1268.

18. Reithmeier T, Graf E, Piroth T, Trippel M, Pinsker MO, Nikkhah G. BCNU for recurrent glioblastoma multiforme: efficacy, toxicity and prognostic factors. BMC Cancer. 2010;10(1):30. https://doi.org/10.1186/1471-2407-10-30.

19. Brandes AA, Tosoni A, Amistà P, et al. How effective is BCNU in recurrent glioblastoma in the modern era? Neurology. 2004;63(7):1281. https://doi.org/10.1212/01.WNL.0000140495.33615.CA.

20. Wick W, Puduvalli VK, Chamberlain MC, et al. Phase III study of enzastaurin compared with lomustine in the treatment of recurrent intracranial glioblastoma. J Clin Oncol. 2010;28(7):1168–74. https://doi.org/10.1200/JCO.2009.23.2595.

21. Batchelor TT, Mulholland P, Neyns B, et al. Phase III randomized trial comparing the efficacy of cediranib as monotherapy, and in combination with lomustine, versus lomustine alone in patients with recurrent glioblastoma. J Clin Oncol. 2013;31(26):3212.

22. Taal W, Oosterkamp HM, Walenkamp AM, et al. Single-agent bevacizumab or lomustine versus a combination of bevacizumab plus lomustine in patients with recurrent glioblastoma (BELOB trial): a randomised controlled phase 2 trial. Lancet Oncol. 2014;15(9):943–53.

23. Brandes AA, Carpentier AF, Kesari S, et al. A phase II randomized study of galunisertib monotherapy or galunisertib plus lomustine compared with lomustine monotherapy in patients with recurrent glioblastoma. Neuro Oncol. 2016;18(8):1146–56.

24. Wick W, Gorlia T, Bendszus M, et al. Lomustine and bevacizumab in progressive glioblastoma. N Engl J Med. 2017;377(20):1954–63.

25. Duerinck J, Du Four S, Bouttens F, et al. Randomized phase II trial comparing axitinib with the combination of axitinib and lomustine in patients with recurrent glioblastoma. J Neurooncol. 2018;136(1):115–25.

26. Lombardi G, De Salvo GL, Brandes AA, et al. Regorafenib compared with lomustine in patients with relapsed glioblastoma (REGOMA): a multi-centre, open-label, randomised, controlled, phase 2 trial. Lancet Oncol. 2019;20(1):110–9. https://doi.org/10.1016/S1470-2045(18)30675-2.

27. Van Den Bent M, Eoli M, Sepulveda JM, et al. INTELLANCE 2/EORTC 1410 randomized phase II study of Depatux-M alone and with temozolomide vs temozolomide or lomustine in recurrent EGFR amplified glioblastoma. Neuro Oncol. 2020;22(5):684–93.

28. Medical Research Council Brain Tumor Working Party. Randomized trial of procarbazine, lomustine, and vincristine in the adjuvant treatment of high-grade astrocytoma: a Medical Research Council trial. J Clin Oncol. 2001;19(2):509–18. https://doi.org/10.1200/JCO.2001.19.2.509.

29. Brada M, Stenning S, Gabe R, et al. Temozolomide versus procarbazine, lomustine, and vincristine in recurrent high-grade glioma. J Clin Oncol. 2010;28(30):4601–8. https://doi.org/10.1200/JCO.2009.27.1932.

30. Cairncross G, Wang M, Shaw E, et al. Phase III trial of chemoradiotherapy for anaplastic oligodendroglioma: long-term results of RTOG 9402. J Clin Oncol. 2013;31(3):337–43. https://doi.org/10.1200/JCO.2012.43.2674.

31. van den Bent MJ, Brandes AA, Taphoorn MJB, et al. Adjuvant procarbazine, lomustine, and vincristine chemotherapy in newly diagnosed anaplastic oligodendroglioma: long-term follow-up of EORTC brain tumor group study 26951. J Clin Oncol. 2013;31(3):344–50. https://doi.org/10.1200/JCO.2012.43.2229.

32. Buckner JC, Shaw EG, Pugh SL, et al. Radiation plus procarbazine, CCNU, and vincristine in low-grade glioma. N Engl J Med. 2016;374(14):1344–55. https://doi.org/10.1056/NEJMoa1500925.

33. Brandes AA, Tosoni A, Franceschi E, et al. Fotemustine as second-line treatment for recurrent or progressive glioblastoma after concomitant and/or adjuvant temozolomide: a phase II trial of Gruppo Italiano Cooperativo di Neuro-Oncologia (GICNO). Cancer Chemother Pharmacol. 2009;64(4):769–75. https://doi.org/10.1007/s00280-009-0926-8.

34. Addeo R, Caraglia M, De Santi MS, et al. A new schedule of fotemustine in temozolomide-pretreated patients with relapsing glioblastoma. J Neurooncol. 2011;102(3):417–24. https://doi.org/10.1007/s11060-010-0329-z.

35. Soffietti R, Trevisan E, Bertero L, et al. Bevacizumab and fotemustine for recurrent glioblastoma: a phase II study of AINO (Italian Association of Neuro-Oncology). J Neurooncol. 2014;116(3):533–41. https://doi.org/10.1007/s11060-013-1317-x.

36. Friedman HS, Prados MD, Wen PY, et al. Bevacizumab alone and in combination with irinotecan in recurrent glioblastoma. J Clin Oncol. 2009;27(28):4733–40. https://doi.org/10.1200/JCO.2008.19.8721.

37. Raizer JJ, Giglio P, Hu J, et al. A phase II study of bevacizumab and erlotinib after radiation and temozolomide in MGMT unmethylated GBM patients. J Neurooncol. 2016;126(1):185–92. https://doi.org/10.1007/s11060-015-1958-z.

38. Lassen U, Sorensen M, Gaziel TB, Hasselbalch B, Poulsen HS. Phase II study of bevacizumab and temsirolimus combination therapy for recurrent glioblastoma multiforme. Anticancer Res. 2013;33(4):1657.

39. Gilbert MR, Pugh SL, Aldape K, et al. NRG oncology RTOG 0625: a randomized phase II trial of bevacizumab with either irinotecan or dose-dense temozolomide in recurrent glioblastoma. J Neurooncol. 2017;131(1):193–9. https://doi.org/10.1007/s11060-016-2288-5.

40. Wirsching HG, Roelcke U, Weller J, et al. MRI and 18FET-PET predict survival benefit from bevacizumab plus radiotherapy in patients with isocitrate dehydrogenase wild-type glioblastoma: results from the randomized ARTE trial. Clin Cancer Res. 2021;27(1):179–88. https://doi.org/10.1158/1078-0432.CCR-20-2096.

41. Wirsching HG, Tabatabai G, Roelcke U, et al. Bevacizumab plus hypofractionated radiotherapy versus radiotherapy alone in elderly patients with glioblastoma: the randomized, open-label, phase II ARTE trial. Ann Oncol. 2018;29(6):1423–30. https://doi.org/10.1093/annonc/mdy120.

42. Batchelor TT, Sorensen AG, di Tomaso E, et al. AZD2171, a pan-VEGF receptor tyrosine kinase inhibitor, normalizes tumor vasculature and alleviates edema in glioblastoma patients. Cancer Cell. 2007;11(1):83–95. https://doi.org/10.1016/j.ccr.2006.11.021.

43. Emblem KE, Mouridsen K, Bjornerud A, et al. Vessel architectural imaging identifies cancer patient responders to anti-angiogenic therapy. Nat Med. 2013;19(9):1178–83. https://doi.org/10.1038/nm.3289.

44. Nayak L, de Groot J, Wefel JS, et al. Phase I trial of aflibercept (VEGF trap) with radiation therapy and concomitant and adjuvant temozolomide in patients with high-grade gliomas. J Neurooncol. 2017;132(1):181–8. https://doi.org/10.1007/s11060-016-2357-9.

45. de Groot JF, Lamborn KR, Chang SM, et al. Phase II study of aflibercept in recurrent malignant glioma: a North American brain tumor consortium study. J Clin Oncol. 2011;29(19):2689–95. https://doi.org/10.1200/JCO.2010.34.1636.

46. Cher L, Nowak A, Iatropoulos G, et al. ACTR-75. A multicenter, 3-ARM, open-label, phase IIA clinical trial to evaluate safety and efficacy of tanibirumab (VEGFR2 MAB), in patients with recurrent GBM assessed with K-trans and initial area under the gadolinium concentration-time curve (IAUGC). Neuro Oncol. 2017;19(Suppl_6):vi17. https://doi.org/10.1093/neuonc/nox168.062.

47. Pignatti F, van den Bent M, Curran D, et al. Prognostic factors for survival in adult patients with cerebral low-grade glioma. J Clin Oncol. 2002;20(8):2076–84. https://doi.org/10.1200/JCO.2002.08.121.

48. Donovan LE, Lassman AB. Chemotherapy treatment and trials in low-grade gliomas. Neurosurg Clin N Am. 2019;30(1):103–9. https://doi.org/10.1016/j.nec.2018.08.007.

49. van den Bent M, Afra D, de Witte O, et al. Long-term efficacy of early versus delayed radiotherapy for low-grade astrocytoma and oligodendroglioma in adults: the EORTC 22845 randomised trial. Lancet. 2005;366(9490):985–90. https://doi.org/10.1016/S0140-6736(05)67070-5.

50. Cairncross JG, Macdonald DR, Ramsay DA. Aggressive oligodendroglioma: a chemosensitive tumor. Neurosurgery. 1992;31(1):78. https://journals.lww.com/neurosurgery/fulltext/1992/07000/aggressive_oligodendroglioma__a_chemosensitive.11.aspx.

51. Schaff LR, Lassman AB. Indications for treatment: is observation or chemotherapy alone a reasonable approach in the management of low-grade gliomas? Semin Radiat Oncol. 2015;25(3):203–9. https://doi.org/10.1016/j.semradonc.2015.02.008.

52. Baumert BG, Hegi ME, van den Bent MJ, et al. Temozolomide chemotherapy versus radiotherapy in high-risk low-grade glioma (EORTC 22033-26033): a randomised, open-label, phase 3 intergroup study. Lancet Oncol. 2016;17(11):1521–32. https://doi.org/10.1016/S1470-2045(16)30313-8.

53. Wahl M, Phillips JJ, Molinaro AM, et al. Chemotherapy for adult low-grade gliomas: clinical outcomes by molecular subtype in a phase II study of adjuvant temozolomide. Neuro Oncol. 2017;19(2):242–51. https://doi.org/10.1093/neuonc/now176.

54. Rudà R, Pellerino A, Pace A, et al. Efficacy of initial temozolomide for high-risk low grade gliomas in a phase II AINO (Italian Association for Neuro-Oncology) study: a post-hoc analysis within molecular subgroups of WHO 2016. J Neurooncol. 2019;145(1):115–23. https://doi.org/10.1007/s11060-019-03277-x.

55. van den Bent MJ. Chemotherapy for low-grade glioma: when, for whom, which regimen? Curr Opin Neurol. 2015;28(6):633. https://journals.lww.com/co-neurology/fulltext/2015/12000/chemotherapy_for_low_grade_glioma__when,_for_whom,.15.aspx.

56. Hafazalla K, Sahgal A, Jaja B, Perry JR, Das S. Procarbazine, CCNU and vincristine (PCV) versus temozolomide chemotherapy for patients with low-grade glioma: a systematic review. Oncotarget. 2018;9(72). Published online 2018. Accessed 1 Jan 2018. https://www.oncotarget.com/article/25890/text/.

57. Lassman AB, Hoang-Xuan K, Polley MYC, et al. Joint final report of EORTC 26951 and RTOG 9402: phase III trials with procarbazine, lomustine, and vincristine chemotherapy for anaplastic oligodendroglial tumors. J Clin Oncol. 2022;40(23):2539–45. https://doi.org/10.1200/JCO.21.02543.

58. Lassman AB, Iwamoto FM, Cloughesy TF, et al. International retrospective study of over 1000 adults with anaplastic oligodendroglial tumors. Neuro Oncol. 2011;13(6):649–59. https://doi.org/10.1093/neuonc/nor040.

59. Mikkelsen T, Doyle T, Anderson J, et al. Temozolomide single-agent chemotherapy for newly diagnosed anaplastic oligodendroglioma. J Neurooncol. 2009;92(1):57–63. https://doi.org/10.1007/s11060-008-9735-x.

60. Jaeckle KA, Ballman KV, van den Bent M, et al. CODEL: phase III study of RT, RT + TMZ, or TMZ for newly diagnosed 1p/19q codeleted oligodendroglioma. Analysis from the initial study design. Neuro Oncol. 2021;23(3):457–67. https://doi.org/10.1093/neuonc/noaa168.

61. Lassman AB, Cloughesy TF. Early results from the CODEL trial for anaplastic oligodendrogliomas: is temozolomide futile? Neuro Oncol. 2021;23(3):347–9. https://doi.org/10.1093/neuonc/noab006.

62. Wick W, Hartmann C, Engel C, et al. NOA-04 randomized phase III trial of sequential radiochemotherapy of anaplastic glioma with procarbazine, lomustine, and vincristine or temozolomide. J Clin Oncol. 2009;27(35):5874–80. https://doi.org/10.1200/JCO.2009.23.6497.

63. Wick W, Roth P, Hartmann C, et al. Long-term analysis of the NOA-04 randomized phase III trial of sequential radiochemotherapy of anaplastic glioma with PCV or temozolomide. Neuro Oncol. 2016;18(11):1529–37. https://doi.org/10.1093/neuonc/now133.

64. Han S, Liu Y, Cai SJ, et al. IDH mutation in glioma: molecular mechanisms and potential therapeutic targets. Br J Cancer. 2020;122(11):1580–9. https://doi.org/10.1038/s41416-020-0814-x.

65. Yan H, Parsons DW, Jin G, et al. IDH1 and IDH2 mutations in gliomas. N Engl J Med. 2009;360(8):765–73. https://doi.org/10.1056/NEJMoa0808710.

66. Mellinghoff IK, Ellingson BM, Touat M, et al. Ivosidenib in isocitrate dehydrogenase 1-mutated advanced glioma. J Clin Oncol. 2020;38(29):3398–406. https://doi.org/10.1200/JCO.19.03327.

67. Konteatis Z, Artin E, Nicolay B, et al. Vorasidenib (AG-881): a first-in-class, brain-penetrant dual inhibitor of mutant IDH1 and 2 for treatment of glioma. ACS Med Chem Lett. 2020;11(2):101–7. https://doi.org/10.1021/acsmedchemlett.9b00509.

68. Mellinghoff IK, Penas-Prado M, Peters KB, et al. Vorasidenib, a dual inhibitor of mutant IDH1/2, in recurrent or progressive glioma; results of a first-in-human phase I trial. Clin Cancer Res. 2021;27(16):4491–9. https://doi.org/10.1158/1078-0432.CCR-21-0611.

69. Mellinghoff IK, Lu M, Wen PY, et al. Vorasidenib and ivosidenib in IDH1-mutant low-grade glioma: a randomized, perioperative phase 1 trial. Nat Med. 2023;29(3):615–22. https://doi.org/10.1038/s41591-022-02141-2.

70. Mellinghoff IK, Van Den Bent MJ, Clarke JL, et al. INDIGO: a global, randomized, double-blind, phase III study of vorasidenib (VOR; AG-881) vs placebo in patients (pts) with residual or recurrent grade II glioma with an isocitrate dehydrogenase 1/2 (IDH1/2) mutation. J Clin Oncol. 2020;38(15_Suppl):TPS2574. https://doi.org/10.1200/JCO.2020.38.15_suppl.TPS2574.

71. Mellinghoff IK, van den Bent MJ, Blumenthal DT, et al. Vorasidenib in IDH1- or IDH2-mutant low-grade glioma. N Engl J Med. 2023;389:589. Published online 4 Jun 2023. https://doi.org/10.1056/NEJMoa2304194.

72. Chen H, Judkins J, Thomas C, et al. Mutant IDH1 and seizures in patients with glioma. Neurology. 2017;88(19):1805. https://doi.org/10.1212/WNL.0000000000003911.

73. Carstam L, Rydén I, Jakola AS. Seizures in patients with IDH-mutated lower grade gliomas. J Neurooncol. 2022;160:403. Published online 18 Oct 2022. https://doi.org/10.1007/s11060-022-04158-6.

74. Correia CE, Umemura Y, Flynn JR, Reiner AS, Avila EK. Pharmacoresistant seizures and IDH mutation in low-grade gliomas. Neurooncol Adv. 2021;3(1):vdab146. https://doi.org/10.1093/noajnl/vdab146.

75. Phan K, Ng W, Lu VM, et al. Association between IDH1 and IDH2 mutations and preoperative seizures in patients with low-grade versus high-grade glioma: a systematic review and meta-analysis. World Neurosurg. 2018;111:e539–45. https://doi.org/10.1016/j.wneu.2017.12.112.

76. Drumm MR, Wang W, Sears TK, et al. Postoperative risk of IDH-mutant glioma–associated seizures and their potential management with IDH-mutant inhibitors. J Clin Invest. 2023;133(12) https://doi.org/10.1172/JCI168035.

77. Vo AH, Ambady P, Spencer D. The IDH1 inhibitor ivosidenib improved seizures in a patient with drug-resistant epilepsy from IDH1 mutant oligodendroglioma. Epilepsy Behav Rep. 2022;18:100526. https://doi.org/10.1016/j.ebr.2022.100526.

78. Barthel FP, Wesseling P, Verhaak RGW. Reconstructing the molecular life history of gliomas. Acta Neuropathol. 2018;135(5):649–70. https://doi.org/10.1007/s00401-018-1842-y.

79. Picca A, Berzero G, Di Stefano AL, Sanson M. The clinical use of IDH1 and IDH2 mutations in gliomas. Expert Rev Mol Diagn. 2018;18(12):1041–51. https://doi.org/10.1080/14737159.2018.1548935.

80. Normanno N, De Luca A, Bianco C, et al. Epidermal growth factor receptor (EGFR) signaling in cancer. Gene. 2006;366(1):2–16. https://doi.org/10.1016/j.gene.2005.10.018.

81. Frederick L, Wang XY, Eley G, James CD. Diversity and frequency of epidermal growth factor receptor mutations in human glioblastomas. Cancer Res. 2000;60(5):1383–7.

82. Neyns B, Sadones J, Joosens E, et al. Stratified phase II trial of cetuximab in patients with recurrent high-grade glioma. Ann Oncol. 2009;20(9):1596–603. https://doi.org/10.1093/annonc/mdp032.

83. Hasselbalch B, Lassen U, Hansen S, et al. Cetuximab, bevacizumab, and irinotecan for patients with primary glioblastoma and progression after radiation therapy and temozolomide: a phase II trial. Neuro Oncol. 2010;12(5):508–16. https://doi.org/10.1093/neuonc/nop063.

84. Westphal M, Heese O, Steinbach JP, et al. A randomised, open label phase III trial with nimotuzumab, an anti-epidermal growth factor receptor monoclonal antibody in the treatment of newly diagnosed adult glioblastoma. Eur J Cancer. 2015;51(4):522–32. https://doi.org/10.1016/j.ejca.2014.12.019.

85. Nitta Y, Shimizu S, Shishido-Hara Y, Suzuki K, Shiokawa Y, Nagane M. Nimotuzumab enhances temozolomide-induced growth suppression of glioma cells expressing mutant EGFR in vivo. Cancer Med. 2016;5(3):486–99. https://doi.org/10.1002/cam4.614.

86. Phillips AC, Boghaert ER, Vaidya KS, et al. ABT-414, an antibody–drug conjugate targeting a tumor-selective EGFR epitope. Mol Cancer Ther. 2016;15(4):661–9. https://doi.org/10.1158/1535-7163.MCT-15-0901.

87. Clarke JL, Molinaro AM, Phillips JJ, et al. A single-institution phase II trial of radiation, temozolomide, erlotinib, and bevacizumab for initial treatment of glioblastoma. Neuro Oncol. 2014;16(7):984–90. https://doi.org/10.1093/neuonc/nou029.

88. Peereboom DM, Ahluwalia MS, Ye X, et al. NABTT 0502: a phase II and pharmacokinetic study of erlotinib and sorafenib for patients with progressive or recurrent glioblastoma multiforme. Neuro Oncol.

2013;15(4):490–6. https://doi.org/10.1093/neuonc/nos322.

89. Chakravarti A, Wang M, Robins HI, et al. RTOG 0211: a phase 1/2 study of radiation therapy with concurrent gefitinib for newly diagnosed glioblastoma patients. Int J Radiat Oncol Biol Phys. 2013;85(5):1206–11. https://doi.org/10.1016/j.ijrobp.2012.10.008.

90. Robinson GW, Gajjar AJ, Gauvain KM, et al. Phase 1/1B trial to assess the activity of entrectinib in children and adolescents with recurrent or refractory solid tumors including central nervous system (CNS) tumors. J Clin Oncol. 2019;37(15_Suppl):10009. https://doi.org/10.1200/JCO.2019.37.15_suppl.10009.

91. Reardon DA, Nabors LB, Mason WP, et al. Phase I/randomized phase II study of afatinib, an irreversible ErbB family blocker, with or without protracted temozolomide in adults with recurrent glioblastoma. Neuro Oncol. 2015;17(3):430–9. https://doi.org/10.1093/neuonc/nou160.

92. Sepúlveda-Sánchez JM, Vaz MÁ, Balañá C, et al. Phase II trial of dacomitinib, a pan–human EGFR tyrosine kinase inhibitor, in recurrent glioblastoma patients with EGFR amplification. Neuro Oncol. 2017;19(11):1522–31. https://doi.org/10.1093/neuonc/nox105.

93. Jimenez-Pascual A, Siebzehnrubl FA. Fibroblast growth factor receptor functions in glioblastoma. Cells. 2019;8(7) https://doi.org/10.3390/cells8070715.

94. Lasorella A, Sanson M, Iavarone A. FGFR-TACC gene fusions in human glioma. Neuro Oncol. 2017;19(4):475–83. https://doi.org/10.1093/neuonc/now240.

95. Schmieder R, Hoffmann J, Becker M, et al. Regorafenib (BAY 73-4506): antitumor and antimetastatic activities in preclinical models of colorectal cancer. Int J Cancer. 2014;135(6):1487–96.

96. Abou-Elkacem L, Arns S, Brix G, et al. Regorafenib inhibits growth, angiogenesis, and metastasis in a highly aggressive, orthotopic colon cancer model. Mol Cancer Ther. 2013;12(7):1322–31.

97. Wilhelm S, Dumas J, Adnane L, et al. A new oral multikinase inhibitor of angiogenic, stromal and oncogenic receptor tyrosine kinases with potent preclinical antitumor activity. Int J Cancer. 2011;129(1):245–55.

98. Zopf D, Fichtner I, Bhargava A, et al. Pharmacologic activity and pharmacokinetics of metabolites of regorafenib in preclinical models. Cancer Med. 2016;5(11):3176–85.

99. Grothey A, Van Cutsem E, Sobrero A, et al. Regorafenib monotherapy for previously treated metastatic colorectal cancer (CORRECT): an international, multicentre, randomised, placebo-controlled, phase 3 trial. Lancet. 2013;381(9863):303–12.

100. Demetri GD, Reichardt P, Kang YK, et al. Efficacy and safety of regorafenib for advanced gastrointestinal stromal tumours after failure of imatinib and sunitinib (GRID): an international, multicentre, randomised, placebo-controlled, phase 3 trial. Lancet. 2013;381(9863):295–302.

101. Bruix J, Qin S, Merle P, et al. Regorafenib for patients with hepatocellular carcinoma who progressed on sorafenib treatment (RESORCE): a randomised, double-blind, placebo-controlled, phase 3 trial. Lancet. 2017;389(10064):56–66.

102. Lombardi G, Caccese M, Padovan M, et al. Regorafenib in recurrent glioblastoma patients: a large and monocentric real-life study. Cancers. 2021;13(18) https://doi.org/10.3390/cancers13184731.

103. Kebir S, Rauschenbach L, Radbruch A, et al. Regorafenib in patients with recurrent high-grade astrocytoma. J Cancer Res Clin Oncol. 2019;145(4):1037–42. https://doi.org/10.1007/s00432-019-02868-5.

104. Zeiner PS, Kinzig M, Divé I, et al. Regorafenib CSF penetration, efficacy, and MRI patterns in recurrent malignant glioma patients. J Clin Med. 2019;8(12) https://doi.org/10.3390/jcm8122031.

105. Tzaridis T, Gepfner-Tuma I, Hirsch S, et al. Regorafenib in advanced high-grade glioma: a retrospective bicentric analysis. Neuro Oncol. 2019;21(7):954–5. https://doi.org/10.1093/neuonc/noz071.

106. Treiber H, von der Brelie C, Malinova V, Mielke D, Rohde V, Chapuy CI. Regorafenib for recurrent high-grade glioma: a unicentric retrospective analysis of feasibility, efficacy, and toxicity. Neurosurg Rev. 2022;45:3201. Published online 20 Jun 2022. https://doi.org/10.1007/s10143-022-01826-z.

107. Werner JM, Wolf L, Tscherpel C, et al. Efficacy and tolerability of regorafenib in pretreated patients with progressive CNS grade 3 or 4 gliomas. J Neurooncol. 2022;159:309. Published online 18 Jun 2022. https://doi.org/10.1007/s11060-022-04066-9.

108. Rudà R, Bruno F, Pellerino A, et al. Observational real-life study on regorafenib in recurrent glioblastoma: does dose reduction reduce toxicity while maintaining the efficacy? J Neurooncol. 2022;160(2):389–402. https://doi.org/10.1007/s11060-022-04155-9.

109. Srinivasa K, Cross KA, Dahiya S. BRAF alteration in central and peripheral nervous system tumors. Front Oncol. 2020;10:1883. https://doi.org/10.3389/fonc.2020.574974.

110. Halle BR, Johnson DB. Defining and targeting BRAF mutations in solid tumors. Curr Treat Options in Oncol. 2021;22(4):30. https://doi.org/10.1007/s11864-021-00827-2.

111. Lassaletta A, Zapotocky M, Mistry M, et al. Therapeutic and prognostic implications of BRAF V600E in pediatric low-grade gliomas. J Clin Oncol. 2017;35(25):2934–41. https://doi.org/10.1200/JCO.2016.71.8726.

112. Schindler G, Capper D, Meyer J, et al. Analysis of BRAF V600E mutation in 1,320 nervous system tumors reveals high mutation frequencies in

pleomorphic xanthoastrocytoma, ganglioglioma and extra-cerebellar pilocytic astrocytoma. Acta Neuropathol. 2011;121(3):397–405.

113. Wen PY, Stein A, van den Bent M, et al. Dabrafenib plus trametinib in patients with BRAFV600E-mutant low-grade and high-grade glioma (ROAR): a multicentre, open-label, single-arm, phase 2, basket trial. Lancet Oncol. 2022;23(1):53–64. https://doi.org/10.1016/S1470-2045(21)00578-7.

114. Kaley T, Touat M, Subbiah V, et al. BRAF inhibition in BRAF(V600)-mutant gliomas: results from the VE-BASKET study. J Clin Oncol. 2018;36(35):3477–84. https://doi.org/10.1200/JCO.2018.78.9990.

115. Schreck KC, Grossman SA, Pratilas CA. BRAF mutations and the utility of RAF and MEK inhibitors in primary brain tumors. Cancers. 2019;11(9) https://doi.org/10.3390/cancers11091262.

116. Lim SY, Menzies AM, Rizos H. Mechanisms and strategies to overcome resistance to molecularly targeted therapy for melanoma. Cancer. 2017;123(S11):2118–29.

117. Xing H, Song Y, Zhang Z, Koch PD. Clinical characteristics of BRAF V600E gene mutation in patients of epilepsy-associated brain tumor: a meta-analysis. J Mol Neurosci. 2021;71:1815. Published online 31 Mar 2021. https://doi.org/10.1007/s12031-021-01837-3.

118. Curatolo P, Bombardieri R, Jozwiak S. Tuberous sclerosis. Lancet. 2008;372(9639):657–68. https://doi.org/10.1016/S0140-6736(08)61279-9.

119. Ebrahimi-Fakhari D, Franz DN. Pharmacological treatment strategies for subependymal giant cell astrocytoma (SEGA). Expert Opin Pharmacother. 2020;21(11):1329–36. https://doi.org/10.1080/14656566.2020.1751124.

120. Krueger DA, Wilfong AA, Holland-Bouley K, et al. Everolimus treatment of refractory epilepsy in tuberous sclerosis complex. Ann Neurol. 2013;74(5):679–87. https://doi.org/10.1002/ana.23960.

121. Cepeda C, Levinson S, Yazon VW, et al. Cellular antiseizure mechanisms of everolimus in pediatric tuberous sclerosis complex, cortical dysplasia, and non–mTOR-mediated etiologies. Epilepsia Open. 2018;3(S2):180–90. https://doi.org/10.1002/epi4.12253.

122. Faivre S, Kroemer G, Raymond E. Current development of mTOR inhibitors as anticancer agents. Nat Rev Drug Discov. 2006;5(8):671–88. https://doi.org/10.1038/nrd2062.

123. Franz DN, Belousova E, Sparagana S, et al. Efficacy and safety of everolimus for subependymal giant cell astrocytomas associated with tuberous sclerosis complex (EXIST-1): a multicentre, randomised, placebo-controlled phase 3 trial. Lancet. 2013;381(9861):125–32. https://doi.org/10.1016/S0140-6736(12)61134-9.

124. Franz DN, Belousova E, Sparagana S, et al. Long-term use of everolimus in patients with tuberous sclerosis complex: final results from the EXIST-1 study. PLoS One. 2016;11(6):e0158476. https://doi.org/10.1371/journal.pone.0158476.

125. Krueger DA, Wilfong AA, Mays M, et al. Long-term treatment of epilepsy with everolimus in tuberous sclerosis. Neurology. 2016;87(23):2408. https://doi.org/10.1212/WNL.0000000000003400.

126. Curatolo P, Franz DN, Lawson JA, et al. Adjunctive everolimus for children and adolescents with treatment-refractory seizures associated with tuberous sclerosis complex: post-hoc analysis of the phase 3 EXIST-3 trial. Lancet Child Adolesc Health. 2018;2(7):495–504. https://doi.org/10.1016/S2352-4642(18)30099-3.

127. French JA, Lawson JA, Yapici Z, et al. Adjunctive everolimus therapy for treatment-resistant focal-onset seizures associated with tuberous sclerosis (EXIST-3): a phase 3, randomised, double-blind, placebo-controlled study. Lancet. 2016;388(10056):2153–63. https://doi.org/10.1016/S0140-6736(16)31419-2.

128. Mizuguchi M, Ikeda H, Kagitani-Shimono K, et al. Everolimus for epilepsy and autism spectrum disorder in tuberous sclerosis complex: EXIST-3 substudy in Japan. Brain Dev. 2019;41(1):1–10. https://doi.org/10.1016/j.braindev.2018.07.003.

129. Fogarasi A, De Waele L, Bartalini G, et al. EFFECTS: an expanded access program of everolimus for patients with subependymal giant cell astrocytoma associated with tuberous sclerosis complex. BMC Neurol. 2016;16(1):126. https://doi.org/10.1186/s12883-016-0658-4.

130. Bobeff K, Krajewska K, Baranska D, et al. Maintenance therapy with everolimus for subependymal giant cell astrocytoma in patients with tuberous sclerosis—final results from the EMINENTS study. Front Neurol. 2021;12:518. https://doi.org/10.3389/fneur.2021.581102.

131. Gambella A, Senetta R, Collemi G, et al. NTRK fusions in central nervous system tumors: a rare, but worthy target. Int J Mol Sci. 2020;21(3) https://doi.org/10.3390/ijms21030753.

132. Albert CM, Davis JL, Federman N, Casanova M, Laetsch TW. TRK fusion cancers in children: A clinical review and recommendations for screening. J Clin Oncol. 2018;37(6):513–24. https://doi.org/10.1200/JCO.18.00573.

133. Ferguson SD, Zhou S, Huse JT, et al. Targetable gene fusions associate with the IDH wild-type astrocytic lineage in adult gliomas. J Neuropathol Exp Neurol. 2018;77(6):437–42. https://doi.org/10.1093/jnen/nly022.

134. Liu D, Offin M, Harnicar S, Li BT, Drilon A. Entrectinib: an orally available, selective tyrosine kinase inhibitor for the treatment of NTRK, ROS1, and ALK fusion-positive solid tumors. Ther Clin Risk Manag. 2018;14:1247–52. https://doi.org/10.2147/TCRM.S147381.

135. Drilon A, Siena S, Ou SHI, et al. Safety and antitumor activity of the multitargeted pan-TRK,

ROS1, and ALK inhibitor entrectinib: combined results from two phase I trials (ALKA-372-001 and STARTRK-1). Cancer Discov. 2017;7(4):400. https://doi.org/10.1158/2159-8290.CD-16-1237.

136. Drilon A, Laetsch TW, Kummar S, et al. Efficacy of larotrectinib in TRK fusion–positive cancers in adults and children. N Engl J Med. 2018;378(8):731–9. https://doi.org/10.1056/NEJMoa1714448.

137. Drilon AE, DuBois SG, Farago AF, et al. Activity of larotrectinib in TRK fusion cancer patients with brain metastases or primary central nervous system tumors. J Clin Oncol. 2019;37(15_Suppl):2006. https://doi.org/10.1200/JCO.2019.37.15_suppl.2006.

138. Drilon A, Nagasubramanian R, Blake JF, et al. A next-generation TRK kinase inhibitor overcomes acquired resistance to prior TRK kinase inhibition in patients with TRK fusion–positive solid tumors. Cancer Discov. 2017;7(9):963. https://doi.org/10.1158/2159-8290.CD-17-0507.

139. Drilon A, Ou SHI, Cho BC, et al. Repotrectinib (TPX-0005) is a next-generation ROS1/TRK/ALK inhibitor that potently inhibits ROS1/TRK/ALK solvent-front mutations. Cancer Discov. 2018;8(10):1227. https://doi.org/10.1158/2159-8290.CD-18-0484.

Radiation Oncology in Glioblastoma (GBM)

7

Isacco Desideri, Valerio Nardone, Ilaria Morelli, Federico Gagliardi, and Giuseppe Minniti

Highlights

- **Glioblastoma Prevalence and Prognostic Factors**: Glioblastoma (GBM) is a common, aggressive brain tumor with a dismal prognosis. The extent of tumor resection, age at diagnosis, and Karnofsky performance status are critical prognostic factors.
- **Standard GBM Treatment**: Standard GBM treatment includes radiotherapy with concurrent temozolomide (TMZ) and maintenance TMZ. The effectiveness of TMZ is influenced by MGMT promoter methylation status.

- **Emerging Immunotherapy**: Immunotherapy, particularly immune-checkpoint inhibitors (ICIs), is being explored in GBM treatment. While promising, larger trials are needed to confirm its efficacy.
- **Radiosensitization Techniques**: Radiosensitization approaches aim to make cancer cells more susceptible to radiation therapy by targeting tumor hypoxia, interfering with DNA damage repair, and enhancing apoptotic pathways.
- **Advanced Imaging and Targeted Therapies**: Advanced imaging techniques like MRI and PET scans are vital for precise target volume definition in radiation therapy. Additionally, novel therapies, such as tumor-treating fields (TTFields) or nano-technologies, offer potential avenues for improving GBM patient outcomes.

7

I. Desideri · I. Morelli
Department of Experimental and Clinical Biomedical Sciences, "Mario Serio" University of Florence, Florence, Italy
e-mail: isacco.desideri@unifi.it; ilaria.morelli@unifi.it

V. Nardone (✉) · F. Gagliardi
Department of Precision Medicine, University of Campania "L. Vanvitelli", Naples, Italy
e-mail: valerio.nardone@unicampania.it; Federico.gagliardi@student.unicampania.it

G. Minniti
Department of Radiological, Oncological and Pathological Sciences, "Sapienza" University of Rome, Rome, Italy
e-mail: Giuseppe.minniti@uniroma1.it

7.1 Introduction

Glioblastoma (GBM) is the most common glioma type, with its incidence ranging from 0.59 to 3.69 per 100,000 persons. Anaplastic astrocytoma and GBM are most common among those aged 75–84, while oligodendroglioma and oligoastrocytomas prevail in the 35–44 age group [1].

Overall survival (OS) after glioma diagnosis varies by grade. GBM has the poorest survival, with <5% surviving 5 years after diagnosis. Molecular markers such as IDH1/2 mutation, G-CIMP status, MGMT methylation, and 1p19q deletion impact survival [2].

According to the 2021 WHO classification of Central Nervous System (CNS) tumors, the diagnosis of glioblastoma is restricted only to isocitrate dehydrogenase (IDH) wild type. The previously IDH-mutated glioblastoma is reclassified as IDH-mutated astrocytoma grade 4. IDH wild-type diffuses astrocytic tumors in adults without the histologic features of glioblastoma but with one or more of three genetic parameters (TERT promoter mutation, EGFR gene amplification, or combined gain of entire chromosome 7 and loss of entire chromosome 10 [+7/−10]) will also be classified as glioblastomas [3].

Key prognostic factors for GBM include extent of tumor resection, age at diagnosis, and Karnofsky performance status (KPS). The EORTC/NCIC trial in 2004 established concurrent temozolomide with postoperative radiation as the standard care for primary GBM, resulting in improved median survival [4].

GBM has an infiltrative nature, and surgical resection usually is not curative due to postoperative residual tumor cells that contribute to recurrence. Radiation therapy (RT) is a crucial part of GBM treatment, current guidelines recommend RT as an adjuvant treatment after surgical resection or as a primary option for unresectable GBMs [5].

Several case series in the 1960s and 1970s indicated improved survival with postoperative RT.

The Brain Tumor Study Group (BTSG) initiated randomized studies in the 1970s that solidified postoperative RT as the standard of care for GBM. The BTSG 66-01 study randomized patients after tumor resection to mithramycin or no chemotherapy, with whole-brain radiotherapy (WBRT) allowed. Patients who received adjuvant WBRT demonstrated a significant survival advantage compared to those who didn't receive RT [6].

A subsequent study, BTSG 72-01, evaluated the role of nitrosoureas plus RT. Patients receiving postoperative WBRT with nitrosourea had the longest median survival. Both studies suggested a trend towards improved survival, especially in the chemotherapy plus RT group [7].

Optimal radiation doses for treating GBM have been extensively studied and there was evidence of improved survival with increasing radiation doses, but further escalation beyond 60 Gy did not consistently provide substantial benefits in terms of survival outcomes [8].

Later, studies demonstrated that multicentric involvement is rare. Hochberg and Pruitt's study showed that GBM relapse mostly occurred near the primary site, supporting a shift toward involved-field radiotherapy (IFRT) [9].

Toxicity associated with high WBRT doses requested the transition to IFRT, defined as treating the tumor and a 3 cm margin, rendered similar outcomes to WBRT in several studies.

BTCG 80-01 compared WBRT (6020 cGy) to WBRT (4300 cGy) followed by IFRT boost (1720 cGy), showing no significant survival differences. IFRT became the standard for treating GBM [10, 11].

7.2   Understanding Glioblastoma

Molecular profiling has revealed common mutations and core pathways in sporadic GBM. There are three main glioblastoma subgroups based on gene expression and DNA methylation patterns: proneural, classical, and mesenchymal. These subgroups are marked by specific genetic alterations and clinical characteristics, accounting for most glioblastomas [12–15].

The proneural gene expression/receptor tyrosine kinase (RTK) I/LGm6 DNA methylation group is characterized by amplifications of cyclin-dependent kinase 4 (CDK4) and platelet-derived growth factor alpha (PDGFRα) and is most common in relatively younger adults.

The classical gene expression/classic-like/ RTK II DNA methylation group shows a high frequency of EGFR amplifications and homozygous loss of CDKN2A/B.

The mesenchymal/mesenchymal-like subtype is characterized by an abundance of tumors with a loss of neurofibromatosis type 1 (NF1) and a high tumor infiltration by macrophages.

However, the clinical utility of these subtypes remains unclear. They are not predictive of treatment response to current therapies, and the assignment of a subtype can be challenging due to the presence of multiple subtypes within the same tumor and subtype "switching" during disease progression [16].

In 2008, collaborative research using whole exome sequencing identified a common mutation in the metabolic gene IDH1 in 12% of glioblastoma. This mutation is present in about 80% of grade 2–3 gliomas and secondary GBMs [17].

Mutations in IDH2 are rarer and mutually exclusive with IDH1 mutations. These mutations involve a single amino acid change in IDH1 at arginine 132 (R132) or the corresponding position in IDH2 (R172) [18].

Initially, it was believed that mutant IDH had a dominant-negative function by forming heterodimers with wild-type IDH1, inhibiting its activity. However, recent in vitro studies showed that mutated IDH1 can convert α-ketoglutarate (α-KG) into $R(-)$-2-hydroxyglutarate (2-HG). This discovery led to the idea that mutant IDH acts as an oncogene and 2-HG functions as an "oncometabolite" [19].

New evidence indicates that 2-HG competitively inhibits various α-KG-dependent dioxygenases, including histone demethylases. This inhibition affects processes like DNA hydroxylation. The Cancer Genome Atlas (TCGA) profiling demonstrated that IDH mutation correlates with increased promoter methylation, known as the G-CIMP phenotype. This phenotype often leads to the silencing of associated genes. Recent studies suggest that the G-CIMP hypermethylation phenotype in diffuse gliomas is primarily a result of the IDH mutation itself, rather than being directly associated with it [20].

Blood vessel formation in gliomas often involves angiogenesis, primarily driven by vascular endothelial growth factor (VEGF). VEGF is significantly overexpressed in brain tumors, and its expression increases with tumor grade [21].

In some cases, glioma cells can transform into malignant endothelial cells. The stop of angiogenesis, inhibiting VEGF signaling, has been suggested to potentially increase glioma invasiveness, although this idea remains controversial [22].

The invasion of normal brain tissue is characteristic in diffuse gliomas and contributes to their resistance to surgery alone. Gliomas migrate along structures as white matter tracks, neuronal pathways, blood vessels, and subpial spaces, as outlined by Scherer's secondary structures [23].

The secretion of various proteases, including matrix metalloproteases (MMPs), membrane-type matrix metalloproteases (MT-MMPs), and adamalysins (ADAMS) helps glioma migration.

Factors like TGF-beta and NF-κB regulated the expression and secretion of these proteases [24].

7.3 Standard Radiotherapy for Glioblastoma

After maximal safe resection of newly diagnosed glioblastoma, the standard treatment typically involves radiotherapy (RT) concurrently with temozolomide (TMZ) (75 mg/m^2/day for 6 weeks) followed by maintenance TMZ (150–200 mg/m^2/day for 5 days during six 28-day cycles) [4, 25, 26]. The effectiveness of TMZ is influenced by the MGMT promoter methylation status, and in cases of MGMT unmethylated tumors, TMZ may be omitted, especially in clinical trial contexts or when TMZ risks outweigh its benefits [27, 28]. The addition of tumor-treating fields (TTF), utilizing low-intensity, intermediate-frequency (200 kHz) alternating electric fields, has extended survival by approximately 4.9 months in some studies during adjuvant TMZ [29]. Neither dose-dense TMZ regimens nor the incorporation of bevacizumab has shown additional survival benefits [30–34]. A recent small randomized phase III trial explored an intensified lomustine-TMZ regimen for MGMT promoter methylated glioblastoma, demonstrating an increased median overall survival (OS) from 31.4 to 48.1 months when combined with radiotherapy [35]. However, the regimen's role remains uncertain due to sample size limitations and potential hematologic toxicities [35, 36].

Regarding radiotherapy considerations, most guidelines recommend delivering RT at approximately 60 Gy in 30 fractions of 2 Gy each, based on target delineation using immediate post-surgical MRI [37]. The European Organisation for Research and Treatment of Cancer (EORTC) advises a single-phase RT delivery of 60 Gy at 2 Gy per fraction, while the Radiation Therapy Oncology Group (RTOG) approach entails an initial larger volume encompassing the fluid-attenuated inversion recovery (FLAIR) abnormality with a 2-cm margin, receiving 46 Gy in 23 fractions of 2 Gy, along with an additional 14 Gy directed at the resection cavity and any residual enhancing tumor [37]. Special attention is given to minimizing radiation exposure to structures at risk of therapy-induced damage, including ophthalmic and optic structures, brainstem, cervical cord, cochlea, and, when feasible, temporal lobes and/or hippocampi [25, 38]. Variations of these approaches have been proposed to reduce irradiation of normal brain tissue, although there is ongoing debate concerning the optimal RT volume and margin expansions, with advanced imaging methods like perfusion/diffusion MR, MRS, and amino acid Positron Emission Tomography (PET) still under investigation to provide clarity [38, 39]. Previous dose-escalation efforts have mostly failed, but contemporary trials explore whether RT dose-escalation, especially when combined with TMZ, may benefit certain patients [40].

Traditional treatment volumes for GBM are primarily based on postoperative-enhanced MRI scans, aiming to encompass the entire gross tumor volume (GTV), including the resection cavity and any remaining enhancing tumor tissue. This initial GTV is then expanded to form a clinical target volume (CTV), with variations in margin size.

- The European Organisation for Research and Treatment of Cancer (EORTC) suggests a CTV margin of 2–3 cm and a 3–5 mm planning target volume (PTV) expansion.
- In contrast, the Radiation Therapy Oncology Group (RTOG) employs a larger initial volume based on the T2 or FLAIR abnormality on postoperative MRI, with a 2 cm CTV margin and 3–5 mm PTV margin. This is followed by a "boost" phase with a more restricted volume, defined by the contrast-enhanced T1 abnormality on MRI while maintaining a 2-cm CTV margin and a 3–5 mm PTV margin [37].

Studies investigating patterns of GBM recurrence have consistently shown that a significant majority of recurrences occur within 2–3 cm of the surgical cavity. This observation has influenced the development of the conventional treatment volumes described above. The rationale behind CTV margins stems from the belief that areas of T1 contrast enhancement represent regions of high tumor cell density, while areas of T2 or FLAIR abnormality correspond to more diffusely infiltrating disease [39].

Smaller treatment volumes have been explored to challenge the conventional approach. For instance, the Department of Radiation Oncology at MD Anderson Cancer Center employs an alternative treatment volume specification that includes the resection cavity and any contrast-enhancing residual disease with a 2-cm margin, deliberately excluding peritumoral edema [41]. This is followed by a 5-mm PTV expansion, treated to 50 Gy in 2 Gy fractions, with an additional 10 Gy in five fractions to the resection cavity and a 5-mm PTV expansion. This represents a smaller volume compared to RTOG specifications. A study comparing this approach to the RTOG criteria showed no difference in recurrence patterns but demonstrated an improved mean overall survival and quality of life outcomes [41, 42]. In this context, a large retrospective review from Wake Forest, examining RT outcomes with different CTV expansions (5-, 10-, and 15- to 20-mm CTV margins) using modern RT techniques with concurrent and adjuvant TMZ, found no significant difference in treatment patterns of failure [42]. The New Approaches to Brain Tumor Therapy consortium has used 5-mm margins in various phase II studies, resulting in significant improvements in survival over the chemoRT arm of the Stupp trial [43]. One hypothesis supporting the use of smaller CTV margins is that more limited irradiated volumes may limit the occurrence of lymphopenia, which has been associated with improved survival. This suggests that smaller treatment volumes could potentially improve patient outcomes [39].

One challenge with conventional imaging is distinguishing true tumor tissue from edema. Advanced imaging modalities, such as PET tracers, may offer promise in enhancing GBM treatment planning and are further discussed in the next paragraphs.

The development of precise targeting techniques using advanced imaging modalities, such as PET tracers, DTI, and others, holds significant promise for improving GBM treatment outcomes. These techniques allow for the identification of tumor regions not visible on conventional imaging and may result in more effective treatment volumes [44].

More recently, ESTRO-EANO has provided an updated guideline for target delineation and radiotherapy treatment in glioblastoma [45]. The ESTRO-EANO guidelines present significant advances over previous standards for glioblastoma target delineation. They recommend defining the Gross Tumor Volume (GTV) on MRI as the T1 contrast-enhancing tumor or the resection cavity plus any remaining contrast-enhancing tumor. A 15 mm margin around the GTV is advised to create the Clinical Target Volume (CTV), with adjustments for anatomical barriers, excluding edema but considering T2/FLAIR signal abnormalities. The guidelines propose a single CTV definition based on postoperative contrast-enhanced T1 abnormalities, using isotropic margins without the need for a cone-down. The Planning Target Volume (PTV) margin should be no greater than 3 mm when employing Image-Guided Radiation Therapy (IGRT). These guidelines enhance precision and accuracy in glioblastoma treatment planning, incorporating modern imaging techniques and tailored margin definitions.

In conclusion, the landscape of GBM treatment planning is evolving, with efforts focused on optimizing treatment volumes to improve outcomes. The incorporation of advanced imaging modalities and the exploration of smaller CTV margins, coupled with the potential of combined RT and immunotherapy strategies, offer promising avenues for enhancing the management of this challenging disease. Further research is needed to refine these approaches and translate them into clinical practice effectively.

7.4 How to Increase the Therapeutic Ratio: Radiosensitizers and Radioprotectors

Radiosensitizing agents, commonly employed to enhance the efficacy of radiotherapy in various cancer treatments, have exhibited promising potential in augmenting the therapeutic benefits of radiotherapy. A recent comprehensive review has undertaken the analysis of multiple studies, each investigating distinct mechanisms of radiosensitization [46]. The different agents can be classified according to a different mechanism of action (see Table 7.1), as follows:

7.4.1 Targeting Tumor Hypoxia

Several strategies are employed to mitigate the impact of tumor hypoxia, a phenomenon where oxygen-deprived cancer cells become resistant to radiation therapy. The first approach involves using drugs to optimize perfusion and tissue oxygenation during radiotherapy, with earlier studies showing promise in increasing time to progression and overall survival. However, subsequent trials with nitroimidazoles like misonidazole and etanidazole did not demonstrate significant improvements in survival and led to the exploration of other strategies [47–49]. Hyperbaric oxygen was initially tested but faced challenges with setup difficulties, leading to investigations of its effects when combined with radiation [50–54]. Nicotinamide and carbogen were also explored for higher tissue oxygenation but resulted in high treatment toxicity, discouraging their use [55–58]. Tipifarnib, a farnesyltransferase inhibitor, was studied in combination with radiation, showing potential in early trials, but further research in

Table 7.1 A straightforward overview of the different radiosensitization approaches, the agents used, and their respective mechanisms of action in glioblastoma treatment

Approach	Agent	Mechanism of action
Targeting tumor hypoxia	Nitroimidazoles (e.g., misonidazole, etanidazole), hyperbaric oxygen, nicotinamide, carbogen, tipifarnib, efaproxiral, tirapazamine	Improve tissue oxygenation and perfusion to overcome hypoxia
Interfering with repair of radiation-induced damage	Halogenated pyrimidines (BUdR, IUdR), PARP inhibitors, motexafin gadolinium (MGd), difluoromethylornithine (DFMO)	Inhibit repair of radiation-induced DNA damage, either by enhancing DNA damage or disrupting repair mechanisms
Enhancing apoptotic pathways	Recombinant interferon-alpha2a, lovastatin, boron neutron capture therapy (BNCT), 5-Aminolevulinic acid (5-ALA)	Promote radiation-induced apoptosis through various pathways
Radiosensitizing effects of chemotherapeutic drugs	Temozolomide, nitrosoureas (ACNU, BCyNU, CCNU), procarbazine, taxanes, 5-fluorouracil, capecitabine, gemcitabine, platinum derivatives, bevacizumab	Enhance radiation therapy efficacy through various mechanisms within these chemotherapeutic agents

glioma treatment was limited [59–61]. Efaproxiral, an allosteric hemoglobin modifier, demonstrated good tolerance in phase I and II trials but did not provide a marked improvement in survival [62]. Tirapazamine, a compound that can be reduced to hydroxy radicals in hypoxic cells, was tested with conventional fractionated radiotherapy, but no significant benefit in overall survival was observed [39, 63]. While some approaches showed promise, further investigations and larger randomized controlled studies are needed to determine their efficacy in overcoming tumor hypoxia in glioblastoma treatment.

7.4.2 Interfering with Repair of Radiation-Induced Damage

Various radiosensitizing approaches aim to interfere with the repair of radiation-induced damage, especially DNA damage, by preventing or disrupting cellular repair mechanisms. The halogenated pyrimidines bromodeoxyuridine (BUdR) and iododeoxyuridine (IUdR) act as antimetabolites, making dividing cells more vulnerable to primary or secondary radiation-induced DNA damage, such as single- or double-strand breaks or secondary damage from free radicals [64, 65]. Early research showed comparable survival in trials combining BUdR with conventionally fractionated radiation and IUdR with hyperfractionated

radiation, but photosensitivity and dermatologic side effects were reported with BUdR. Intra-arterial infusion was explored to mitigate side effects but did not significantly improve survival, and intravenous concepts also did not reveal clear evidence of a survival benefit, with hematological toxicity remaining a concern. Halogenated pyrimidines as radiosensitizers for glioma treatment were abandoned due to insufficient profitability [66, 67]. PARP inhibitors, which target poly(ADP-ribose) polymerase proteins involved in DNA damage repair, have been investigated for radiosensitizing and chemosensitizing properties [68–72]. While some studies showed acceptable tolerability, they resulted in increased hematotoxicity, and overall survival benefits were not consistently observed. Motexafin gadolinium (MGd), a compound generating reactive oxygen species and interfering with repair mechanisms, was tested in glioma treatment, showing potential in terms of tumor tissue effectiveness [73, 74]. However, follow-up trials combining MGd with standard therapy did not lead to significant survival benefits. Difluoromethylornithine (DFMO), a polyamine synthesis inhibitor, has been explored as a radiosensitizer, with large phase III trials showing little side effects but no significant impact on progression-free or overall survival [75]. Further research and evidence are required to establish the efficacy of this approach in glioblastoma treatment.

7.4.3 Enhancing Apoptotic Pathways

Advances in understanding cellular mechanisms, signaling pathways, and interactions have expanded the potential targets in oncology for radiosensitization, particularly those involving apoptotic pathways. Recombinant interferon-alpha2a, known for its immunomodulatory and antiangiogenic properties, can enhance radiosensitivity by promoting radiation-induced apoptosis through pathways such as p53 activation. Clinical trials investigating interferon-alpha2a combined with conventional fractionated radiotherapy showed feasibility but did not establish a survival benefit compared to other treatments [76]. Lovastatin, a lipid-lowering drug, influences radiation sensitivity by enhancing apoptotic pathways, primarily those involving p53. A single trial evaluated its benefit when combined with ionizing radiation, with no long-term results or follow-up investigations reported. Subsequent analyses did not find a significant impact of statin co-medication on patient outcomes [77–79]. Boron neutron capture therapy (BNCT) involves the infusion of stabilized boron-10 compounds before neutron irradiation, aiming to increase radiation-induced apoptosis. Several study groups explored this concept as a potential treatment for malignant glioma, optimizing dose delivery, monitoring, and various combinations. While some studies showed promise and histopathologic proof of treatment response, BNCT did not surpass standard therapy with photon irradiation and concurrent chemotherapy with TMZ. Further research is needed, especially in larger randomized trials [80–85]. 5-Aminolevulinic acid (5-ALA), primarily used in resective surgery for tumor visualization, has radiosensitizing potential. In vitro and rodent models have demonstrated increased cell death after photon irradiation, attributed to mitochondrial oxidative stress and reactive oxygen species production. However, human patient trials are currently lacking [86–88]. In conclusion, these radiosensitization strategies have shown potential in enhancing radiation-induced apoptosis, but further research, particularly with human patients, is required to validate their efficacy in glioblastoma treatment.

7.4.4 Radiosensitizing Effects of Chemotherapeutic Drugs in Glioblastoma Treatment

Several chemotherapeutic drugs have exhibited radiosensitizing potential in the context of glioblastoma treatment. While they are primarily employed for their cytoreductive properties, their ability to enhance the efficacy of radiation therapy makes them noteworthy in the overall treatment strategy. As an alkylating chemotherapeutic drug, temozolomide has become a cornerstone in systemic adjuvant therapy for glioblastoma multiforme. By methylating radiation-induced DNA lesions, particularly on the O6 atom of adenine, temozolomide can stabilize the damage, resulting in a heightened response to concomitant radiation therapy [89]. Alkylating substances such as ACNU, BCyNU, and CCNU have the ability to cross-link DNA and operate both cell-cycles dependently and independently [90]. Notably, their activity is most pronounced in the late S phase, which is the most radioresistant phase of the cell cycle [91]. This makes nitrosoureas particularly valuable in the context of radiation therapy, as they target radioresistant cells. They have been explored for use in recurrent glioma and other glioma subtypes, such as oligodendroglioma, often in combination with the PCV regimen [92]. Notably, a combination of CCNU and TMZ with radiation demonstrated improved overall survival in MGMT-methylated glioblastoma patients [35]. As part of the PCV combination regimen in glioma treatment, procarbazine has shown radiosensitizing qualities, particularly in hypoxic cells, which is attributed to the redox potential of its structure [93]. While the PCV combination is highly effective for grade 2 and 3 gliomas, especially the oligodendroglial subtype [94], its use in glioblastoma treatment appears to be less effective when compared to other regimens [35, 92]. Targeting the assembly of the mitotic spindle, the taxane family of chemotherapeutic drugs leads to G2/M cell cycle arrest, a phase that has been found to exhibit increased sensitivity to ionizing radiation [95]. Paclitaxel, in particular, was initially investigated extensively for its potential in glioblastoma treatment. Some early results appeared promising, especially in combination with high fractional doses, as an alternative treatment for older patients or those with reduced performance status [96, 97]. However, the overall benefit did not surpass that of other treatment regimens, leading to a reevaluation of its use. 5-Fluorouracil and its oral prodrug capecitabine, both members of the antimetabolite family, have been studied for their radiosensitizing potential in combination with radiation therapy. They target and eliminate radioresistant cells in the S phase, similar to nitrosoureas [98]. 5-FU has been used in glioma treatment in combination with other chemotherapeutic agents [99, 100] as well as radiosensitizers [101]. There is ongoing research into the continuous application of 5-FU through locally applied microspheres, which presents a novel approach with potential benefits in glioma treatment, along with inherent radiosensitization [102]. Gemcitabine, a deoxynucleoside analog, exhibits radiosensitizing qualities stemming from multiple mechanisms, including the reduction of DNA repair, the lowering of thresholds for apoptotic pathways, and the redistribution of cells in the cell cycle [103]. It is capable of penetrating the blood-tumor barrier in human glioma and has shown activity in both MGMT-methylated and -unmethylated tumors [104]. Although various phase I and II trials have explored combination therapy with gemcitabine, none have succeeded in improving survival outcomes [105, 106]. Current research is exploring novel drug conjugates and alternative methods of intratumoral delivery of gemcitabine, such as injectable hydrogel, in preclinical glioma settings [107]. Platinum-based chemotherapeutic agents like cisplatin and carboplatin can synergize with ionizing radiation by inhibiting nonhomologous end joining, leading to the stabilization of radiation-induced damage [108]. While the use of platinum-based therapy concurrently with radiation has been a method to enhance therapeutic efficacy in various malignancies, the combination has not led to significant improvements in survival for glioma patients. Moreover, the use of platinum derivatives has been associated with increased treatment toxicity, which limits the applicable dose and, consequently, their effectiveness [109]. Efforts to circumvent this

obstacle, such as with liposomal-coated drugs, have not yet reached clinical testing [110]. Glioblastoma multiforme is characterized by a high degree of vascular proliferation, which reduces therapy effectiveness due to inadequate vascularization, leading to tumor hypoxia and insufficient distribution of chemotherapeutic agents [111]. Bevacizumab, a monoclonal antibody targeting vascular endothelial growth factor A, addresses this challenge by reducing tumor angiogenesis. This results in improved perfusion, decreased hypoxia, and lower radioresistance [112]. Despite phase II trials having shown promising results [113], recent phase III trials have not found a survival benefit [34]. As a result, the role of anti-VEGF therapy in combined modality treatment remains unclear, and its use is restricted to second-line treatment of recurrent glioma, with varying approval statuses depending on the country [25].

All these categories encompass various strategies to enhance the effectiveness of radiation therapy in glioblastoma treatment, ranging from alleviating tumor hypoxia and interfering with DNA repair mechanisms to promoting apoptosis and combining chemotherapy drugs with radiation. Each approach contributes to the complex landscape of radiosensitization, offering hope for improved outcomes in the battle against this challenging brain cancer.

7.5 Advanced Imaging in Radiotherapy Planning

7.5.1 Role of MRI, PET, and Functional Imaging in Target Delineation

Intensity-modulated radiotherapy (IMRT) and, more specifically, volumetric-modulated arc therapy (VMAT) have been recently introduced in clinical practice for radiotherapy planning and delivery. These sophisticated techniques allow limited exposure of normal brain volume to moderate-high radiation doses, thus minimizing the adverse effects of treatment. They also enable selected dose distributions to critical brain structures, such as optic chiasm and brainstem.

Therefore, accurate delineation of tumor volumes and organs at risk is mandatory. Target delineation can exploit new imaging diagnostic techniques, such as magnetic resonance imaging (MRI) and functional imaging with different variety of PET tracers.

During planning CT, patients are usually immobilized with a 3-point thermoplastic mask in a flat position with neutral head. A CT scan should be acquired from the vertex to the lower border of vertebral body C3, with 2 mm slice thickness maximum. In the target delineation process, current guidelines recommend fusing post-operative contrast-enhanced T1-weighted and T2/FLAIR sequences MRI, in order to provide better target delineation.

The latest published ESTRO-EANO guidelines [45] suggest a new MRI within 2 weeks prior the start of radiation therapy, due to the high probability of volume changes. A new MRI is mandatory for those who undergo subtotal or partial resection. In case of contraindications to MRI, intravenous contrast administered during the planning CT scan could help in identifying any residual disease. If amino acid PET/CT or PET/MRI is used to provide a better target definition, the same maximum interval of 2 weeks is recommended.

Then image registration follows in the treatment planning process. MRI fusion with planning CT scan is facilitated by the presence of rigid bony anatomical markers and by limited movement of the brain and its accuracy is confirmed by matching standard anatomical references (clinoid processes, bony sella, tentorium cerebelli, and vertebral artery) [114].

The precise fusion between MRI and CT scans should be carefully monitored; in case of discrepancies in terms of degrees of head extension between different imaging techniques, the selection of peculiar regions of interest instead of the whole head is recommended.

7.5.2 The Role of MRI in Target Volume Delineation

MRI plays a crucial role in CNS target delineation both in primary and metastatic setting. Its superior soft-tissue resolution and the capacity for functional imaging (diffusion-weighted imaging (DWI), perfusion imaging, blood oxygenation level-dependent) account for the superiority of MRI over all other forms of cross-sectional imaging in this regard [114].

The clinical utility of MRI in treatment planning for brain tumors has its roots as early as 1992 when Thornton demonstrated that CT-defined fields needed to be enlarged to also incorporate MRI tumor volumes across all histologies and greatest for low-grade astrocytomas [115].

In resected tumors, gross tumor volume (GTV) delineation should be based on tumor resection cavity plus any residual contrast-enhancement on T1-weighted post-operative MRI. As many contrast-enhancing areas may be referred to gliosis or post-surgical infarction, immediate post-operative MRI scans should be checked to exclude these areas from target volume. Also, peritumoral edema should not be included.

New current guidelines (Table 7.2) suggest a GTV 1.5 cm-expansion in all directions to generate clinical target volume (CTV) which could

Table 7.2 Current guidelines for glioblastoma target delineation and differences from previous guidelines

Article	Year	GTV	FLAIR	PET	CTV	PTV
Niyazi et al. [37]	2016	Cavity + contrast-enhanced T1	Optional inclusion of edema	Lack of definite evidence	20 mm	3–5 mm
Niyazi et al. [45]	2023	Cavity + T1 contrast enhancement, optionally PET-based BTV, or FLAIR alteration clearly visualized as tumor	Exclude vasogenic edema, if FLAIR indicates presence of non contrast-enhancing tumor, include with variable/no margin	Amino acid PET is a valuable tool for target delineation, even if not validated by current guidelines	15 mm isotropic expansion	3 mm advised

account for the risk of tumor recurrences with limited treatment-related adverse events.

The role of T2-weighted and Fluid Attenuated Inversion Recovery (FLAIR) sequences for planning purposes is still debated. Hyperintense signals are often attributable to edema, ischemic changes, or gliosis, rather than to tumor infiltration, and can vary over time. Therefore, their inclusion in tumor target delineation could lead to larger tumor volume which could possibly exceed the tolerance of normal brain volume. Nonetheless, T2/FLAIR signal changes may reflect tumor infiltration as well (especially when involving cortex or deep grey nuclei or in case of ventricular compression or thickening of the corpus callosum). In this regard, pre-operative T2/FLAIR sequences could help in the determination of edema vs. tumor infiltration, and, in the latter case, signals on T2/FLAIR should be integrated into the delineation of CTV.

Stall et al. outlined the importance of FLAIR sequence for planning purposes, as FLAIR volumes were significantly higher than those based on T2-weighted sequences without affecting dose to OARs and GTV at recurrence overlapped most with FLAIR PTV [116].

The gadolinium-enhancing lesion on T1-weighted MRI reflects areas involved by a breakdown of the blood–brain barrier. This may not be a reliable indicator of an active tumor if we consider both non-enhancing tumor tissue and contrast-enhancing necrosis. Magnetic Resonance-Spectroscopy Imaging (MRSI) provides information about tumor activity based on the levels of cellular metabolites [117]; an assessment of the degree of alteration in metabolite levels may help differentiate normal from abnormal tissue in patients suspected of harboring a high-grade glioma. Gliomas usually present a markedly high resonance in the spectral region of Choline (Cho) and/or a low N-acetylaspartate (NAA) resonance, with an increased Cho/NAA ratio. When comparing differences between contrast-enhancing (CE) lesion on T1-weight MRI, T2/FLAIR, and metabolic lesions for GBM, the volume of Cho/NAA abnormality is often larger than the contrast-enhancing area and the margins of FLAIR abnormality. In the context

of RT planning, MRSI may thus help in improving microscopic disease coverage and preventing marginally recurrent disease [118–121]. Many studies evaluated dose-escalation techniques according to MRSI, providing heterogeneous dose distribution within the tumor (with higher doses to areas defined by higher Cho/NAA ratio) and minimizing the dose to the surrounding healthy brain tissue [122–124].

However, MRSI should be used only in the setting of prospective trials and it is not recommended by current guidelines [45]. Further investigation is warranted to exploit the potential of MRSI in radiation treatment planning and to standardize the analysis of MRSI spectra.

Diffusion MR imaging (dMRI) probes molecular water diffusion within tissues, thus providing microscopic details about the structure of both normal and pathologic tissue [125]. Apparent diffusion coefficient (ADC) quantifies the mean diffusivity of water molecules within each voxel (mm²/s) and determines tumor hypercellularity and brain glioma grade [126]. Lower ADC corresponds to areas of hypercellularity; higher b-value DWI may identify non-enhancing hypercellular components in GBM and could be adopted for PFS prediction and for RT volume definition, due to extension beyond FLAIR abnormalities [127].

Diffusion tensor imaging (DTI) is an MRI technique that uses anisotropic diffusion to estimate the axonal (white matter) organization of the brain. **Fiber tractography (FT)** is a 3D reconstruction technique to assess neural tracts using data collected by diffusion tensor imaging. Since invasive glioma cells migrate along white matter fiber tracts, DTI and tractography could play a role in target delineation volume [128, 129], as DTI abnormalities define the extent of peritumoral infiltration beyond what is apparent on conventional MRI [130]. This could represent an advantage in the case of non-enhancing tumors and diffusely infiltrating low-grade gliomas. In two retrospective evidence, a DTI-CTV was obtained from GTV by adding DTI abnormalities. In both series, DTI-PTV size was smaller than conventional volume but nonetheless still inclusive of areas of tumor recurrence and with

Table 7.3 Main features of MRI advanced techniques and adoption for target delineation in glioblastoma patients

	Magnetic resonance-spectroscopy imaging (MRSI)	Diffusion-weighted (DWI) and diffusion tensor imaging (DTI) MRI	Perfusion-weighted MRI (PWI)	Quantitative blood-oxygen-level-dependent (qBOLD) MRI
MRI sequences for target delineation	Markedly high resonance in the spectral region of Choline (Cho) and/or a low N-acetylaspartate (NAA) resonance, with increased Cho/NAA ratio The volume of Cho/NAA abnormality is often larger than the contrast-enhancing area and the margins of FLAIR abnormality	Lower ADC corresponds to areas of hypercellularity and higher b-value DWI could be adopted for RT volume definition, due to extension beyond FLAIR abnormalities DTI abnormalities define the extent of peritumoral infiltration beyond what is apparent on conventional MRI	Relative cerebral blood volume (rCBV) is the most validated perfusion parameter to predict tumor grade and malignancy and, as it often extends beyond areas of contrast-enhancement on T1-weighted imaging, it could play a role in RT planning	qBOLD MRI could prove useful in non-invasively characterize hypoxic microenvironment in a clinical setting, and possibly, in RT planning

greater sparing of normal brain tissue [131, 132]. The PRaM-GBM is a prospective multicenter study that aims at establishing a DTI-based prediction model for GBM recurrence after treatment and for adequate treatment planning.

Perfusion-weighted imaging (PWI) accounts for blood flow, vascular permeability, and, therefore, for neo-angiogenesis-associated changes in brain gliomas. Relative cerebral blood volume (rCBV) is the most validated perfusion parameter to predict tumor grade and malignancy [133] and, as it often extends beyond areas of contrast-enhancement on T1-weighted imaging, it could play a role in RT planning [134, 135], even if not validated by currently available guideline.

MRI techniques could also contribute to hypoxia imaging, along with PET tracers, with the advantage of higher temporal resolution, repeatability, and independence from vascularization and biodistribution.

Quantitative blood-oxygen-level-dependent (qBOLD) MRI infers quantitative metrics (oxygen-extraction fraction (OEF) and cerebral metabolic rate of oxygen ($CMRO_2$)) regarding blood oxygenation thanks to the intrinsic paramagnetic properties of deoxy-hemoglobin [136]. High-grade gliomas showed lower OEF, higher $CMRO_2$, and higher neovascularization markers [137]. Stadlbauer et al. have combined the

qBOLD-derived oxygen metabolism biomarkers with quantitative metrics of neovascularization derived from PWI and identified two different metabolic phenotypes for newly diagnosed GBM: a glycolytic phenotype with functional neovasculature and a necrotic/hypoxic phenotype with a high proportion of dysfunctional neovasculature and more aggressive tumor behavior [137]. qBOLD MRI could then prove useful in non-invasively characterizing hypoxic microenvironment in a clinical setting, and possibly, in RT planning.

The main features of MRI advanced techniques for GBM target delineation are summarized in Table 7.3.

7.5.3 The Role of Functional Imaging in Target Volume Delineation (Table 7.4)

The most used PET tracer in clinical practice is 2-deoxy-2-[^{18}F]fluoroglucose (FDG). Due to the high glucose metabolism in the brain, the role of FDG PET is limited. New radiolabeled amino acids exhibit low uptake in normal brain and permit better brain tumor visualization due to their high tumor-to-background signal. Commonly used tracers are methyl-^{11}C-l-methionine (MET), 2-[^{18}F]fluoroethyl)-l-tyrosine

Table 7.4 Role of amino acid PET for target tumor delineation

	MET	FET	FDOPA
Aminoacid PET for target delineation	BTV larger than the volume based on contrast-enhancement on MRI in WHO grade III/IV gliomas	BTV larger than the volume based on contrast-enhancement on MRI in WHO grade III/IV gliomas FET and MET PET provide comparable results	BTV larger than the volume based on contrast-enhancement on MRI in WHO grade III/IV gliomas FDOPA seems to be comparable to MET and FET PET

(FET), 3,4-dihydroxy-6-[^{18}F]fluoro-l-phenylalanine (FDOPA), α-^{11}C-methyl-l-tryptophan (AMT), anti-1-amino-3-[^{18}F]-fluorocyclobutane-1-carboxylic acid (FACBC or fluciclovine) [138]. The afore-mentioned tracers can cross intact blood–brain barrier via transport system L, thus permitting delineation of tumor extent beyond contrast enhancement on MRI [139] and helping in tumor volume definition in those cases of non-enhancing glioma on MRI.

18F-Fluoromisonidazole (FMISO) can detect intra-tumoral hypoxia and it could have a potential role in "selected radiation delivering", with higher doses to the most hypoxic tumor subvolumes [140].

Conventional MRI sequences have intrinsic limitations, as they cannot precisely distinguish between edema, gliosis, or enhancing tumor infiltration. Therefore, radiolabeled amino acids, which can detect metabolic active tumor more reliably than MRI, could play a crucial role in target delineation during radiotherapy planning. Indeed, a biological tumor volume (BTV) could represent the real tumor extent more accurately than the MRI-based volume (Fig. 7.1).

MET PET has been investigated in tumor target delineation in comparison to conventional MRI and in most studies it was reported that BTV was larger than the volume based on contrast-enhancement on MRI, thus emphasizing the limits of conventional anatomic imaging [44, 142, 143].

Regarding FET PET, much clinical evidence reported significant discordance between FET PET-based BTV and MRI-based GTV, with poor spatial congruence [144–146]. Munck et al. in their prospective trial analyzing grade III–IV gliomas showed that approximately 90% of FET PET-based tumor volume would be included in a

CTV based on MRI-contrast enhanced GTV with 2 cm-expansion [147].

BTVs could then represent both the real tumor extent and the areas at greater risk of recurrence.

FDOPA, along with MET PET and FET PET, could help in the delineation of more accurate larger tumor volumes than the ones based on MRI-contrast enhancement [148, 149].

MET, FET, and FDOPA yield similar results in terms of target volume delineation [44, 150, 151].

Current guidelines state that PET is not part of standard imaging for GBM delineation but, if used, PET scans should be obtained at least 2 weeks after neurosurgery. BTV should be defined by uptake above a threshold of 1.6–1.8 of mean standard uptake volume (SUV) in the background [152]. Other centers use a threshold of 1.8 × background activity for estimation of BTV [153]. Review and manual editing with respect to the MRI is required [45]. At the moment changes in margins when amino acids PET is used are not recommended, but FET PET could prove useful in the future.

PET/MRI is a hybrid imaging technology that incorporates morphological and functional imaging [154].

In the future, it could help in tumor target delineation by optimizing co-registration of brain images, reducing scanning time, and limiting exposure to additional radiation doses.

7.5.4 MRI-Linac

The traditional platforms for image-guided radiotherapy (IGRT) involve computed tomography (CT). The integration of a compatible MRI scanner with a linear accelerator (linac) device has successfully led to an MR-linear accelerator (MR-Linac),

Fig. 7.1 The extent of increased FET uptake (left image; red contour transferred onto MR images) is considerably larger than the contrast enhancement (left side) and the extent of the signal hyperintensity on the T2-weighted MR image (right side). (Adapted from Brighi et al. [141] under Creative Commons Attribution (CC BY) license (https://creativecommons.org/licenses/by/4.0/))

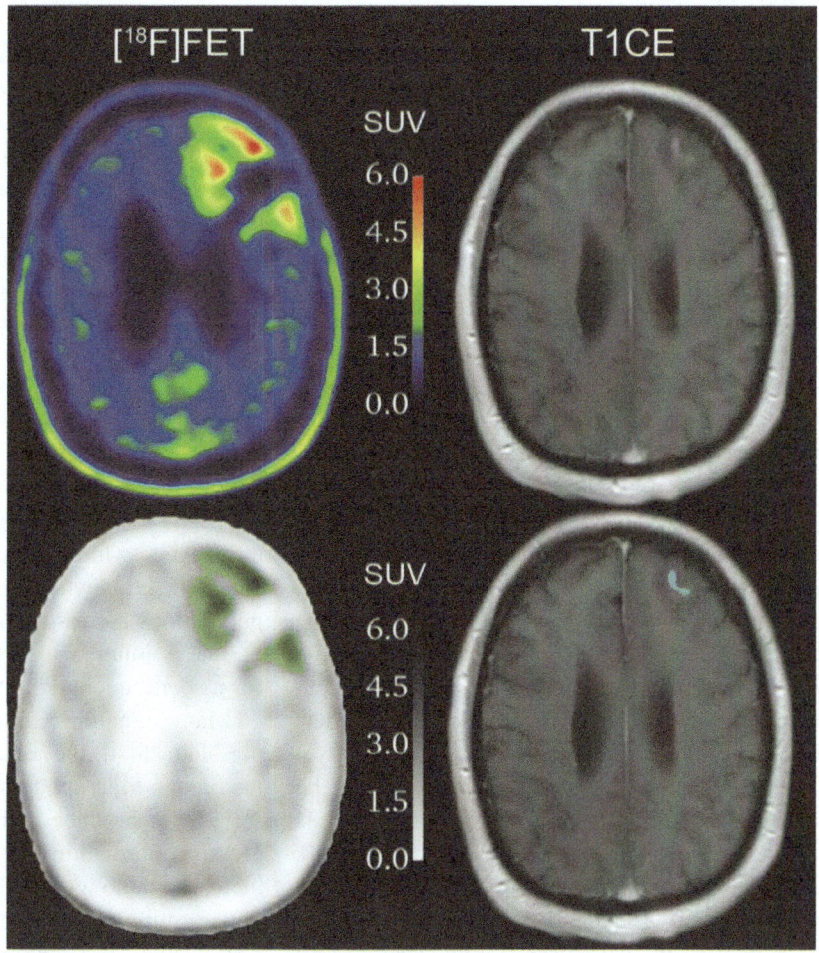

which had been introduced in clinical practice with the name of MRI-guided radiotherapy (MRgRT) [155, 156]. Compared to conventional CT-based image-guidance, MRI allows clinicians to better identify target volumes and critical structures with potentially less involvement of organs at risk, due to its optimal soft tissue contrast [157].

In regard to brain tumors, the volumes of resection cavity, residual tumor, and edema can undergo substantial changes during treatment, potentially leading to inaccurate treatment volumes. Resonance image-guided-radiotherapy (MR-IGRT) could then allow for the detection of structural changes with daily MRIs during treatment. This could lead to enhanced adapted treatment, better local control and decreased radiation-induced neurotoxicity with maximum sparing of the OARs [158, 159].

Patient positioning is different from conventional linac treatments due to the small gantry size and the need to include MRI-coils in the immobilization process. In the setting of brain and head and neck cancer, the use of thermoplastic masks remains the gold standard to prevent motion and guarantee reproducible positioning [160].

The optimal MRI for RT planning should provide images with uniform signal intensity, lack of artifacts and high geometric accuracy [161]. Also, image quality should be comparable with referent diagnostic MRI to be integrated in the clinical workflow. The latter could offer set-up and registration error minimization but, since MRI voxel intensities are not associated with electron density of tissues as in CT, dose calculation on MRI needs a conversion to a synthetic-CT (synCT). Different strategies are available for synCT generation.

Many studies in GBM patients that underwent adjuvant RT showed significant changes of target volume between post-operative MRIs and repeated MRIs performed during RT course with volumetric and/or geometric variations of disease and target volumes. Repeated MRIs could improve doses to the OARs or target coverage [162–164]. In most series most lesions progressively shrinked during radiotherapy, although expansion was reported in a fraction of the cases. Adaptive radiotherapy based on serial MRI could improve doses to the OARs particularly in case of volume reduction and guarantee adequate coverage in case of volumetric increase [165].

During RT glioblastoma undergoes many physiologic changes; multiparametric functional sequences could then be exploited in MRgRT devices for treatment assessment. For example, MRI perfusion and diffusion parameters may be affected by chemoradiation treatment and MRI linac could therefore provide a more frequent data evaluation of over the course of radiotherapy. Spectroscopy has not been implemented yet on MRI-Linac; it could hypothetically be acquired on a 1.5 T MRgRT system, though it is still debated whether Cho/NAA MRSI on a 1.5 T MRgRT system might have proper resolution and spectral quality for adaptive RT [166].

However, in real-world setting MRI is still limited available to perform dedicated simulation MRI and repeated MRI during treatment course. The current standard is represented by simulation CT scan and CT-based IGRT cannot precisely detect most of tissue changes during treatment. Therefore, the exploit of MRI-linac could overcome these limits, allowing daily replanning based on the actual anatomy.

7.6 Immunotherapy and Radiotherapy Combinations

7.6.1 GBM Microenvironment

The brain has historically been considered an immunologically different and privileged environment protected by the blood–brain barrier (BBB), lacking antigen presenting cells (APCs) and closed off to circulating lymphocytes [167]. Therefore, Central Nervous System (CNS) provides a perfect microenvironment for tumor growth and proliferation.

This assumption has been reconsidered in recent years, due to the detection of a lymphatic drainage system in the brain and to the discovery of the role of migroglia/macrophage cells as able to present antigens and to activate lymphocytes in case of BBB breakdown [168].

Rather than an immune-distinct site, GBM should be considered as an immune-suppressive microenvironment (Fig. 7.2), characterized by the combination of two different types of cells: microglia (CNS-resident macrophages) and monocytes, which travel through the blood and enters the brain when BBB is damaged. Both cell populations are responsible for the development of GBM immunosuppressive environment and for its consequent definition as "cold tumor".

Many signaling pathways lead to immunosuppression; first, the release of various soluble mediators. Macrophages and tumoral cells themselves can produce and secret the immunosuppressive interleukin-10 (IL-10), whose levels are increased amongst GBM patients [169]. Also, transforming-growth factor beta (TGF-β), responsible for T-cells inhibition, is secreted by microglia in GBM patients [170], as well as prostaglandin E2 [171].

GBM cells can escape immune responses thanks to the surface expression of Immune-Checkpoint molecules (ICs). Programmed-death ligand 1 (PDL-1) is upregulated in GBM microenvironment and it can induce exhaustion and anergy of T-cell response [172, 173]. The expression of CD95 ligand by GBM cells can induce apoptosis in infiltrating lymphocytes [174]. CTLA-4 is also an important IC; it competes with CD28 for binding to costimulatory molecules (CD80 and CD86) on antigen-presenting cells, thereby precluding the activation of T cells [173, 175].

GBM also can escape the immune system due to direct interaction between GBM tumoral cells and immune system cells. GBM indeed suppresses natural killer (NK) cells by inducing their

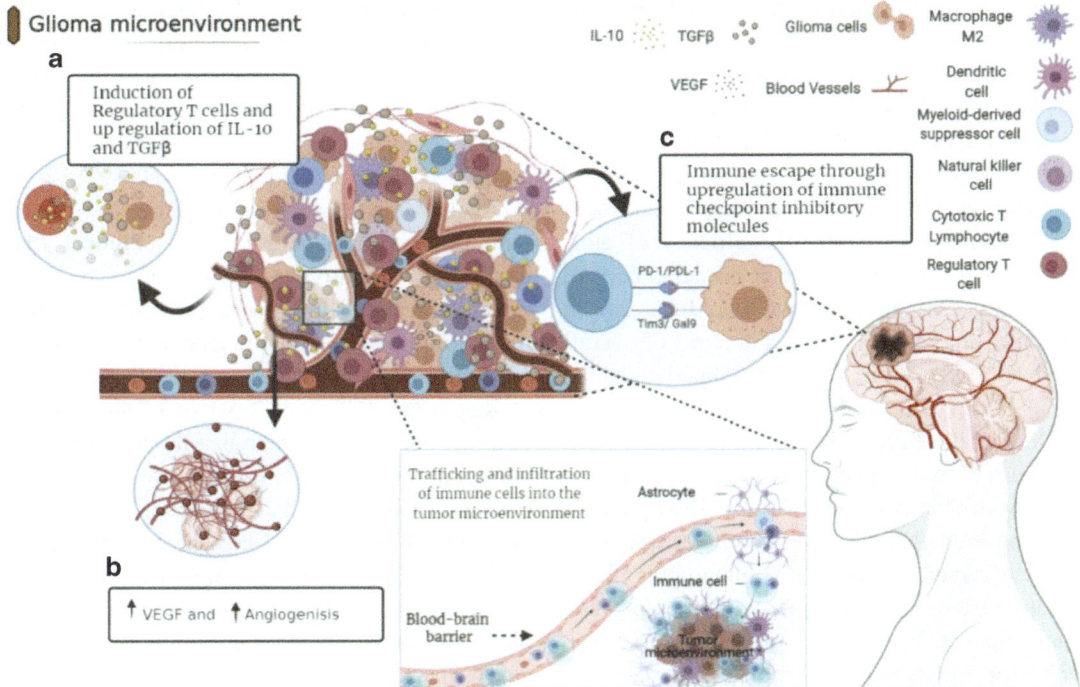

Fig. 7.2 Immunosuppressive GBM microenvironment. (**a**) Tumor cells release soluble mediators (IL-1, TGF-β) which contribute to immunosuppression. (**b**) Angiogenesis is a pathologic hallmark of glioblastoma mainly mediated by vascular endothelial growth factor (VEGF). (**c**) Immune checkpoints (ICs) on tumor cells surface suppress T cell response. (From Ghouzlani et al. [183] distributed under the terms of the Creative Commons Attribution License (CC BY))

apoptosis via tumor necrosis factor receptor superfamily member 6 (TNFRSF6) or PD-L1 [176–178]. GBM is also characterized by a T cell depletion, at the basis of which some studies have suggested an M2-like phenotype of GBM myeloid cells [179–181].

Since immunotherapy is critically dependent on the availability of pre-existing tumor immunity, a cold microenvironment like the one assessed in GBM patients may raise questions in the adoption of immunotherapy in this setting. Moreover, for a long time it was thought that immune-checkpoint inhibitors (ICIs) could not be adopted in clinical practice due to the impermeability of BBB and the large molecular size of monoclonal antibody (150 kDa) [182].

However, this consensus must be reconsidered. ICIs have indeed demonstrated the ability to cross BBB thanks to two different mechanisms: by binding on peripheral lymphocytes which act as a vehicle and by direct crossing BBB. Once penetrated, ICIs can promote immunomodulation of the tumor microenvironment [182].

7.6.2 Immune-Checkpoint Inhibitors (ICIs) in GBM

As afore-mentioned, GBM cells express on their surface ICs that can interact with their complementary receptors on immune cells, thus resulting in the blockade of immune response. Immune-checkpoint inhibitors have then recently emerged as a possible therapeutic approach able to prevent the interaction between GBM cells ICs and their receptors and the consequent inactivation of immune response [183].

The main targets in GBM are represented by PD-1/PDL-1, CTLA-4/CD80 or CD86, TIM-3/GAL-9 [184].

Park et al. evaluated the combined effect of anti-PD-1 and temozolomide in an orthotopic GBM murine model and proved a synergistic anti-tumoral efficacy [185]. Unfortunately, most clinical studies of anti-PD-1/PDL-1 monotherapy in GBM have failed to show clinical efficacy.

The first large-scale randomized controlled phase III trial comparing the efficacy of anti-PD-1 agent nivolumab with bevacizumab in recurrent GBM patients showed no difference in outcomes among the two arms in terms of overall survival (OS) and treatment-related adverse events [186].

Despite the failure of second line trial, anti-PD1 drugs were tested in first line in the CheckMate-498. In this trial, 560 GBM patients with non-methylated MGMT promoter were randomly assigned to receive nivolumab plus radiotherapy or temozolomide plus radiotherapy. The study did not meet its primary endpoint (OS), with a longer OS in standard arm [187], and considering that the population included only non-methylated MGMT patients the results were really disappointing. Subsequently, the study CheckMate-548 evaluated the addition of nivolumab to standard chemoradiation treatment in GBM patients with MGMT promoter methylation or indeterminate status. Again, nivolumab did not improve survival [188].

Pembrolizumab, as well, did not prolong survival when used as a single agent. In Keynote 28 pembrolizumab was investigated in 26 GBM recurrent patients with reported limited survival benefits [189].

Anti-PDL-1 antibodies durvalumab and atezolizumab were also investigated as single agents in the management of GBM patients. In a phase I trial addressing 16 recurrent GBM patients, atezolizumab did not improve survival, except for three patients reporting IDH or POLE mutations [190]. A phase II trial evaluating durvalumab in 5 GBM cohorts published preliminary results from subgroups with partially clinical benefits. In the arm involving 30 recurrent GBM patients on durvalumab monotherapy, the overall disease control rate was 60.0%, median OS was 28.9 weeks and the median PFS was 13.9 weeks [191].

Avelumab is an IgG1 monoclonal antibody targeting PD-L1. In a phase II study of avelumab concurrently added to the first monthly temozolomide cycle in newly diagnosed GBM patients, the addition of immunotherapy was not associated with a benefit on survival [192].

Avelumab was also investigated in association with oral axitinib in a phase II clinical trial involving 54 recurrent GBM patients. The combinations resulted in an acceptable toxicity profile but did not meet the prespecified endpoint of 6-months PFS [193].

Regarding CTLA-4/CD80 or CD86 interaction, the agent ipilimumab is a monoclonal antibody that binds to CTLA-4 receptors and blocks the inhibition of T cells that occurs through this molecule. CheckMate 143, the first phase III study involving immunotherapy in GBM setting, initially evaluated the combination ipilimumab plus nivolumab. However, the combination approach showed increased toxicity and was suspended [194]. In a phase I study the authors investigated intracerebral administration of ipilimumab and nivolumab in combination with nivolumab intravenously administered in 27 recurrent GBM patients who had undergone maximal safe resection. Although preliminary findings appeared promising [195], it is crucial to exercise caution due to the numerous past failures with combination approaches.

GAL-9 is highly expressed in GBM cells and its binding with TIM-3, a membrane protein on CD4+/CD8+ surface, leads to T cell apoptosis and to the inactivation of immune response. As a consequence, TIM3 has recently become a potential target for ICIs [196].

Immunotherapy has been investigated also in the neoadjuvant setting, as able to counteract the immunosuppressive microenvironment of high-grade gliomas.

In a phase II study by Schalper et al., neoadjuvant nivolumab resulted in a local immunomodulatory effect of treatment [197]. Neoadjuvant pembrolizumab was associated with better survival outcomes in 35 recurrent GBM patients, with a converted tumor gene expression profile [198].

In comparison to other diseases, it can be seen as somewhat illusory to expect ICIs therapy to be effective in treating GBM, as its current efficacy is unsatisfactory and warrants further research.

In this regard, many factors can influence the efficacy of ICIs, including PD-L1 expression by tumor cells, tumor-infiltrating lymphocytes (TILs), tumor-infiltrating myeloid cells (TIMs), tumor mutation burden (TMB), microsatellite instability (MSI), mismatch repair (MMR) system status and POLE mutation status [199].

Eighty-eight percent of patients with newly diagnosed GBM and 72.2% of patients with recurrent GBM have high PD-1 expression [200] and this could be a challenge for further studies.

Many specific GBM subtypes may benefit more from CI therapies; a higher TMB, higher MSI, MMR system deficiency (MMRD) and germline POLE mutation usually are associated with better efficacy.

TMB quantitatively reflects the quantity of tumor mutations; however, there is no consensus yet for the precise definition of "hypermutation", since different thresholds have been reported for pan-cancer analysis. In relation to GBM, several different criteria were used in published studies to define TMB [201–204].

Better efficacy to ICIs is associated to phenotype MMRD; GBM with MMRD indeed demonstrated higher TMB. In preliminary studies, GBM patients with deficient DNA mismatch repair ability had significant radiologic and clinical responses to nivolumab and pembrolizumab [203, 205].

7.6.3 ICIs Safety Profile

For what concerns tolerability and safety profile, ICIs are usually manageable. In the CheckMate 143, the most common adverse events related to nivolumab included fatigue, diarrhea, headache, increased lipase level and nausea. Ipilimumab, on the other hand, reported increased adverse events and led to trial discontinuation. Amongst neurological adverse events, headaches and seizures were the most reported [194]. Brain ICI-related pseudoprogression is worth mentioning. Pseudo-progression is attributable to a locally stimulated immune response and it results in the radiologic features of progression with enhancement and edema [206]. Therefore, initial imaging features at immunotherapy start cannot exclude subsequent clinical benefit according to the Immunotherapy Response Assessment in Neuro-Oncology (iRANO) criteria [207]. In clinical practice, it is of extreme importance to distinguish pseudo-progression from true progression and treatment failure.

7.6.4 Synergy Between ICIs and RT

Radiation therapy (RT), one of the cornerstones in the treatment of GBM, can act as an immuno-modulating agent. "Immunogenic modulation" is the definition of all radiation-induced molecular alterations that make the tumor more responsive to cytotoxic-T-cell-mediated destruction [208]. RT, indeed, can promote adaptive immune response against tumors by induction of immunologic cell death, antigen presentation, and dendritic cells maturation; it can also modulate CD8 T cell responses by inducing T cell tumor infiltration and T cell and NK-cell recognition of tumor-associated antigens (TAAs).

Therefore, combining RT and immunotherapy can have a synergistic effect in the immunomodulation process. RT promotes the releasing of tumor antigens and of pro-inflammatory signals; it contributes to cross-presentation of tumor associated antigens by dendritic cells to T-cells; RT may damage BBB thus facilitating diffusion of systemic agents into CNS. Immunotherapy on the other hand can reduce tumor hypoxia and increase radiosensitivity [209].

Adding immunotherapy to the standard of care for GBM could then have a biological rationale and preclinical studies in GBM models suggest the efficacy of this combination [210]. Unfortunately, the association of anti-PD-1 therapy and RT with and without temozolomide has been explored in two main phase III clinical trials, without success.

In the Checkmate 498, 560 newly diagnosed GBM patients without MGMT promoter methylation were randomly assigned in a 1:1 ratio to standard RT (60 Gy) plus nivolumab (240 mg every 2 weeks for eight cycles, then 480 mg every 4 weeks) or to standard chemoradiation treatment with concomitant and subsequent TMZ. As median OS (mOS) was 13.4 months with NIVO + RT and 14.9 months with TMZ + RT ($p = 0.0037$), the primary end point was not met. In regard to safety profile, any-grade treatment-related adverse events (TRAEs) were reported in 72.7% of patients treated with NIVO + RT and 75.6% of patients treated with TMZ + RT [187].

In the Checkmate 548, the efficacy of nivolumab (240 mg every 2 weeks for eight cycles, then 480 mg every 4 weeks) plus standard chemoradiation with temozolomide-based therapy was compared to placebo plus standard chemoradiation in a population of 716 newly-diagnosed GBM with MGMT promoter methylation assessed. Also in this case, results did not favor the addition of immunotherapy to standard treatment for GBM (mOS 28.9 months in NIVO + RTCT vs. 32.1 months in PBO + RTCT) [188].

In summary, when considering both trials, the outcomes were disheartening, revealing an even shorter overall survival (OS) in the experimental immunotherapy group when compared to the standard treatment approaches.

Immunotherapy and stereotactic radiotherapy (SBRT) combination has also been the subject of other small-scale phase I trials involving recurrent GBM.

In a recent phase I study of pembrolizumab and bevacizumab concomitantly administered with hypofractionated stereotactic RT (30 Gy in 5 fractions) in patients with recurrent GBM/anaplastic glioma, the association resulted safe and well tolerated and prompted further investigation [211].

Also, the anti-PD-L1 monoclonal antibody durvalumab has been investigated in combination with hypofractionated stereotactic RT in a small sample of six patients with recurrent GBM. In this phase I study, the treatment regimen was well tolerated with median PFS and OS of 2.3 months and 16.7 months, respectively [212].

In conclusion, the performance of immunotherapy in the treatment of GBM has thus far proven to be rather underwhelming, necessitating further exploration to bridge the knowledge gap concerning the immune system's role in the brain. Currently, outside the realm of clinical trials, the use of immunotherapy in GBM management cannot be endorsed. Large-scale clinical trial data are scarce, and a majority of the published findings have yielded unfavorable results, showing no substantial improvements in survival rates. Nevertheless, smaller-scale studies indicate the importance of persevering in the face of GBM's unique immunosuppressive microenvironment. Furthermore, it is imperative to investigate potential biomarkers, such as TMB, MMRD, and POLE mutation status, to better predict the responsiveness to immunotherapy.

7.7 Management of Elderly GBM Patients

Glioblastoma (GBM) is the most common malignancy among Central Nervous System (CNS) primary tumors and it accounts for most gliomas (57.7%). Its incidence rate increases with advancing age and patients older than 65 years account for more than half of all newly diagnosed GBM cases. Median age at diagnosis is 65 years [213].

Management of elderly patients can be demanding due to their poorer performance status, multiple co-morbidities, dismal disease prognosis, and increased adverse events from combined treatment strategy (surgery, radiotherapy and chemotherapy) [214]. Moreover, the definition of "elderly" patients is not clearly assessed yet [215], with current available evidence referring to those above 65 years [216–218] or 60 years [219, 220].

Also, many older patients have been excluded from clinical trials because age has been historically considered an adverse prognostic factor [221–224], probably due to its correlation with more aggressive tumor biology.

7.7.1 Molecular Features of Elderly GBM

Molecular characteristics of elderly GBM patients are not entirely known, but many genetic factors may negatively impact the prognosis [225].

A sub-analysis of 272 GBM patients from The Cancer Genome Atlas (TCGA) showed that GBM in elderly population had a significantly lower rate of the glioma-CpG island methylator phenotype (G-CIMP) which correlates with isocitrate dehydrogenase (*IDH*)-mutant lower-grade gliomas and with the *O*-6-methylguanine-DNA methyltransferase promoter (*MGMT*p) methylation, the strongest predictive factor for response to chemotherapy with alkylating agents [226, 227]. It also showed that survival of patients with G-CIMP was significantly longer than that of older patients without the G-CIMP phenotype and that age was an independent adverse prognostic factor even among G-CIMP negative GBM [20]. A significantly lower prevalence of IDH-mutant tumors among elderly was confirmed by Ostrom et al. [228] who also reported amongst 4512 GBM patients a single nucleotide polymorphism (SNP) for two loci in 7p11.2 located near EGFR gene (strongly associated with risk for developing GBM) in those older than 54 years.

This contributes to the evidence that *IDH*-mutant high-grade astrocytomas (formerly known as "secondary GBMs") are separate entities from GBMs with evolution from lower-grade astrocytomas and different genetic and molecular features. The new 2021 WHO Classification of brain tumors identifies a new class of astrocytomas *IDH*-mutant grade 4, while the diagnosis of glioblastoma *IDH*-mutant is not allowed anymore [3].

An analysis from 425 GBM patients from TCGA demonstrated that in older (≥70 years) population with G-CIMP negative phenotype some genes with biological role in tumorigenesis (i.e., tumor suppressors or involved in tumor growth pathways) can be downregulated or upregulated. It also showed significant differences among age groups for what concerns miRNA expression, differentially methylated genes (DMG) and differentially altered genes (DAG) [229].

Furthermore, in elderly patients with IDH-wild type GBM, *PTEN* deletions and *CDK4* amplification prevailed significantly and a trend for higher representation of *PDGFR* amplified/gained tumors was seen; likewise, mutation of *TERT* promoter was slightly prevalent among elderly patients [230].

7.7.2 Clinical Features and Prognostic Assessment in Elderly GBM

Management of elderly patients is more challenging due to multiple comorbidities and the risk of increased side effects from combined treatment strategies; therefore, the assessment of prognostic factors is of primary importance for the selection of the most suitable therapeutic approach.

Karnofsky Performance Status (KPS) allows patients to be classified as to their functional impairment with scores from 100 (= *patient able to carry on normal activity and work; no special care needed*) to 0 (= *dead*).

Pre-operative and post-operative KPS have been evaluated as prognostic factors in many series. Some studies reported that pre-operative KPS is survival predictor in GBM elderly population [231–233]. Other found no correlation between pre-operative KPS and overall survival (OS) or progression-free survival (PFS), but demonstrated that post-operative KPS is associated with prolonged survival [220, 234]. The impact of post-operative KPS on survival was demonstrated also by Pontes et al. [235].

Comorbidities may affect survival in GBM elderly patients, even if this relationship is still unclear. Some studies showed similar prognosis between patients with multiple comorbidities and those with none [220, 236]. On the other hand, evidence is available regarding the role of hyperglycemia [237], lower systolic blood pressure values, and lower serum albumin values [238] in predicting survival outcomes.

The Charlson Comorbidities Index (CCI) is the most common score for the assessment of patient comorbidities in the GBM setting. It includes a wide range of clinical conditions, such as age, myocardial infarction, congestive heart failure, peripheral vascular disease, cerebrovascular accidents, dementia, chronic obstructive pulmonary disease (COPD), connective tissue disease, peptic ulcer disease, liver disease, diabetes mellitus, hemiplegia, chronic kidney failure, solid tumors, blood tumors and acquired immunodeficiency syndrome (AIDS). The final CCI score is used to predict the expected survival and it was investigated in many clinical series, with unclear correlation with survival outcomes. Balducci et al. showed that a CCI < 2 did not correlate with survival [239]; conversely, other studies proved correlation between worse OS and PFS and higher CCI scores [238, 240, 241].

Since surgery is the primary treatment for GBM, the **extent of resection** has been proposed as a prognostic factor, with gross-total resection (GTR) associated with improved OS and PFS, if compared to surgical biopsy only or subtotal resection [242].

A prognostic index based on the most consistent prognostic factors for elderly GBM outcome prediction has not been validated yet.

Scott et al. identified four different prognostic subgroups among GBM population aged more than 70 years, based on age, extent of surgery and KPS [243]. In a large series of elderly GBM patients from the Memorial Sloan Kettering Cancer Center, the **number of tumor lesions** was an additional factor associated with poorer outcome, along with increasing age, worse KPS and subtotal resection [244].

Regarding **MGMT promoter methylation status**, in a series from Schneider et al. the combination of CCI > 2, subtotal resection, unmethylated *MGMT* promoter status, Body Mass Index (BMI) < 30 and clinical frailty (according to the modified Frailty Index (mFI)) was a predictor of worse outcome [245]. In a mono-institutional analysis by Lombardi et al. MGMT methylation status proved as an independent prognostic factor [246].

Liu et al. developed a prognostic index score based on a retrospective analysis of elderly (≥60 years) GBM patients. At univariate analysis age, gender, comorbidities, preoperative KPS < 90 and MGMT promoter methylation were not significantly associated with PFS and OS, whereas total resection, postoperative KPS ≥ 80, Ki67 > 25% and Stupp-protocol treat-

ment were significantly associated with prolonged PFS and OS. At multivariate analysis postoperative KPS ≥ 80, total resection and Stupp-protocol treatment were prognostic factors for PFS and OS [220].

7.7.3 Clinical Management of Elderly GBM Patients

The standard of care in the management of GBM patients is represented by the so-called Stupp-protocol, which consists of extended surgery followed by post-operative radiotherapy over 6 weeks for a Fractionated Total Dose (FTD) of 60 Gy plus concomitant Temozolomide (TMZ) at a daily dose of 75 mg/mq. After 1 month, subsequent adjuvant TMZ is administered for 5 days every 28 days at a daily dose of 150 mg/mq (up to 200 mg/mq) for a total of 6 cycles [4].

The afore-mentioned study excluded patients aged over 70 years, but in the 5-year analysis of the EORTC-NCIC trial [26] a benefit of the combined treatment strategy was observed also in patients older than 60 years.

Due to disease aggressiveness, clinical frailty and dismal prognosis, management of elderly GBM patients still represents a clinical challenge.

7.7.3.1 The Role of Surgery

Surgery is the primary treatment for elderly GBM patients, with surgical extent being relevant for prognostic assessment. Gross-Total Resection (GTR) is warranted, when feasible, since it provides tumor debulking and histopathological diagnosis. The need of extended resections in this setting has been debated for a long time, due to the possible higher risk of post-operative complications.

In a systematic review and meta-analysis of biopsy vs. partial vs. GTR in high-grade glioma patients older than 60 years, Almenawer et al. compared overall survival, KPS, progression-free survival, mortality and morbidity in 12,607 patients from 34 studies. The overall survival was 5.71 months in those undergoing biopsy,

8.68 months for subtotal resection and 14.04 months after gross total resection. Overall resection of any extent reported a significant benefit if compared with biopsy alone, with mean difference in overall survival of 3.88 months and a progressive improvement in clinical outcomes with greater degrees of resection [247]. Chaichana et al. in a retrospective analysis of 40 GBM patients, revealed that GTR confers a significant survival benefit (5.7 vs. 4.0 months, $p = 0.020$) without increased surgery-related morbidities, if compared to those receiving biopsy [232]. The superiority of extended surgery over biopsy regardless of age was demonstrated by other several studies [248–253].

An Italian series of 100 patients proved that aggressive surgical approach is feasible in elderly patients, without differences regarding post-operative KPS, OS and PFS if compared to younger population [254].

Overall, available evidence suggests maximal extension of tumor removal when surgery is feasible, regardless of age. The most appropriate approach should be carefully evaluated, with regards to neurological and geriatric assessment.

7.7.3.2 The Role of Radiotherapy (RT)

Increasing age is usually associated with increasing risk of cognitive side-effects from cranial irradiation; nonetheless radiation therapy has proven feasible in GBM elderly population, both in supportive care [255] and in adjuvant setting.

For what concerns post-operative RT, shorter hypofractionated schedules have been investigated to overcome the limits of prolonged therapies and to support the frailties of older patients [256, 257].

In Roa et al. work of 2004, 100 GBM patients aged 60 or older were randomized to standard adjuvant RT (60 Gy in 30 fractions) or to a hypofractionated regimen (40 Gy in 15 fractions) with no difference in overall survival (5.1 months in the standard arm vs. 5.6 months in the experimental arm) [256].

In 2015 Roa et al. compared the hypofractionated regimen 40 Gy in 15 fractions with an even shorter schedule of 25 Gy in 5 fractions in a population of 98 GBM elderly and/or frail patients.

No differences were found in overall survival (7.9 months in the experimental arm vs. 6.4 months in the standard arm), progression-free survival and quality of life between the two regimens [257].

According to these results and to those of other phase III trials (see below), hypofractionated regimens have become the standard of care in GBM elderly population, with no significant impairment in neurocognitive function and quality of life.

7.7.3.3 The Role of Chemotherapy (CT)

Increasing age has been historically associated with decreasing benefit from chemotherapy and with increased side effects from nitrosourea-based regimens. Single-agent Temozolomide (TMZ) alone has been investigated in the setting of adjuvant treatment as an alternative to radiotherapy due to its feasible oral administration and low toxicity profile [258, 259]. In a phase II study on 70 GBM patients (≥70 years), TMZ was administered as adjuvant monotherapy according to standard schedule (150–200 mg/m^2/daily for 5 days every 28 days) and it showed acceptable tolerance, with improvement in functional status and in overall survival, if compared to supportive care, especially in those *MGMT*p methylation [258].

7.7.3.4 Radiotherapy or Chemotherapy?

Recently, the use of Temozolomide has been evaluated as an alternative to RT in randomized prospective studies. In this context, two main phase III trials are worth mentioning.

Malmström et al. in the NORDIC trial analyzed 342 patients from 28 centers aged ≥60 years (after October 2004 ≥65 years), with Eastern Cooperative Oncology Group (ECOG) Performance Status <2 and who had undergone surgery or biopsy. The different post-operative treatment arms were hypofractionated RT (34 Gy in 10 fractions), standard RT schedule (60 Gy in 30 fractions) and TMZ alone at standard schedule. The poorest survival outcome was associated with conventional RT (median OS 6.0 months) and almost the same results were reported for

TMZ only chemotherapy and hypofractionated RT regimen (8.3 months and 7.5 months, respectively). MGMTp methylation status affected response to TMZ alone (OS 9.7 months in methylated patients vs. 6.8 months in un-methylated ones) [219]. In contrast, MGMTp methylation did not show an impact on patients having RT.

In the NOA-08 trial 412 GBM patients aged ≥65 years were randomly assigned to adjuvant standard regimen RT (60 Gy in 30 fractions) or to adjuvant TMZ at intensified schedule (100 mg/m^2 on days 1–7 every other week). TMZ proved non inferior to standard RT in relation to OS (1-year OS 34.4% vs. 37.4% for TMZ and radiotherapy groups, respectively), but with worse toxicity profile (G2–4 adverse events). Also in this case, MGMTp methylation status provided higher benefit to TMZ, with better event-free survival rates [218].

Overall, Temozolomide is an effective and tolerated treatment for elderly patients with GBM. Response to treatment is significantly associated with *MGMT* promoter methylation status; therefore, in clinical practice, postoperative temozolomide should be considered only in patients with *MGMT* promoter methylated tumors, while its use should not be considered in those with *MGMT* unmethylated tumors [260].

7.7.3.5 And What If… Radiotherapy and Concomitant Chemotherapy?

The tolerability of combined chemoradiation adjuvant treatment seems to be questionable in elderly GBM population. As above-mentioned, the Stupp trial did not include patients aged over 70 years [246] and the EORTC/NCIC trial failed to show a benefit in survival for patients aged more than 65 years treated with combined chemoradiation over radiotherapy alone, due to a lack of statistical power for the small number of elderly patients (60–70 years) included [26].

The association between post-operative TMZ and hypofractionated radiotherapy was investigated in the trial by Perry et al. where 562 patients aged >65 years underwent RT (40 Gy in 15 fractions) with concomitant daily TMZ and

subsequent TMZ up to 12 cycles or hypofractionated RT alone (40 Gy in 15 fractions). A significant OS benefit was found in combined strategy (9.3 months vs. 7.6 months), especially in MGMT-methylated patients where OS reached 13.5 months. Conversely, in patients with *MGMT* unmethylated tumors, a non-significant trend favored the radio-chemotherapy group (median overall survival being 10.0 vs.7.9 months) [214].

The main principles regarding the management of GBM elderly population may be included in the following algorithm (Fig. 7.3).

In elderly patients with good performance status the best treatment strategy is represented by hypofractionated radiotherapy with concomitant TMZ followed by adjuvant TMZ, especially in those with MGMTp methylation status. In those un-methylated, sequential TMZ only can be evaluated after hypofractionated RT completion. In patients with poor KPS, TMZ alone or palliative care may be considered if MGMTp methylation is assessed; otherwise, RT alone (34 Gy in 10 fractions or 25 Gy in 5 fractions) may be a reasonable option.

7.7.4 Recurrent GBM in Elderly

Recurrences in GBM elderly patients raise many questions and patients' limited life expectancy makes it unclear which additional treatment would be the most suitable [261]. KPS is the most determining factor in the salvage therapy selection process. In those with good performance status, surgery and/or radiotherapy provides better survival results.

Re-surgery is associated with greater impairment and mortality, but it should be considered to improve patients' quality of life (i.e., decreasing in intracranial pressure) when feasible (focal disease, not involving eloquent areas, deep structures, or both hemispheres) [262]. Many clinical trials reported that in selected patients (KPS values ≥70) re-surgery reported better survival results, if compared to conservative strategies, without increasing post-operative complication rates [263–266].

Fig. 7.3 Clinical management of elderly patients with glioblastoma. *WT* wild-type, *GTR* gross-total resection, *KPS* Karnofsky Performance Status, *MGMTp* O-6-methylguanine-DNA methyltransferase promoter, *RT* radiotherapy, *TMZ* temozolomide

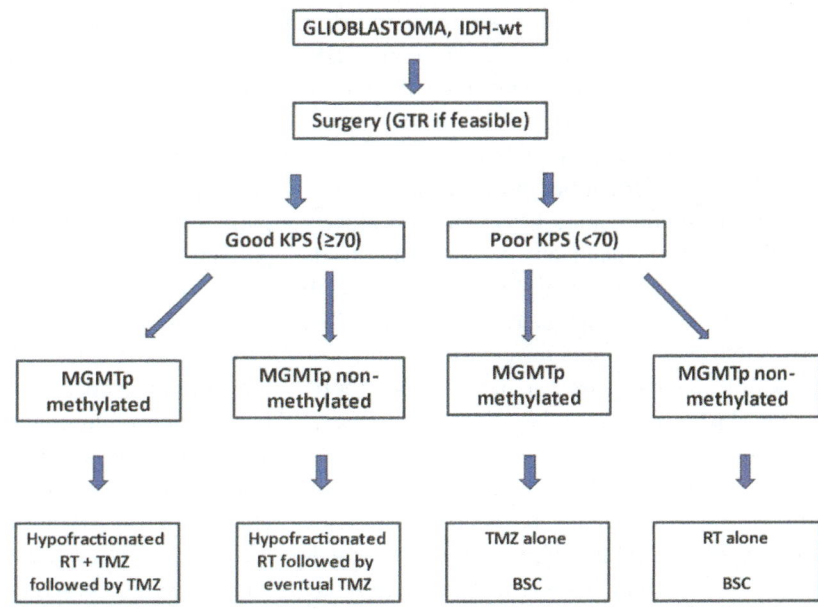

On the other hand, in Goldman's series and Hager's retrospective evaluation, no survival benefit was associated with re-surgery at recurrence [252, 267].

Re-operation provided better survival results also in comparison with temozolomide-based chemotherapy [268, 269] and when compared to re-irradiation [269], even if the latter results are still pending with limited evidence available.

In patients with poor performance status (KPS < 70), re-surgery results in poorer outcomes, probably due to increased post-operative complications. In this context, chemotherapy is preferred over local treatment, with Fotemustine being a valuable therapeutic option [270, 271].

Also, systemic therapy with either Lomustine or Bevacizumab may represent a feasible treatment option at recurrency. Results from RCTs have reported a median survival of 8–10 months when lomustine is administered alone or in combination with other agents [272–274].

The antiangiogenic agent Bevacizumab can be beneficial for patients with recurring enhancing tumors associated with huge cerebral edema, with symptoms relief and steroid-sparing effects [275, 276].

Patients with poor KPS should not be automatically excluded from salvage treatment, with routinely administration of supportive care, since an active therapeutic approach may be suitable for selected elderly and/or frail rGBM patients [269].

7.7.5 New Ongoing Prospectives

Targeted therapies represent an important field of research in the future management of glioblastoma, since standard therapies are poorly effective. Trials investigating safety and efficacy of new targeted agents in elderly GBM patients are currently lacking.

Molecular profiling could contribute to identify prognostic subgroups of elderly GBM who may benefit from new treatments.

Also, new immunotherapy strategies represent an interesting area of research in this setting.

A novel treatment modality for patients with GBM is represented by the tumor-treating fields (TTFields) device, a portable, battery-operated, device that generates TTFields. Results from a prospective phase III trial, comparing TTFields plus temozolomide vs. temozolomide alone after standard chemoradiation in patients with GBM have demonstrated significant longer survival and clinical improvement in those having TTFields plus temozolomide [277].

Extreme hypofractionation by means of stereotactic techniques may be adopted in elderly and poor performance status patients, due to its reduced transport needs and overall costs, with consequent better compliance to treatment [278]. Also, CNS tumoral cells have an intrinsic resistance to fractionated treatment [279]; therefore, a high-dose-per fraction approach may overcome this biological limit. Standard fractionation may have a lymphopenic effect, with long-lasting CD4 count reduction [280]; the adoption of an extreme hypofractionated schedule could represent a less immunosuppressive alternative.

Many fractionation schedules have been explored in clinical practice, starting from 1987 when Souhami et al. treated 15 patients with intracranial tumors with 6 fractions of 7 Gy each [281]. Nowadays, there are still two issues under current debate concerning target volume delineation (and margins) and fractionation schedule. In the former case, a 2-phase (targeting the peritumoral edema first and then the resection cavity plus residual enhancing tumor) or a single phase (resection cavity and residual tumor without edema) process has been adopted in different trials, with heterogeneous expanding margins and without any unified consensus. An aggressive margin restriction should be pursued cautiously due to concerns about pattern-of-failure, but with the advantage of lower exposure of normal brain tissue and decreased neurocognitive side effects. Regarding fractionation schedules, the highest tolerable dose per fraction over the shortest period would be the most biologically effective approach.

Prospective single arms trials have explored hypofractionated radiotherapy to escalate the equivalent dose to greater than 60 Gy over 6 weeks in a series of younger patients [282–287]. Most series adopted concomitant chemotherapy with temolozomide and/or bevacizumab. The

trial by Azoulay et al. [288] adopted a 5-days schedule with a maximum tolerated dose of 40 Gy (BED 72Gy) and with only 5 mm margin expansion and a median PTV of 60 cc. In the update of 2023 [289], *in-field* progression (within the 5-mm margin) occurred in 17 out of 30 patients, *marginal* (between 5 and 20 mm) in 3 patients and *distant* (beyond 20 mm) in 7. Only one patient could have benefitted from greater margin expansion.

In the next future SBRT could be integrated with immune checkpoint inhibitors. Due to its feasibility and immunomodulatory function, this approach deserves further clinical trial evaluation, especially in elderly patients who may benefit the most. Hypofractionation may lead to increased risk of radionecrosis, especially for larger targets; however, in Azoulay and colleagues' phase I/II study only grade 1–2 adverse events were reported. The adoption of bevacizumab might be a necessary component of such an aggressive approach.

Clinical trials evaluating the role of hypofractionated radiotherapy in primary GBM patients are reported in Table 7.5.

Concluding, glioblastoma in elderly patients is characterized by poor prognosis, with scarce treatment-response and increased risk of adverse events from therapy combination. The most appropriate strategy should be considered according to clinical (i.e., performance status) and molecular parameters (i.e., MGMTp methylation), in order to improve survival and quality of life. Current management includes surgery, RT and chemotherapy; elderly patients aged 70 years and older eligible for combined modality treatment should receive a short-course RT with concomitant and adjuvant temozolomide up to 12 cycles. Elderly patients with *MGMT* promoter methylation should be considered for temozolomide alone, especially in case of functional impairment and geriatric syndromes. Un-methylated patients not eligible for combined chemo-radiation should undergo hypofractionated RT. Supportive and palliative care should be considered with large or multifocal tumors and low KPS.

Table 7.5 Prospective clinical trials investigating the potential role of stereotactic body radiotherapy (SBRT) in newly diagnosed glioblastoma treatment

NCT number	Study type	Trial design	Contact and locations	Status
NCT04474353	Interventional, phase I	Safety of Tumor Treating Fields (TTFields) started concurrently with 5 fractions stereotactic radiosurgery (SRS) and temozolomide for newly diagnosed glioblastoma	Aniket Pratapneni, Stanford University	Active, recruiting
NCT03291990	Interventional, early phase I	Pilot study to assess feasibility of 5 fraction hypofractionated stereotactic radiosurgery along with standard temozolomide as a lymphocyte sparing therapy for glioblastoma multiforme	Lawrence Kleinberg, MD, Johns Hopkins (East Baltimore)	Completed
NCT05781321	Interventional, phase II	To demonstrate non-inferior 12-month overall survival (OS) of patients with GBM treated with dose-escalated hypofractionated radiotherapy compared to standard of care	William G. Breen, M.D., Mayo Clinic in Rochester	Recruiting
NCT04547621	Interventional, phase II	This study aims to evaluate the safety and effectiveness of the combination of 30 Gy/5 fx HSRT and 20 Gy/10 fx IMRT adjuvant therapy	Enmin Wang, MD, CyberKnife Center, Department of Neurosurgery, Huashan Hospital	Active, not recruiting

7.8 Conclusions

In conclusion, this chapter offers a comprehensive overview of the current landscape of glioblastoma (GBM) research and treatment strategies, addressing the complex challenges posed by this aggressive brain tumor. While progress has been made in understanding the molecular subgroups of GBM and refining standard radiotherapy protocols, there is a clear need for further research to harness the full potential of advanced imaging techniques, smaller treatment volumes, and radiosensitization methods. Additionally, the integration of immunotherapy into GBM treatment, despite presenting encouraging preclinical data, remains a field where clinical outcomes are yet to be fully realized. The management of elderly GBM patients is an evolving area that requires personalized approaches based on factors like performance status, comorbidities, and molecular features. As we look to the future, the investigation of promising therapies such as tumor-treating fields (TTFields) and targeted treatments, coupled with a deeper understanding of the immune-suppressive microenvironment in GBM, holds great potential. In conclusion, this chapter highlights both the progress achieved and the avenues for further exploration in the quest to improve outcomes for GBM patients.

References

1. Sung H, Ferlay J, Siegel RL, Laversanne M, Soerjomataram I, Jemal A, et al. Global Cancer Statistics 2020: GLOBOCAN estimates of incidence and mortality worldwide for 36 cancers in 185 countries. CA Cancer J Clin. 2021;71(3):209–49.
2. Ostrom QT, Bauchet L, Davis FG, Deltour I, Fisher JL, Langer CE, et al. The epidemiology of glioma in adults: a "state of the science" review. Neuro Oncol. 2014;16(7):896–913.
3. Louis DN. The 2021 WHO Classification of Tumors of the Central Nervous System: a summary. Neuro Oncol. 2021;23(8):1231–51.
4. Stupp R, Mason WP, van den Bent MJ, Weller M, Fisher B, Taphoorn MJ, et al. Radiotherapy plus concomitant and adjuvant temozolomide for glioblastoma. N Engl J Med. 2005;352(10):987–96.
5. Barani IJ, Larson DA. Radiation therapy of glioblastoma. Cancer Treat Res. 2015;163:49–73.
6. Walker MD, Alexander E Jr, Hunt WE, Leventhal CM, Mahaley MS Jr, Mealey J, et al. Evaluation of

mithramycin in the treatment of anaplastic gliomas. J Neurosurg. 1976;44(6):655–67.

7. Walker MD, Alexander E Jr, Hunt WE, MacCarty CS, Mahaley MS Jr, Mealey J Jr, et al. Evaluation of BCNU and/or radiotherapy in the treatment of anaplastic gliomas. A cooperative clinical trial. J Neurosurg. 1978;49(3):333–43.

8. Salazar OM, Rubin P, Feldstein ML, Pizzutiello R. High dose radiation therapy in the treatment of malignant gliomas: final report. Int J Radiat Oncol Biol Phys. 1979;5(10):1733–40.

9. Hochberg FH, Pruitt A. Assumptions in the radiotherapy of glioblastoma. Neurology. 1980;30(9):907–11.

10. Shapiro WR, Green SB, Burger PC, Mahaley MS Jr, Selker RG, VanGilder JC, et al. Randomized trial of three chemotherapy regimens and two radiotherapy regimens and two radiotherapy regimens in postoperative treatment of malignant glioma. Brain Tumor Cooperative Group Trial 8001. J Neurosurg. 1989;71(1):1–9.

11. Shapiro WR, Young DF. Treatment of malignant glioma. A controlled study of chemotherapy and irradiation. Arch Neurol. 1976;33(7):494–50.

12. Behrooz AB, Latifi-Navid H, Nezhadi A, Świat M, Los M, Jamalpoor Z, et al. Molecular mechanisms of microRNAs in glioblastoma pathogenesis. Biochim Biophys Acta Mol Cell Res. 2023;1870(6):119482.

13. Masui K, Mischel PS. Metabolic and epigenetic reprogramming in the pathogenesis of glioblastoma: toward the establishment of "metabolism-based pathology". Pathol Int. 2023;73(11):533–41.

14. Frosina G. Radiotherapy of high-grade gliomas: dealing with a stalemate. Crit Rev Oncol Hematol. 2023;190:104110.

15. Bernhard C, Reita D, Martin S, Entz-Werle N, Dontenwill M. Glioblastoma metabolism: insights and therapeutic strategies. Int J Mol Sci. 2023;24(11):9137.

16. Sturm D, Witt H, Hovestadt V, Khuong-Quang DA, Jones DT, Konermann C, et al. Hotspot mutations in H3F3A and IDH1 define distinct epigenetic and biological subgroups of glioblastoma. Cancer Cell. 2012;22(4):425–37.

17. Yan H, Parsons DW, Jin G, McLendon R, Rasheed BA, Yuan W, et al. IDH1 and IDH2 mutations in gliomas. N Engl J Med. 2009;360(8):765–73.

18. Hartmann C, Meyer J, Balss J, Capper D, Mueller W, Christians A, et al. Type and frequency of IDH1 and IDH2 mutations are related to astrocytic and oligodendroglial differentiation and age: a study of 1,010 diffuse gliomas. Acta Neuropathol. 2009;118(4):469–74.

19. Garber K. Oncometabolite? IDH1 discoveries raise possibility of new metabolism targets in brain cancers and leukemia. J Natl Cancer Inst. 2010;102(13):926–8.

20. Noushmehr H, Weisenberger DJ, Diefes K, Phillips HS, Pujara K, Berman BP, et al. Identification of a CpG island methylator phenotype that defines a distinct subgroup of glioma. Cancer Cell. 2010;17(5):510–22.

21. Chaudhry IH, O'Donovan DG, Brenchley PE, Reid H, Roberts IS. Vascular endothelial growth factor expression correlates with tumour grade and vascularity in gliomas. Histopathology. 2001;39(4):409–15.

22. Keunen O, Johansson M, Oudin A, Sanzey M, Rahim SA, Fack F, et al. Anti-VEGF treatment reduces blood supply and increases tumor cell invasion in glioblastoma. Proc Natl Acad Sci USA. 2011;108(9):3749–54.

23. Peiffer J, Kleihues P. Hans-Joachim Scherer (1906–1945), pioneer in glioma research. Brain Pathol. 1999;9(2):241–5.

24. Lyden D, Hattori K, Dias S, Costa C, Blaikie P, Butros L, et al. Impaired recruitment of bone-marrow-derived endothelial and hematopoietic precursor cells blocks tumor angiogenesis and growth. Nat Med. 2001;7(11):1194–201.

25. Vargas López AJ. Glioblastoma in adults: a Society for Neuro-Oncology (SNO) and European Society of Neuro-Oncology (EANO) consensus review on current management and future directions. Neuro Oncol. 2021;23(3):502–3.

26. Stupp R, Hegi ME, Mason WP, van den Bent MJ, Taphoorn MJ, Janzer RC, et al. Effects of radiotherapy with concomitant and adjuvant temozolomide versus radiotherapy alone on survival in glioblastoma in a randomised phase III study: 5-year analysis of the EORTC-NCIC trial. Lancet Oncol. 2009;10(5):459–66.

27. Hegi ME, Diserens AC, Gorlia T, Hamou MF, de Tribolet N, Weller M, et al. MGMT gene silencing and benefit from temozolomide in glioblastoma. N Engl J Med. 2005;352(10):997–1003.

28. Hegi ME, Stupp R. Withholding temozolomide in glioblastoma patients with unmethylated MGMT promoter—still a dilemma? Neuro Oncol. 2015;17(11):1425–7.

29. Stupp R, Taillibert S, Kanner A, Read W, Steinberg D, Lhermitte B, et al. Effect of tumor-treating fields plus maintenance temozolomide vs maintenance temozolomide alone on survival in patients with glioblastoma: a randomized clinical trial. JAMA. 2017;318(23):2306–16.

30. Gilbert MR, Wang M, Aldape KD, Stupp R, Hegi ME, Jaeckle KA, et al. Dose-dense temozolomide for newly diagnosed glioblastoma: a randomized phase III clinical trial. J Clin Oncol. 2013;31(32):4085–91.

31. Balana C, Vaz MA, Manuel Sepúlveda J, Mesia C, Del Barco S, Pineda E, et al. A phase II randomized, multicenter, open-label trial of continuing adjuvant temozolomide beyond 6 cycles in patients with glioblastoma (GEINO 14-01). Neuro Oncol. 2020;22(12):1851–61.

32. Gramatzki D, Kickingereder P, Hentschel B, Felsberg J, Herrlinger U, Schackert G, et al. Limited role for extended maintenance temozolo-

mide for newly diagnosed glioblastoma. Neurology. 2017;88(15):1422–30.

33. Chinot OL, Wick W, Mason W, Henriksson R, Saran F, Nishikawa R, et al. Bevacizumab plus radiotherapy-temozolomide for newly diagnosed glioblastoma. N Engl J Med. 2014;370(8):709–22.

34. Gilbert MR, Dignam JJ, Armstrong TS, Wefel JS, Blumenthal DT, Vogelbaum MA, et al. A randomized trial of bevacizumab for newly diagnosed glioblastoma. N Engl J Med. 2014;370(8):699–708.

35. Herrlinger U, Tzaridis T, Mack F, Steinbach JP, Schlegel U, Sabel M, et al. Lomustine-temozolomide combination therapy versus standard temozolomide therapy in patients with newly diagnosed glioblastoma with methylated MGMT promoter (CeTeG/NOA-09): a randomised, open-label, phase 3 trial. Lancet. 2019;393(10172):678–88.

36. Stupp R, Lukas RV, Hegi ME. Improving survival in molecularly selected glioblastoma. Lancet. 2019;393(10172):615–7.

37. Niyazi M, Brada M, Chalmers AJ, Combs SE, Erridge SC, Fiorentino A, et al. ESTRO-ACROP guideline "target delineation of glioblastomas". Radiother Oncol. 2016;118(1):35–42.

38. Kruser TJ, Bosch WR, Badiyan SN, Bovi JA, Ghia AJ, Kim MM, et al. NRG brain tumor specialists consensus guidelines for glioblastoma contouring. J Neurooncol. 2019;143(1):157–66.

39. Wernicke AG, Smith AW, Taube S, Mehta MP. Glioblastoma: radiation treatment margins, how small is large enough? Pract Radiat Oncol. 2016;6(5):298–305.

40. Brown PD, Chung C, Liu DD, McAvoy S, Grosshans D, Al Feghali K, et al. A prospective phase II randomized trial of proton radiotherapy vs intensity-modulated radiotherapy for patients with newly diagnosed glioblastoma. Neuro Oncol. 2021;23(8):1337–47.

41. CLIN-RADIATION THERAPY. Neuro Oncol. 2012;14(Suppl_6):vi133–41.

42. Paulsson AK, McMullen KP, Peiffer AM, Hinson WH, Kearns WT, Johnson AJ, et al. Limited margins using modern radiotherapy techniques does not increase marginal failure rate of glioblastoma. Am J Clin Oncol. 2014;37(2):177–81.

43. Grossman SA, Ye X, Piantadosi S, Desideri S, Nabors LB, Rosenfeld M, et al. Survival of patients with newly diagnosed glioblastoma treated with radiation and temozolomide in research studies in the United States. Clin Cancer Res. 2010;16(8):2443–9.

44. Grosu AL, Weber WA, Riedel E, Jeremic B, Nieder C, Franz M, et al. L-(methyl-11C) methionine positron emission tomography for target delineation in resected high-grade gliomas before radiotherapy. Int J Radiat Oncol Biol Phys. 2005;63(1):64–74.

45. Niyazi M, Andratschke N, Bendszus M, Chalmers AJ, Erridge SC, Galldiks N, et al. ESTRO-EANO guideline on target delineation and radiotherapy details for glioblastoma. Radiother Oncol. 2023;184:109663.

46. Pepper NB, Stummer W, Eich HT. The use of radiosensitizing agents in the therapy of glioblastoma multiforme—a comprehensive review. Strahlenther Onkol. 2022;198(6):507–26.

47. Overgaard J. Hypoxic modification of radiotherapy in squamous cell carcinoma of the head and neck—a systematic review and meta-analysis. Radiother Oncol. 2011;100(1):22–32.

48. Fulton DS, Urtasun RC, Shin KH, Geggie PH, Thomas H, Muller PJ, et al. Misonidazole combined with hyperfractionation in the management of malignant glioma. Int J Radiat Oncol Biol Phys. 1984;10(9):1709–12.

49. Asquith JC, Foster JL, Willson RL, Ings R, McFadzean JA. Metronidazole ("Flagyl"). A radiosensitizer of hypoxic cells. Br J Radiol. 1974;47(560):474–81.

50. Beppu T, Kamada K, Yoshida Y, Arai H, Ogasawara K, Ogawa A. Change of oxygen pressure in glioblastoma tissue under various conditions. J Neurooncol. 2002;58(1):47–52.

51. Kohshi K, Kinoshita Y, Terashima H, Konda N, Yokota A, Soejima T. Radiotherapy after hyperbaric oxygenation for malignant gliomas: a pilot study. J Cancer Res Clin Oncol. 1996;122(11):676–8.

52. Beppu T, Kamada K, Nakamura R, Oikawa H, Takeda M, Fukuda T, et al. A phase II study of radiotherapy after hyperbaric oxygenation combined with interferon-beta and nimustine hydrochloride to treat supratentorial malignant gliomas. J Neurooncol. 2003;61(2):161–70.

53. Ogawa K, Yoshii Y, Inoue O, Toita T, Saito A, Kakinohana Y, et al. Phase II trial of radiotherapy after hyperbaric oxygenation with chemotherapy for high-grade gliomas. Br J Cancer. 2006;95(7):862–8.

54. Kohshi K, Yamamoto H, Nakahara A, Katoh T, Takagi M. Fractionated stereotactic radiotherapy using gamma unit after hyperbaric oxygenation on recurrent high-grade gliomas. J Neurooncol. 2007;82(3):297–303.

55. Simon JM, Noël G, Chiras J, Hoang-Xuan K, Delattre JY, Baillet F, et al. Radiotherapy and chemotherapy with or without carbogen and nicotinamide in inoperable biopsy-proven glioblastoma multiforme. Radiother Oncol. 2003;67(1):45–51.

56. Pickles T, Graham P, Syndikus I, Rheaume DE, Duncan GG, Green A, et al. Tolerance of nicotinamide and carbogen with radiation therapy for glioblastoma. Radiother Oncol. 1996;40(3):245–7.

57. Lambin P, Poortmans P, Menten J, Hamers HP. Accelerated radiotherapy with carbogen and nicotinamide (ARCON) in high grade malignant gliomas. Radiother Oncol. 1997;43(3):324.

58. Miralbell R, Mornex F, Greiner R, Bolla M, Storme G, Hulshof M, et al. Accelerated radiotherapy, carbogen, and nicotinamide in glioblastoma multiforme: report of European Organization for Research and Treatment of Cancer trial 22933. J Clin Oncol. 1999;17(10):3143–9.

59. Moyal EC, Laprie A, Delannes M, Poublanc M, Catalaa I, Dalenc F, et al. Phase I trial of tipifarnib (R115777) concurrent with radiotherapy in patients with glioblastoma multiforme. Int J Radiat Oncol Biol Phys. 2007;68(5):1396–401.

60. Lustig R, Mikkelsen T, Lesser G, Grossman S, Ye X, Desideri S, et al. Phase II preradiation R115777 (tipifarnib) in newly diagnosed GBM with residual enhancing disease. Neuro Oncol. 2008;10(6):1004–9.

61. Nghiemphu PL, Ebiana VA, Wen P, Gilbert M, Abrey LE, Lieberman F, et al. Phase I study of sorafenib and tipifarnib for recurrent glioblastoma: NABTC 05-02. J Neurooncol. 2018;136(1):79–86.

62. Kleinberg L, Grossman SA, Carson K, Lesser G, O'Neill A, Pearlman J, et al. Survival of patients with newly diagnosed glioblastoma multiforme treated with RSR13 and radiotherapy: results of a phase II new approaches to brain tumor therapy CNS consortium safety and efficacy study. J Clin Oncol. 2002;20(14):3149–55.

63. Del Rowe J, Scott C, Werner-Wasik M, Bahary JP, Curran WJ, Urtasun RC, et al. Single-arm, open-label phase II study of intravenously administered tirapazamine and radiation therapy for glioblastoma multiforme. J Clin Oncol. 2000;18(6):1254–9.

64. Zimbrick JD, Ward JF, Myers LS Jr. Studies on the chemical basis of cellular radiosensitization by 5-bromouracil substitution in DNA. II. Pulse- and steadystate radiolysis of bromouracil-substituted and unsubstituted DNA. Int J Radiat Biol Relat Stud Phys Chem Med. 1969;16(6):525–34.

65. Kinsella TJ, Dobson PP, Mitchell JB, Fornace AJ Jr. Enhancement of X ray induced DNA damage by pretreatment with halogenated pyrimidine analogs. Int J Radiat Oncol Biol Phys. 1987;13(5):733–9.

66. Jackson D, Kinsella T, Rowland J, Wright D, Katz D, Main D, et al. Halogenated pyrimidines as radiosensitizers in the treatment of glioblastoma multiforme. Am J Clin Oncol. 1987;10(5):437–43.

67. Matsutani M, Kohno T, Nagashima T, Nagayama I, Matsuda T, Hoshino T, et al. Clinical trial of intravenous infusion of bromodeoxyuridine (BUdR) for radiosensitization of malignant brain tumors. Radiat Med. 1988;6(1):33–9.

68. Lesueur P, Chevalier F, El-Habr EA, Junier MP, Chneiweiss H, Castera L, et al. Radiosensitization effect of talazoparib, a parp inhibitor, on glioblastoma stem cells exposed to low and high linear energy transfer radiation. Sci Rep. 2018;8(1):3664.

69. Baxter PA, Su JM, Onar-Thomas A, Billups CA, Li XN, Poussaint TY, et al. A phase I/II study of veliparib (ABT-888) with radiation and temozolomide in newly diagnosed diffuse pontine glioma: a Pediatric Brain Tumor Consortium study. Neuro Oncol. 2020;22(6):875–85.

70. Hanna C, Kurian KM, Williams K, Watts C, Jackson A, Carruthers R, et al. Pharmacokinetics, safety, and tolerability of olaparib and temozolomide for recurrent glioblastoma: results of the phase I OPARATIC trial. Neuro Oncol. 2020;22(12):1840–50.

71. Sim HW, McDonald KL, Lwin Z, Barnes EH, Rosenthal M, Foote MC, et al. A randomized phase II trial of veliparib, radiotherapy, and temozolomide in patients with unmethylated MGMT glioblastoma: the VERTU study. Neuro Oncol. 2021;23(10):1736–49.

72. Lesueur P, Lequesne J, Grellard JM, Dugué A, Coquan E, Brachet PE, et al. Phase I/IIa study of concomitant radiotherapy with olaparib and temozolomide in unresectable or partially resectable glioblastoma: OLA-TMZ-RTE-01 trial protocol. BMC Cancer. 2019;19(1):198.

73. Ford JM, Seiferheld W, Alger JR, Wu G, Endicott TJ, Mehta M, et al. Results of the phase I dose-escalating study of motexafin gadolinium with standard radiotherapy in patients with glioblastoma multiforme. Int J Radiat Oncol Biol Phys. 2007;69(3):831–8.

74. Wu GN, Ford JM, Alger JR. MRI measurement of the uptake and retention of motexafin gadolinium in glioblastoma multiforme and uninvolved normal human brain. J Neurooncol. 2006;77(1):95–103.

75. Prados MD, Wara WM, Sneed PK, McDermott M, Chang SM, Rabbitt J, et al. Phase III trial of accelerated hyperfractionation with or without difluoromethylornithine (DFMO) versus standard fractionated radiotherapy with or without DFMO for newly diagnosed patients with glioblastoma multiforme. Int J Radiat Oncol Biol Phys. 2001;49(1):71–7.

76. Dillman RO, Wiemann M, Oldham RK, Soori G, Bury M, Hafer R, et al. Interferon alpha-2a and external beam radiotherapy in the initial management of patients with glioma: a pilot study of the National Biotherapy Study Group. Cancer Biother. 1995;10(4):265–71.

77. Nübel T, Damrot J, Roos WP, Kaina B, Fritz G. Lovastatin protects human endothelial cells from killing by ionizing radiation without impairing induction and repair of DNA double-strand breaks. Clin Cancer Res. 2006;12(3 Pt 1):933–9.

78. Larner J, Jane J, Laws E, Packer R, Myers C, Shaffrey M. A phase I–II trial of lovastatin for anaplastic astrocytoma and glioblastoma multiforme. Am J Clin Oncol. 1998;21(6):579–83.

79. Happold C, Gorlia T, Nabors LB, Erridge SC, Reardon DA, Hicking C, et al. Do statins, ACE inhibitors or sartans improve outcome in primary glioblastoma? J Neurooncol. 2018;138(1):163–71.

80. Haritz D, Gabel D, Huiskamp R. Clinical phase-I study of Na2B12H11SH (BSH) in patients with malignant glioma as precondition for boron neutron capture therapy (BNCT). Int J Radiat Oncol Biol Phys. 1994;28(5):1175–81.

81. Palmer MR, Goorley JT, Kiger WS, Busse PM, Riley KJ, Harling OK, et al. Treatment planning and dosimetry for the Harvard-MIT Phase I clinical trial of cranial neutron capture therapy. Int J Radiat Oncol Biol Phys. 2002;53(5):1361–79.

82. Takagaki M, Oda Y, Miyatake S, Kikuchi H, Kobayashi T, Sakurai Y, et al. Boron neutron capture therapy: preliminary study of BNCT with sodium borocaptate (Na2B1 2H1 1SH) on glioblastoma. J Neurooncol. 1997;35(2):177–85.

83. Kageji T, Mizobuchi Y, Nagahiro S, Nakagawa Y, Kumada H. Correlation between radiation dose and histopathological findings in patients with gliblastoma treated with boron neutron capture therapy (BNCT). Appl Radiat Isot. 2014;88:20–2.

84. Henriksson R, Capala J, Michanek A, Lindahl SA, Salford LG, Franzén L, et al. Boron neutron capture therapy (BNCT) for glioblastoma multiforme: a phase II study evaluating a prolonged high-dose of boronophenylalanine (BPA). Radiother Oncol. 2008;88(2):183–91.

85. Sander A, Wosniok W, Gabel D. Case numbers for a randomized clinical trial of boron neutron capture therapy for Glioblastoma multiforme. Appl Radiat Isot. 2014;88:16–9.

86. Stummer W, Pichlmeier U, Meinel T, Wiestler OD, Zanella F, Reulen HJ. Fluorescence-guided surgery with 5-aminolevulinic acid for resection of malignant glioma: a randomised controlled multicentre phase III trial. Lancet Oncol. 2006;7(5):392–401.

87. Ueta K, Yamamoto J, Tanaka T, Nakano Y, Kitagawa T, Nishizawa S. 5-Aminolevulinic acid enhances mitochondrial stress upon ionizing irradiation exposure and increases delayed production of reactive oxygen species and cell death in glioma cells. Int J Mol Med. 2017;39(2):387–98.

88. Kitagawa T, Yamamoto J, Tanaka T, Nakano Y, Akiba D, Ueta K, et al. 5-Aminolevulinic acid strongly enhances delayed intracellular production of reactive oxygen species (ROS) generated by ionizing irradiation: quantitative analyses and visualization of intracellular ROS production in glioma cells in vitro. Oncol Rep. 2015;33(2):583–90.

89. Gaber M, Selim H, El-Nahas T. Prospective study evaluating the radiosensitizing effect of reduced doses of temozolomide in the treatment of Egyptian patients with glioblastoma multiforme. Cancer Manag Res. 2013;5:349–56.

90. Weller M, Le Rhun E. How did lomustine become standard of care in recurrent glioblastoma? Cancer Treat Rev. 2020;87:102029.

91. Miller AC, Blakely WF. Inhibition of glutathione reductase activity by a carbamoylating nitrosourea: effect on cellular radiosensitivity. Free Radic Biol Med. 1992;12(1):53–62.

92. Murphy C, Pickles T, Knowling M, Thiesse B. Concurrent modified PCV chemotherapy and radiotherapy in newly diagnosed grade IV astrocytoma. J Neurooncol. 2002;57(3):215–20.

93. Roberts PB. Radiosensitization of E. coli B/r by the cytotoxic agent procarbazine: a hypoxic cell sensitizer preferentially toxic to aerobic cells and easily oxidized. Br J Cancer. 1979;39(6):755–60.

94. Cairncross G, Wang M, Shaw E, Jenkins R, Brachman D, Buckner J, et al. Phase III trial of chemoradiotherapy for anaplastic oligodendroglioma: long-term results of RTOG 9402. J Clin Oncol. 2013;31(3):337–43.

95. Liebmann J, Cook JA, Fisher J, Teague D, Mitchell JB. In vitro studies of Taxol as a radiation sensitizer in human tumor cells. J Natl Cancer Inst. 1994;86(6):441–6.

96. Lederman G, Wronski M, Arbit E, Odaimi M, Wertheim S, Lombardi E, et al. Treatment of recurrent glioblastoma multiforme using fractionated stereotactic radiosurgery and concurrent paclitaxel. Am J Clin Oncol. 2000;23(2):155–9.

97. Ashamalla H, Zaki B, Mokhtar B, Lewis L, Lavaf A, Nasr H, et al. Fractionated stereotactic radiotherapy boost and weekly paclitaxel in malignant gliomas clinical and pharmacokinetics results. Technol Cancer Res Treat. 2007;6(3):169–76.

98. Ojima E, Inoue Y, Watanabe H, Hiro J, Toiyama Y, Miki C, et al. The optimal schedule for 5-fluorouracil radiosensitization in colon cancer cell lines. Oncol Rep. 2006;16(5):1085–91.

99. Shapiro WR, Green SB, Burger PC, Selker RG, VanGilder JC, Robertson JT, et al. A randomized comparison of intra-arterial versus intravenous BCNU, with or without intravenous 5-fluorouracil, for newly diagnosed patients with malignant glioma. J Neurosurg. 1992;76(5):772–81.

100. Grunda JM, Fiveash J, Palmer CA, Cantor A, Fathallah-Shaykh HM, Nabors LB, et al. Rationally designed pharmacogenomic treatment using concurrent capecitabine and radiotherapy for glioblastoma; gene expression profiles associated with outcome. Clin Cancer Res. 2010;16(10):2890–8.

101. Vokes EE, Dolan ME, Krishnasamy S, Mick R, Ratain MJ, Berezin F, et al. 5-Fluorouracil, hydroxyurea and escalating doses of iododeoxyuridine with concomitant radiotherapy for malignant gliomas: a clinical and pharmacologic analysis. Ann Oncol. 1993;4(7):591–5.

102. Larner JM, Phillips CD, Dion JE, Jensen ME, Newman SA, Jane JA. A phase 1–2 trial of superselective carboplatin, low-dose infusional 5-fluorouracil and concurrent radiation for high-grade gliomas. Am J Clin Oncol. 1995;18(1):1–7.

103. Sigmond J, Honeywell RJ, Postma TJ, Dirven CM, de Lange SM, van der Born K, et al. Gemcitabine uptake in glioblastoma multiforme: potential as a radiosensitizer. Ann Oncol. 2009;20(1):182–7.

104. Metro G, Fabi A, Mirri MA, Vidiri A, Pace A, Carosi M, et al. Phase II study of fixed dose rate gemcitabine as radiosensitizer for newly diagnosed glioblastoma multiforme. Cancer Chemother Pharmacol. 2010;65(2):391–7.

105. Weller M, Streffer J, Wick W, Kortmann RD, Heiss E, Küker W, et al. Preirradiation gemcitabine chemotherapy for newly diagnosed glioblastoma. A phase II study. Cancer. 2001;91(2):423–7.

106. Gertler SZ, MacDonald D, Goodyear M, Forsyth P, Stewart DJ, Belanger K, et al. NCIC-CTG phase

II study of gemcitabine in patients with malignant glioma (IND.94). Ann Oncol. 2000;11(3):315–8.

107. Bastiancich C, Lemaire L, Bianco J, Franconi F, Danhier F, Préat V, et al. Evaluation of lauroyl-gemcitabine-loaded hydrogel efficacy in glioblastoma rat models. Nanomedicine (Lond). 2018;13(16):1999–2013.

108. Boeckman HJ, Trego KS, Turchi JJ. Cisplatin sensitizes cancer cells to ionizing radiation via inhibition of nonhomologous end joining. Mol Cancer Res. 2005;3(5):277–85.

109. Buckner JC, Ballman KV, Michalak JC, Burton GV, Cascino TL, Schomberg PJ, et al. Phase III trial of carmustine and cisplatin compared with carmustine alone and standard radiation therapy or accelerated radiation therapy in patients with glioblastoma multiforme: North Central Cancer Treatment Group 93-72-52 and Southwest Oncology Group 9503 Trials. J Clin Oncol. 2006;24(24):3871–9.

110. Elleaume H, Barth RF, Rousseau J, Bobyk L, Balosso J, Yang W, et al. Radiation therapy combined with intracerebral convection-enhanced delivery of cisplatin or carboplatin for treatment of the F98 rat glioma. J Neurooncol. 2020;149(2):193–208.

111. Niyazi M, Harter PN, Hattingen E, Rottler M, von Baumgarten L, Proescholdt M, et al. Bevacizumab and radiotherapy for the treatment of glioblastoma: brothers in arms or unholy alliance? Oncotarget. 2016;7(3):2313–28.

112. McGee MC, Hamner JB, Williams RF, Rosati SF, Sims TL, Ng CY, et al. Improved intratumoral oxygenation through vascular normalization increases glioma sensitivity to ionizing radiation. Int J Radiat Oncol Biol Phys. 2010;76(5):1537–45.

113. Vredenburgh JJ, Desjardins A, Herndon JE II, Marcello J, Reardon DA, Quinn JA, et al. Bevacizumab plus irinotecan in recurrent glioblastoma multiforme. J Clin Oncol. 2007;25(30):4722–9.

114. Srinivasan S, Dasgupta A, Chatterjee A, Baheti A, Engineer R, Gupta T, et al. The promise of magnetic resonance imaging in radiation oncology practice in the management of brain, prostate, and GI malignancies. JCO Glob Oncol. 2022;8:e2100366.

115. Thornton AF Jr, Sandler HM, Ten Haken RK, McShan DL, Fraass BA, La Vigne ML, et al. The clinical utility of magnetic resonance imaging in 3-dimensional treatment planning of brain neoplasms. Int J Radiat Oncol Biol Phys. 1992;24(4):767–75.

116. Stall B, Zach L, Ning H, Ondos J, Arora B, Shankavaram U, et al. Comparison of T2 and FLAIR imaging for target delineation in high grade gliomas. Radiat Oncol. 2010;5:5.

117. Pirzkall A, McKnight TR, Graves EE, Carol MP, Sneed PK, Wara WW, et al. MR-spectroscopy guided target delineation for high-grade gliomas. Int J Radiat Oncol Biol Phys. 2001;50(4):915–28.

118. Chaumeil MM, Lupo JM, Ronen SM. Magnetic resonance (MR) metabolic imaging in glioma. Brain Pathol. 2015;25(6):769–80.

119. Parra NA, Maudsley AA, Gupta RK, Ishkanian F, Huang K, Walker GR, et al. Volumetric spectroscopic imaging of glioblastoma multiforme radiation treatment volumes. Int J Radiat Oncol Biol Phys. 2014;90(2):376–84.

120. Cordova JS, Kandula S, Gurbani S, Zhong J, Tejani M, Kayode O, et al. Simulating the effect of spectroscopic MRI as a metric for radiation therapy planning in patients with glioblastoma. Tomography. 2016;2(4):366–73.

121. Press RH, Zhong J, Gurbani SS, Weinberg BD, Eaton BR, Shim H, et al. The role of standard and advanced imaging for the management of brain malignancies from a radiation oncology standpoint. Neurosurgery. 2019;85(2):165–79.

122. Ken S, Vieillevigne L, Franceries X, Simon L, Supper C, Lotterie JA, et al. Integration method of 3D MR spectroscopy into treatment planning system for glioblastoma IMRT dose painting with integrated simultaneous boost. Radiat Oncol. 2013;8:1.

123. Laprie A, Ken S, Filleron T, Lubrano V, Vieillevigne L, Tensaouti F, et al. Dose-painting multicenter phase III trial in newly diagnosed glioblastoma: the SPECTRO-GLIO trial comparing arm A standard radiochemotherapy to arm B radiochemotherapy with simultaneous integrated boost guided by MR spectroscopic imaging. BMC Cancer. 2019;19(1):167.

124. Gurbani S, Weinberg B, Cooper L, Mellon E, Schreibmann E, Sheriff S, et al. The Brain Imaging Collaboration Suite (BrICS): a cloud platform for integrating whole-brain spectroscopic MRI into the radiation therapy planning workflow. Tomography. 2019;5(1):184–91.

125. Le Bihan D. Looking into the functional architecture of the brain with diffusion MRI. Nat Rev Neurosci. 2003;4(6):469–80.

126. Maier SE, Sun Y, Mulkern RV. Diffusion imaging of brain tumors. NMR Biomed. 2010;23(7):849–64.

127. Pramanik PP, Parmar HA, Mammoser AG, Junck LR, Kim MM, Tsien CI, et al. Hypercellularity components of glioblastoma identified by high b-value diffusion-weighted imaging. Int J Radiat Oncol Biol Phys. 2015;92(4):811–9.

128. Giese A, Bjerkvig R, Berens ME, Westphal M. Cost of migration: invasion of malignant gliomas and implications for treatment. J Clin Oncol. 2003;21(8):1624–36.

129. Jordan K, Morin O, Wahl M, Amirbekian B, Chapman C, Owen J, et al. An open-source tool for anisotropic radiation therapy planning in neuro-oncology using DW-MRI tractography. Front Oncol. 2019;9:810.

130. Sternberg EJ, Lipton ML, Burns J. Utility of diffusion tensor imaging in evaluation of the peritumoral region in patients with primary and metastatic brain tumors. AJNR Am J Neuroradiol. 2014;35(3):439–44.

131. Jena R, Price SJ, Baker C, Jefferies SJ, Pickard JD, Gillard JH, et al. Diffusion tensor imaging: possible

implications for radiotherapy treatment planning of patients with high-grade glioma. Clin Oncol (R Coll Radiol). 2005;17(8):581–90.

132. Berberat J, McNamara J, Remonda L, Bodis S, Rogers S. Diffusion tensor imaging for target volume definition in glioblastoma multiforme. Strahlenther Onkol. 2014;190(10):939–43.

133. Law M, Yang S, Wang H, Babb JS, Johnson G, Cha S, et al. Glioma grading: sensitivity, specificity, and predictive values of perfusion MR imaging and proton MR spectroscopic imaging compared with conventional MR imaging. AJNR Am J Neuroradiol. 2003;24(10):1989–98.

134. Price SJ, Green HA, Dean AF, Joseph J, Hutchinson PJ, Gillard JH. Correlation of MR relative cerebral blood volume measurements with cellular density and proliferation in high-grade gliomas: an image-guided biopsy study. AJNR Am J Neuroradiol. 2011;32(3):501–6.

135. Mardaleishvili K, Orkodashvili G. Use of perfusion MRI for determination of irradiation volumes in radiotherapy of patients with brain glioma. Georgian Med News. 2018;278:30–3.

136. Christen T, Schmiedeskamp H, Straka M, Bammer R, Zaharchuk G. Measuring brain oxygenation in humans using a multiparametric quantitative blood oxygenation level dependent MRI approach. Magn Reson Med. 2012;68(3):905–11.

137. Stadlbauer A, Zimmermann M, Kitzwögerer M, Oberndorfer S, Rössler K, Dörfler A, et al. MR imaging-derived oxygen metabolism and neovascularization characterization for grading and IDH gene mutation detection of gliomas. Radiology. 2017;283(3):799–809.

138. Langen KJ, Galldiks N, Hattingen E, Shah NJ. Advances in neuro-oncology imaging. Nat Rev Neurol. 2017;13(5):279–89.

139. Galldiks N, Niyazi M, Grosu AL, Kocher M, Langen KJ, Law I, et al. Contribution of PET imaging to radiotherapy planning and monitoring in glioma patients—a report of the PET/RANO group. Neuro Oncol. 2021;23(6):881–93.

140. Bekaert L, Valable S, Lechapt-Zalcman E, Ponte K, Collet S, Constans JM, et al. [18F]-FMISO PET study of hypoxia in gliomas before surgery: correlation with molecular markers of hypoxia and angiogenesis. Eur J Nucl Med Mol Imaging. 2017;44(8):1383–92.

141. Brighi C, Puttick S, Woods A, Keall P, Tooney PA, Waddington DEJ, Sproule V, Rose S, Fay M. Comparison between [68Ga]Ga-PSMA-617 and [18F]FET PET as imaging biomarkers in adult recurrent glioblastoma. Int J Mol Sci. 2023;24(22):16208.

142. Matsuo M, Miwa K, Tanaka O, Shinoda J, Nishibori H, Tsuge Y, et al. Impact of [11C]methionine positron emission tomography for target definition of glioblastoma multiforme in radiation therapy planning. Int J Radiat Oncol Biol Phys. 2012;82(1):83–9.

143. Mahasittiwat P, Mizoe JE, Hasegawa A, Ishikawa H, Yoshikawa K, Mizuno H, et al. l-[METHYL-(11)C]

methionine positron emission tomography for target delineation in malignant gliomas: impact on results of carbon ion radiotherapy. Int J Radiat Oncol Biol Phys. 2008;70(2):515–22.

144. Lohmann P, Stavrinou P, Lipke K, Bauer EK, Ceccon G, Werner JM, et al. FET PET reveals considerable spatial differences in tumour burden compared to conventional MRI in newly diagnosed glioblastoma. Eur J Nucl Med Mol Imaging. 2019;46(3):591–602.

145. Weber DC, Zilli T, Buchegger F, Casanova N, Haller G, Rouzaud M, et al. [(18)F]Fluoroethyltyrosine-positron emission tomography-guided radiotherapy for high-grade glioma. Radiat Oncol. 2008;3:44.

146. Niyazi M, Geisler J, Siefert A, Schwarz SB, Ganswindt U, Garny S, et al. FET-PET for malignant glioma treatment planning. Radiother Oncol. 2011;99(1):44–8.

147. Munck Af Rosenschold P, Costa J, Engelholm SA, Lundemann MJ, Law I, Ohlhues L, et al. Impact of [18F]-fluoro-ethyl-tyrosine PET imaging on target definition for radiation therapy of high-grade glioma. Neuro Oncol. 2015;17(5):757–63.

148. Pafundi DH, Laack NN, Youland RS, Parney IF, Lowe VJ, Giannini C, et al. Biopsy validation of 18F-DOPA PET and biodistribution in gliomas for neurosurgical planning and radiotherapy target delineation: results of a prospective pilot study. Neuro Oncol. 2013;15(8):1058–67.

149. Kosztyla R, Chan EK, Hsu F, Wilson D, Ma R, Cheung A, et al. High-grade glioma radiation therapy target volumes and patterns of failure obtained from magnetic resonance imaging and 18F-FDOPA positron emission tomography delineations from multiple observers. Int J Radiat Oncol Biol Phys. 2013;87(5):1100–6.

150. Lapa C, Linsenmann T, Monoranu CM, Samnick S, Buck AK, Bluemel C, et al. Comparison of the amino acid tracers 18F-FET and 18F-DOPA in high-grade glioma patients. J Nucl Med. 2014;55(10):1611–6.

151. Becherer A, Karanikas G, Szabó M, Zettinig G, Asenbaum S, Marosi C, et al. Brain tumour imaging with PET: a comparison between [18F]fluorodopa and [11C]methionine. Eur J Nucl Med Mol Imaging. 2003;30(11):1561–7.

152. Pauleit D, Floeth F, Hamacher K, Riemenschneider MJ, Reifenberger G, Müller HW, et al. O-(2-[18F]fluoroethyl)-L-tyrosine PET combined with MRI improves the diagnostic assessment of cerebral gliomas. Brain. 2005;128(Pt 3):678–87.

153. Jansen NL, Suchorska B, Wenter V, Eigenbrod S, Schmid-Tannwald C, Zwergal A, et al. Dynamic 18F-FET PET in newly diagnosed astrocytic low-grade glioma identifies high-risk patients. J Nucl Med. 2014;55(2):198–203.

154. Antoch G, Bockisch A. Combined PET/MRI: a new dimension in whole-body oncology imaging? Eur J Nucl Med Mol Imaging. 2009;36(Suppl 1):S113–20.

155. Corradini S, Alongi F, Andratschke N, Belka C, Boldrini L, Cellini F, et al. MR-guidance in clinical

reality: current treatment challenges and future perspectives. Radiat Oncol. 2019;14(1):92.

156. Hall WA, Paulson ES, van der Heide UA, Fuller CD, Raaymakers BW, Lagendijk JJW, et al. The transformation of radiation oncology using real-time magnetic resonance guidance: a review. Eur J Cancer. 2019;122:42–52.

157. Snyder JE, St-Aubin J, Yaddanapudi S, Boczkowski A, Dunkerley DAP, Graves SA, et al. Commissioning of a 1.5T Elekta Unity MR-linac: a single institution experience. J Appl Clin Med Phys. 2020;21(7):160–72.

158. Mehta S, Gajjar SR, Padgett KR, Asher D, Stoyanova R, Ford JC, et al. Daily tracking of glioblastoma resection cavity, cerebral edema, and tumor volume with MRI-guided radiation therapy. Cureus. 2018;10(3):e2346.

159. Stewart J, Sahgal A, Lee Y, Soliman H, Tseng CL, Detsky J, et al. Quantitating interfraction target dynamics during concurrent chemoradiation for glioblastoma: a prospective serial imaging study. Int J Radiat Oncol Biol Phys. 2021;109(3):736–46.

160. Cuccia F, Alongi F, Belka C, Boldrini L, Hörner-Rieber J, McNair H, et al. Patient positioning and immobilization procedures for hybrid MR-Linac systems. Radiat Oncol. 2021;16(1):183.

161. Guerini AE, Nici S, Magrini SM, Riga S, Toraci C, Pegurri L, et al. Adoption of hybrid MRI-Linac systems for the treatment of brain tumors: a systematic review of the current literature regarding clinical and technical features. Technol Cancer Res Treat. 2023;22:15330338231199286.

162. Şenkesen Ö, Tezcanlı E, Abacıoğlu MU, Özen Z, Çöne D, Küçücük H, et al. Limited field adaptive radiotherapy for glioblastoma: changes in target volume and organ at risk doses. Radiat Oncol J. 2022;40(1):9–19.

163. Shukla D, Huilgol NG, Trivedi N, Mekala C. T2 weighted MRI in assessment of volume changes during radiotherapy of high grade gliomas. J Cancer Res Ther. 2005;1(4):235–8.

164. Tyyger M, Bhaumik S, Nix M, Currie S, Nallathambi C, Speight R, et al. Volumetric and dosimetric impact of post-surgical MRI-guided radiotherapy for glioblastoma: a pilot study. BJR Open. 2021;3(1):20210067.

165. Kim TG, Lim DH. Interfractional variation of radiation target and adaptive radiotherapy for totally resected glioblastoma. J Korean Med Sci. 2013;28(8):1233–7.

166. Maziero D, Straza MW, Ford JC, Bovi JA, Diwanji T, Stoyanova R, et al. MR-guided radiotherapy for brain and spine tumors. Front Oncol. 2021;11:626100.

167. Bianconi A. Updates in glioblastoma immunotherapy: an overview of the current clinical and translational scenario. Biomedicines. 2023;11(6):1520.

168. Louveau A. Structural and functional features of central nervous system lymphatic vessels. Nature. 2015;523(7560):337–41.

169. Huettner C, Paulus W, Roggendorf W. Messenger RNA expression of the immunosuppressive cytokine IL-10 in human gliomas. Am J Pathol. 1995;146(2):317–22.

170. Lim M, Xia Y, Bettegowda C, Weller M. Current state of immunotherapy for glioblastoma. Nat Rev Clin Oncol. 2018;15(7):422–42.

171. Jiang J, Qiu J, Li Q, Shi Z. Prostaglandin E2 signaling: alternative target for glioblastoma? Trends Cancer. 2017;3(2):75–8.

172. Nduom EK. PD-L1 expression and prognostic impact in glioblastoma. Neuro Oncol. 2016;18(2):195–205.

173. Davidson TB. Expression of PD-1 by T cells in malignant glioma patients reflects exhaustion and activation. Clin Cancer Res. 2019;25(6):1913–22.

174. Gratas C. Fas ligand expression in glioblastoma cell lines and primary astrocytic brain tumors. Brain Pathol. 1997;7(3):863–9.

175. Liu F, Huang J, Liu X, Cheng Q, Luo C, Liu Z. CTLA-4 correlates with immune and clinical characteristics of glioma. Cancer Cell Int. 2020;20:7.

176. Hulse RE, Swenson WG, Kunkler PE, White DM, Kraig RP. Monomeric IgG is neuroprotective via enhancing microglial recycling endocytosis and TNF-α. J Neurosci. 2008;28(47):12199–211.

177. Dovedi SJ. Acquired resistance to fractionated radiotherapy can be overcome by concurrent PD-L1 blockade. Cancer Res. 2014;74(19):5458–68.

178. Derer A. Chemoradiation increases PD-L1 expression in certain melanoma and glioblastoma cells. Front Immunol. 2016;7:610.

179. Szulzewsky F. Glioma-associated microglia/macrophages display an expression profile different from M1 and M2 polarization and highly express Gpnmb and Spp1. PLoS One. 2015;10(2):0116644.

180. Zhou W. Periostin secreted by glioblastoma stem cells recruits M2 tumour-associated macrophages and promotes malignant growth. Nat Cell Biol. 2015;17(2):170–82.

181. Komohara Y, Ohnishi K, Kuratsu J, Takeya M. Possible involvement of the M2 anti-inflammatory macrophage phenotype in growth of human gliomas. J Pathol. 2008;216(1):15–24.

182. Bussel MTJ, Beijnen JH, Brandsma D. Intracranial antitumor responses of nivolumab and ipilimumab: a pharmacodynamic and pharmacokinetic perspective, a scoping systematic review. BMC Cancer. 2019;19(1):519.

183. Ghouzlani A, Kandoussi S, Tall M, Reddy KP, Rafii S, Badou A. Immune checkpoint inhibitors in human glioma microenvironment. Front Immunol. 2021;12:679425.

184. Pinheiro SLR. Immunotherapy in glioblastoma treatment: current state and future prospects. World J Clin Oncol. 2023;14(4):138–59.

185. Park J. Effect of combined anti-PD-1 and temozolomide therapy in glioblastoma. Oncoimmunology. 2019;8(1):1525243.

186. Reardon DA. Effect of nivolumab vs bevacizumab in patients with recurrent glioblastoma: the CheckMate

143 phase 3 randomized clinical trial. JAMA Oncol. 2020;6(7):1003–10.

187. Omuro A. Radiotherapy combined with nivolumab or temozolomide for newly diagnosed glioblastoma with unmethylated MGMT promoter: an international randomized phase III trial. Neuro Oncol. 2023;25(1):123–34.

188. Lim M. Phase III trial of chemoradiotherapy with temozolomide plus nivolumab or placebo for newly diagnosed glioblastoma with methylated MGMT promoter. Neuro Oncol. 2022;24(11):1935–49.

189. Ott PA. T-cell-inflamed gene-expression profile, programmed death ligand 1 expression, and tumor mutational burden predict efficacy in patients treated with pembrolizumab across 20 cancers: KEYNOTE-028. J Clin Oncol. 2019;37(4):318–27.

190. Lukas RV. Clinical activity and safety of atezolizumab in patients with recurrent glioblastoma. J Neurooncol. 2018;140(2):317–28.

191. Reardon DA. Phase 2 study to evaluate safety and efficacy of MEDI4736 (durvalumab [DUR]) in glioblastoma (GBM) patients: an update. J Clin Oncol. 2017;35(15_Suppl):2042.

192. Jacques FH. Avelumab in newly diagnosed glioblastoma. Neurooncol Adv. 2021;3(1):118.

193. Awada G. Axitinib plus avelumab in the treatment of recurrent glioblastoma: a stratified, open-label, single-center phase 2 clinical trial (GliAvAx). J Immunother Cancer. 2020;8(2):001146.

194. Reardon DA. OS10.3 randomized phase 3 study evaluating the efficacy and safety of nivolumab vs bevacizumab in patients with recurrent glioblastoma: CheckMate 143. Neuro Oncol. 2017;19(Suppl_3):21.

195. Duerinck J. Intracerebral administration of CTLA-4 and PD-1 immune checkpoint blocking monoclonal antibodies in patients with recurrent glioblastoma: a phase I clinical trial. J Immunother Cancer. 2021;9(6):002296.

196. Liu Z. Expression of the galectin-9-Tim-3 pathway in glioma tissues is associated with the clinical manifestations of glioma. Oncol Lett. 2016;11(3):1829–34.

197. Schalper KA. Neoadjuvant nivolumab modifies the tumor immune microenvironment in resectable glioblastoma. Nat Med. 2019;25(3):470–6.

198. Cloughesy TF. Neoadjuvant anti-PD-1 immunotherapy promotes a survival benefit with intratumoral and systemic immune responses in recurrent glioblastoma. Nat Med. 2019;25(3):477–86.

199. Yang T, Kong Z, Ma W. PD-1/PD-L1 immune checkpoint inhibitors in glioblastoma: clinical studies, challenges and potential. Hum Vaccin Immunother. 2021;17(2):546–53.

200. Berghoff AS. Programmed death ligand 1 expression and tumor-infiltrating lymphocytes in glioblastoma. Neuro Oncol. 2015;17(8):1064–75.

201. Hodges TR. Mutational burden, immune checkpoint expression, and mismatch repair in glioma: implications for immune checkpoint immunotherapy. Neuro Oncol. 2017;19(8):1047–57.

202. Campbell BB. Comprehensive analysis of hypermutation in human cancer. Cell. 2017;171(5):1042–56. e10.

203. Bouffet E. Immune checkpoint inhibition for hypermutant glioblastoma multiforme resulting from germline biallelic mismatch repair deficiency. J Clin Oncol. 2016;34(19):2206–11.

204. Johnson A. Comprehensive genomic profiling of 282 pediatric low- and high-grade gliomas reveals genomic drivers, tumor mutational burden, and hypermutation signatures. Oncologist. 2017;22(12):1478–90.

205. Lombardi G. Pembrolizumab (Pem) in recurrent high-grade glioma (HGG) patients (PTS) with mismatch repair deficiency (MMRd): an observational study. J Clin Oncol. 2019;37(15_Suppl):2043.

206. Nayak L. The Neurologic Assessment in Neuro-Oncology (NANO) scale: a tool to assess neurologic function for integration into the Response Assessment in Neuro-Oncology (RANO) criteria. Neuro Oncol. 2017;19(5):625–35.

207. Okada H. Immunotherapy response assessment in neuro-oncology: a report of the RANO working group. Lancet Oncol. 2015;16(15):534–42.

208. Loi M. Radiotherapy in the age of cancer immunology: current concepts and future developments. Crit Rev Oncol Hematol. 2017;112:1–10.

209. Spiotto M, Fu Y-X, Weichselbaum RR. The intersection of radiotherapy and immunotherapy: mechanisms and clinical implications. Sci Immunol. 1266;1(3):EAAG1266.

210. Zeng J. Anti-PD-1 blockade and stereotactic radiation produce long-term survival in mice with intracranial gliomas. Int J Radiat Oncol Biol Phys. 2013;86(2):343–9.

211. Sahebjam S. Hypofractionated stereotactic re-irradiation with pembrolizumab and bevacizumab in patients with recurrent high-grade gliomas: results from a phase I study. Neuro Oncol. 2021;23(4):677–86.

212. Pouessel D. Hypofractionated stereotactic re-irradiation and anti-PDL1 durvalumab combination in recurrent glioblastoma: STERIMGLI phase I results. Oncologist. 2023;28(9):825–17.

213. Ostrom QT. CBTRUS Statistical Report: primary brain and other central nervous system tumors diagnosed in the United States in 2012–2016. Neuro Oncol. 2019;21(Suppl 5):1–100.

214. Perry JR. Short-course radiation plus temozolomide in elderly patients with glioblastoma. N Engl J Med. 2017;376(11):1027–37.

215. Zarnett OJ. Treatment of elderly patients with glioblastoma: a systematic evidence-based analysis. JAMA Neurol. 2015;72(5):589–96.

216. Hoffermann M, Bruckmann L, Mahdy AK, Asslaber M, Payer F, Campe G. Treatment results and outcome in elderly patients with glioblastoma multiforme—a retrospective single institution analysis. Clin Neurol Neurosurg. 2015;128:60–9.

217. Youssef M. Treatment strategies for glioblastoma in older patients: age is just a number. J Neurooncol. 2019;145(2):357–64.

218. Wick W. Temozolomide chemotherapy alone versus radiotherapy alone for malignant astrocytoma in the elderly: the NOA-08 randomised, phase 3 trial. Lancet Oncol. 2012;13(7):707–15.

219. Malmström A. Temozolomide versus standard 6-week radiotherapy versus hypofractionated radiotherapy in patients older than 60 years with glioblastoma: the Nordic randomised, phase 3 trial. Lancet Oncol. 2012;13(9):916–26.

220. Liu J. Prognostic and predictive factors in elderly patients with glioblastoma: a single-center retrospective study. Front Aging Neurosci. 2022;13:777962.

221. Gulati S, Jakola AS, Johannesen TB, Solheim O. Survival and treatment patterns of glioblastoma in the elderly: a population-based study. World Neurosurg. 2012;78(5):518–26.

222. Dehcordi SR. Survival prognostic factors in patients with glioblastoma: our experience. J Neurosurg Sci. 2012;56(3):239–45.

223. Yang P. Management and survival rates in patients with glioma in China (2004–2010): a retrospective study from a single-institution. J Neurooncol. 2013;113(2):259–66.

224. Straube C. A balanced score to predict survival of elderly patients newly diagnosed with glioblastoma. Radiat Oncol. 2020;15(1):97.

225. Bruno F. Glioblastoma in the elderly: review of molecular and therapeutic aspects. Biomedicines. 2022;10(3):644.

226. Weller M. MGMT promoter methylation in malignant gliomas: ready for personalized medicine? Nat Rev Neurol. 2010;6(1):39–51.

227. Malta TM. Glioma CpG island methylator phenotype (G-CIMP): biological and clinical implications. Neuro Oncol. 2018;20(5):608–20.

228. Ostrom QT. Age-specific genome-wide association study in glioblastoma identifies increased proportion of 'lower grade glioma'-like features associated with younger age. Int J Cancer. 2018;143(10):2359–66.

229. Bozdag S. Age-specific signatures of glioblastoma at the genomic, genetic, and epigenetic levels. PLoS One. 2013;8(4):62982.

230. Fukai J. Molecular characteristics and clinical outcomes of elderly patients with IDH-wildtype glioblastomas: comparative study of older and younger cases in Kansai Network cohort. Brain Tumor Pathol. 2020;37(2):50–9.

231. Chaichana KL. Factors associated with survival for patients with glioblastoma with poor pre-operative functional status. J Clin Neurosci. 2013;20(6):818–23.

232. Chaichana KL. Supratentorial glioblastoma multiforme: the role of surgical resection versus biopsy among older patients. Ann Surg Oncol. 2011;18(1):239–45.

233. Marina O. Treatment outcomes for patients with glioblastoma multiforme and a low Karnofsky Performance Scale score on presentation to a tertiary care institution: Clinical article. J Neurosurg. 2011;115(2):220–9.

234. Chambless LB, Kistka HM, Parker SL, Hassam-Malani L, McGirt MJ, Thompson RC. The relative value of postoperative versus preoperative Karnofsky Performance Scale scores as a predictor of survival after surgical resection of glioblastoma multiforme. J Neurooncol. 2015;121(2):359–64.

235. Pontes LB, et al. Patterns of care and outcomes in elderly patients with glioblastoma in Sao Paulo, Brazil: a retrospective study. J Geriatr Oncol. 2013;4(4):388–93.

236. Voisin MR, Sasikumar S, Zadeh G. Predictors of survival in elderly patients undergoing surgery for glioblastoma. Neurooncol Adv. 2021;3(1):vdab083.

237. Montemurro N, Perrini P, Rapone B. Clinical risk and overall survival in patients with diabetes mellitus, hyperglycemia and glioblastoma multiforme. A review of the current literature. Int J Environ Res Public Health. 2020;17(22):8501.

238. Liu W. The association between common clinical characteristics and postoperative morbidity and overall survival in patients with glioblastoma. Oncologist. 2019;24(4):529–36.

239. Balducci M. Impact of age and co-morbidities in patients with newly diagnosed glioblastoma: a pooled data analysis of three prospective mono-institutional phase II studies. Med Oncol. 2012;29(5):3478–83.

240. Fiorentino A. Comorbidity assessment and adjuvant radiochemotherapy in elderly affected by glioblastoma. Med Oncol. 2012;29(5):3467–71.

241. Ening G, Osterheld F, Capper D, Schmieder K, Brenke C. Charlson comorbidity index: an additional prognostic parameter for preoperative glioblastoma patient stratification. J Cancer Res Clin Oncol. 2015;141(6):1131–7.

242. Li X-Z. Prognostic implications of resection extent for patients with glioblastoma multiforme: a meta-analysis. J Neurosurg Sci. 2017;61(6):631–9.

243. Scott JG. Recursive partitioning analysis of prognostic factors for glioblastoma patients aged 70 years or older. Cancer. 2012;118(22):5595–600.

244. Iwamoto FM, Cooper AR, Reiner AS, Nayak L, Abrey LE. Glioblastoma in the elderly: the Memorial Sloan-Kettering Cancer Center Experience (1997–2007). Cancer. 2009;115(16):3758–66.

245. Schneider M. Newly diagnosed glioblastoma in geriatric (65+) patients: impact of patients frailty, comorbidity burden and obesity on overall survival. J Neurooncol. 2020;149(3):421–7.

246. Lombardi G. Validation of the comprehensive geriatric assessment as a predictor of mortality in elderly glioblastoma patients. Cancers (Basel). 2019;11(10):1509.

247. Almenawer SA. Biopsy versus partial versus gross total resection in older patients with high-grade glioma: a systematic review and meta-analysis. Neuro Oncol. 2015;17(6):868–81.

248. Vuorinen V, Hinkka S, Färkkilä M, Jääskeläinen J. Debulking or biopsy of malignant glioma in elderly people—a randomised study. Acta Neurochir. 2003;145(1):5–10.

249. Ewelt C, Goeppert M, Rapp M, Steiger H-J, Stummer W, Sabel M. Glioblastoma multiforme of the elderly: the prognostic effect of resection on survival. J Neurooncol. 2011;103(3):611–8.

250. Babu R. Glioblastoma in the elderly: the effect of aggressive and modern therapies on survival. J Neurosurg. 2016;124(4):998–1007.

251. Karsy M. Surgical treatment of glioblastoma in the elderly: the impact of complications. J Neurooncol. 2018;138(1):123–32.

252. Hager J. Impact of resection on overall survival of recurrent Glioblastoma in elderly patients. Clin Neurol Neurosurg. 2018;174:21–5.

253. Liu Z-Y. Competing risk model to determine the prognostic factors and treatment strategies for elderly patients with glioblastoma. Sci Rep. 2021;11(1):9321.

254. Barbagallo GMV. High grade glioma treatment in elderly people: is it different than in younger patients? Analysis of surgical management guided by an intraoperative multimodal approach and its impact on clinical outcome. Front Oncol. 2020;10:631255.

255. Keime-Guibert F. Radiotherapy for glioblastoma in the elderly. N Engl J Med. 2007;356(15):1527–35.

256. Roa W. Abbreviated course of radiation therapy in older patients with glioblastoma multiforme: a prospective randomized clinical trial. J Clin Oncol. 2004;22(9):1583–8.

257. Roa W. International Atomic Energy Agency randomized phase III study of radiation therapy in elderly and/or frail patients with newly diagnosed glioblastoma multiforme. J Clin Oncol. 2015;33(35):4145–50.

258. Pérez-Larraya JG. Temozolomide in elderly patients with newly diagnosed glioblastoma and poor performance status: an ANOCEF phase II trial. J Clin Oncol. 2011;29(22):3050–5.

259. Chinot O-L. Phase II study of temozolomide without radiotherapy in newly diagnosed glioblastoma multiforme in an elderly populations. Cancer. 2004;100(10):2208–14.

260. Minniti G, Lombardi G, Paolini S. Glioblastoma in elderly patients: current management and future perspectives. Cancers (Basel). 2019;11(3):336.

261. Prajapati HP, Singh DK. Recurrent glioblastoma in elderly: options and decision for the treatment. Surg Neurol Int. 2022;13:397.

262. Ringel F. Clinical benefit from resection of recurrent glioblastomas: results of a multicenter study including 503 patients with recurrent glioblastomas undergoing surgical resection. Neuro Oncol. 2016;18(1):96–104.

263. Nuñez MTF. Resection of recurrent glioblastoma multiforme in elderly patients: a pseudo-randomized analysis revealed clinical benefit. J Neurooncol. 2020;146(2):381–7.

264. Young JS, Chmura SJ, Wainwright DA, Yamini B, Peters KB, Lukas RV. Management of glioblastoma in elderly patients. J Neurol Sci. 2017;380:250–5.

265. Chen Y-R. National trends for reoperation in older patients with glioblastoma. World Neurosurg. 2018;113:179–89.

266. Zanello M. Recurrent glioblastomas in the elderly after maximal first-line treatment: does preserved overall condition warrant a maximal second-line treatment? J Neurooncol. 2017;135(2):285–97.

267. Goldman DA, Reiner AS, Diamond EL, DeAngelis LM, Tabar V, Panageas KS. Lack of survival advantage among re-resected elderly glioblastoma patients: a SEER-Medicare study. Neurooncol Adv. 2021;3(1):159.

268. Kim HR. Outcome of salvage treatment for recurrent glioblastoma. J Clin Neurosci. 2015;22(3):468–73.

269. Socha J. Outcome of treatment of recurrent glioblastoma multiforme in elderly and/or frail patients. J Neurooncol. 2016;126(3):493–8.

270. Paccapelo A. A retrospective pooled analysis of response patterns and risk factors in recurrent malignant glioma patients receiving a nitrosourea-based chemotherapy. J Transl Med. 2012;10:90.

271. Perry JR, Rizek P, Cashman R, Morrison M, Morrison T. Temozolomide rechallenge in recurrent malignant glioma by using a continuous temozolomide schedule: the 'rescue' approach. Cancer. 2008;113(8):2152–7.

272. Batchelor TT, Phase III. Randomized trial comparing the efficacy of cediranib as monotherapy, and in combination with lomustine, versus lomustine alone in patients with recurrent glioblastoma. J Clin Oncol. 2013;31(26):3212–8.

273. Taal W. Single-agent bevacizumab or lomustine versus a combination of bevacizumab plus lomustine in patients with recurrent glioblastoma (BELOB trial): a randomised controlled phase 2 trial. Lancet Oncol. 2014;15(9):943–53.

274. Wick W. Lomustine and bevacizumab in progressive glioblastoma. N Engl J Med. 2017;377(20):1954–63.

275. Friedman HS. Bevacizumab alone and in combination with irinotecan in recurrent glioblastoma. J Clin Oncol. 2009;27(28):4733–40.

276. Kreisl TN. Phase II trial of single-agent bevacizumab followed by bevacizumab plus irinotecan at tumor progression in recurrent glioblastoma. J Clin Oncol. 2009;27(5):740–5.

277. Mehta M, Wen P, Nishikawa R, Reardon D, Peters K. Critical review of the addition of tumor treating fields (TTFields) to the existing standard of care for newly diagnosed glioblastoma patients. Crit Rev Oncol Hematol. 2017;111:60–5.

278. Kotecha R, Mehta MP. Extreme hypofractionation for newly diagnosed glioblastoma: rationale, dose, techniques, and outcomes. Neuro Oncol. 2020;22(8):1062–4.

279. Gao X, McDonald JT, Hlatky L, Enderling H. Acute and fractionated irradiation differentially modulate glioma stem cell division kinetics. Cancer Res. 2013;73(5):1481–90.

280. Grossman SA, Ye X, Lesser G, Sloan A, Carraway H, Desideri S, et al. Immunosuppression in patients with high-grade gliomas treated with radiation and temozolomide. Clin Cancer Res. 2011;17(16):5473–80.

281. Souhami L, Olivier A, Podgorsak EB, Villemure JG, Pla M, Sadikot AF. Fractionated stereotactic radiation therapy for intracranial tumors. Cancer. 1991;68(10):2101–8.

282. Floyd NS, Woo SY, Teh BS, Prado C, Mai WY, Trask T, et al. Hypofractionated intensity-modulated radiotherapy for primary glioblastoma multiforme. Int J Radiat Oncol Biol Phys. 2004;58(3):721–6.

283. Iuchi T, Hatano K, Kodama T, Sakaida T, Yokoi S, Kawasaki K, et al. Phase 2 trial of hypofractionated high-dose intensity modulated radiation therapy with concurrent and adjuvant temozolomide for newly diagnosed glioblastoma. Int J Radiat Oncol Biol Phys. 2014;88(4):793–800.

284. Ney DE, Carlson JA, Damek DM, Gaspar LE, Kavanagh BD, Kleinschmidt-DeMasters BK, et al. Phase II trial of hypofractionated intensity-modulated radiation therapy combined with temozolomide and bevacizumab for patients with newly diagnosed glioblastoma. J Neurooncol. 2015;122(1):135–43.

285. Chen C, Damek D, Gaspar LE, Waziri A, Lillehei K, Kleinschmidt-DeMasters BK, et al. Phase I trial of hypofractionated intensity-modulated radiotherapy with temozolomide chemotherapy for patients with newly diagnosed glioblastoma multiforme. Int J Radiat Oncol Biol Phys. 2011;81(4):1066–74.

286. Omuro A, Beal K, Gutin P, Karimi S, Correa DD, Kaley TJ, et al. Phase II study of bevacizumab, temozolomide, and hypofractionated stereotactic radiotherapy for newly diagnosed glioblastoma. Clin Cancer Res. 2014;20(19):5023–31.

287. Reddy K, Damek D, Gaspar LE, Ney D, Waziri A, Lillehei K, et al. Phase II trial of hypofractionated IMRT with temozolomide for patients with newly diagnosed glioblastoma multiforme. Int J Radiat Oncol Biol Phys. 2012;84(3):655–60.

288. Azoulay M, Chang SD, Gibbs IC, Hancock SL, Pollom EL, Harsh GR, et al. A phase I/II trial of 5-fraction stereotactic radiosurgery with 5-mm margins with concurrent temozolomide in newly diagnosed glioblastoma: primary outcomes. Neuro Oncol. 2020;22(8):1182–9.

289. Mendoza MG, Azoulay M, Chang SD, Gibbs IC, Hancock SL, Pollom EL, et al. Patterns of progression in patients with newly diagnosed glioblastoma treated with 5-mm margins in a phase 1/2 trial of 5-fraction stereotactic radiosurgery with concurrent and adjuvant temozolomide. Pract Radiat Oncol. 2023;13(3):e239–e45.

Heavy Ion Therapy in Brain Tumors

Giulia Riva, Lucia Pia Ciccone, Alberto Iannalfi,
and Ester Orlandi

8.1 Physical and Biological Properties of Heavy Ions

In the field of high-precision radiotherapy (RT), heavy ion therapy (or particle therapy or charged particle therapy) marks a new era. Among various types of charged particles, protons and carbon ions have been most widely employed for cancer therapy in the world.

The rationale for the clinical application of particle beam therapy in the treatment of human cancer was elucidated by a physicist named Dr. Robert Wilson in 1946.

The physical advantages of particle therapy are due to the favorable depth–dose distribution compared to conventional photons which minimizes the collateral damage to normal tissues. While photons deposit the largest amount of dose near the entrance continuing to deposit significant dose beyond the target, in the case of particle therapy (such as protons and carbon ions) the energy deposited per unit track increases with depth, reaching a sharp and narrow maximum peak close, called the "Bragg peak" (Fig. 8.1), to the end of the range. The Bragg peak of carbon ions is higher and sharper than protons, and there is less lateral dose scatter, although there is some distal dose beyond the target due to nuclear fragmentation.

To cover a tumor of known shape and diameter, the medical physicist could combine a distribution of heavy ion energies to allow for a flat, high-dose region that would sufficiently cover the target lesion while sparing surrounding normal tissues. Therefore, the Bragg peak has to be widened, creating a spread-out Bragg peak (SOBP).

In past years, a SOBP was generally achieved through passive scattering of a monoenergetic beam. Passive scattering is a dose delivery system in which a broad monoenergetic beam is used to treat a tumor. The energy variation is obtained with compensating filters of different depths and the shape is controlled with patient-specific collimators.

Conversely, nowadays, almost all newly created radiation therapy centers use pencil-beam scanning (PBS), a dose-delivery system in particle therapy in which the beam is concentrated in spots of a few millimeters of diameter and scanned through a 2D tumor slice, and intensity-modulated proton therapy (IMPT), in which the intensity of each pencil beam is modified to achieve a better target coverage.

Another advantage of particle therapy is related to the high linear energy transfer (LET) of the charged particles around the Bragg peak. LET is commonly used for expressing the radiation quality of particle beams. As charged parti-

G. Riva · L. P. Ciccone · A. Iannalfi · E. Orlandi (✉)
Radiation Oncology Unit, Clinical Department,
National Center for Oncological Hadrontherapy
(CNAO), Pavia, Italy
e-mail: ester.orlandi@cnao.it

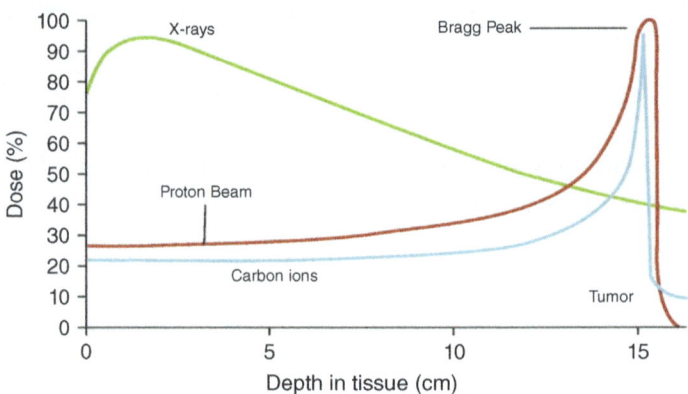

Fig. 8.1 The "Bragg peak"of charged particles. (From Kong, L., Yang, J., Lu, J.J. (2022). Particle Therapy for Head and Neck Sarcomas. In: Kim, E., Parvathaneni, U., Welliver, M.X. (eds) Radiation Therapy for Sarcomas and Skin Cancers. Practical Guides in Radiation Oncology. Springer, Cham with permission)

cles traverse a medium, they continuously scatter and lose energy. The amount of energy transferred to the material traversed per unit distance, known as linear energy transfer (LET), increases as particles slow down until their energy is fully depleted and they come to a sudden stop. Mostly, LET is used qualitatively, i.e., a high LET is associated with increased relative biological effectiveness (RBE).

For protons, the RBE, based on the average of multiple experiments, has been assumed to have a constant value of 1.1 for all cancers and normal tissues, and, therefore, their advantage is limited to the sparing of the normal tissue due to the Bragg peak. However, recent observations demonstrated a continuous increase in RBE along a proton path and a rapid increase in RBE in the region of the Bragg peak, reaching the highest value of 1.7.

For heavier ions, such as carbon ions, LET is considerably higher than that of protons, but it can no longer be approximated by a constant value. This leads to a higher RBE, where damage caused by carbon ions is clustered in the DNA, producing more complex DNA double-strand breaks and overwhelming the cellular repair systems. Due to these peculiar distinctive radiobiological hallmarks carbon ion therapy (CIRT) offers exerting two- to threefold higher superior RBE in comparison to photons and protons against intrinsic radioresistant tumors. In addition, carbon ions are characterized by a reduced dependence on fractionation, cell-cycle phases, and tissue oxygenation status and they enhance apoptosis in radioresistant cancer stem cells. All these hallmarks render CIRT more effective in the treatment of radioresistant tumors.

8.2 Heavy Ions Radiotherapy for Brain and Skull Base Tumors

Brain and skull base tumors comprise very different and rare entities. Most of them are challenging lesions in terms of clinical management because of their anatomical location and the close vicinity of critical structures such as the brainstem, spinal cord, and anterior optic pathways. Therefore, resection with a sufficient surgical margin of skull base or brain tumors is not always feasible.

A variety of conditions that arise within the central nervous system and in the skull base may benefit from particle beam therapy.

In low-grade tumors, proton therapy should be considered in challenging cases for tumor volume and involvement of critical neural structures.

Dosimetric studies and predictive normal tissue complication probability (NTCP) models provide evidence of superior capability in particle therapy.

Primarily, in terms of sparing critical and minimizing risk of radio-induced toxicity with particular reference to sparing radiation dose exposure of hippocampi and brain volume and consequent better preservation of neurocognitive function [1–4].

In radioresistant tumors, such as chordoma, sarcoma, and previously irradiated recurrent tumors, particle therapy permits to deliver high biologically effective doses with low or however acceptable toxicity.

8.2.1 Chordoma and Chondrosarcoma

Chordomas are malignant bone tumors that originate from embryonic notochord remnant cells sited while chondrosarcomas are a heterogeneous group of slow-growing neoplasms originating from cartilage-producing cells in areas of enchondral ossification [5]. Intracranial chordoma and chondrosarcoma are located in skull base regions.

Although these lesions are distinct clinicopathological entities and vary significantly in their clinical outcome, management is quite similar: when complete resection is not possible, maximal safe resection is desirable, followed subsequently by radiation treatment.

Chordomas and chondrosarcomas are relatively radioresistant and respond best to high radiation doses above 70 Gy (Fig. 8.2).

It presents a challenge when using photon therapy because of the close proximity to dose-limiting neural structures (i.e., brainstem, spinal cord, and optic structures) which tolerate lower doses than those prescribed.

For this reason, most of the recent publications come from particle therapy facilities with protons, carbon ions, or both (Table 8.1) [6–14].

Both proton and carbon ion radiation therapy have been successfully used in the treatment of skull base chordoma and chondrosarcoma. In the last 15 years, different institutions have consistently reported local control rates in excess of 70% for chordoma [6–11], while a recent review on chondrosarcomas treated with proton therapy by Amichetti et al. reported 5-year and 10-year

LC rates in patients with chondrosarcomas of the skull base of 75–99% and 98%, respectively [15].

Protons have a longer treatment history and have been applied in multiple centers over the past 20–25 years, therefore the long-term follow-up data makes protons the standard against which carbon ions have to be measured.

The rationale to expect an improvement in large-tumor control with carbon ions is based on the increased efficacy of their high linear-energy transfer against the hypoxic and radioresistant tumor clones. The potential advantage of carbon ions in midsize tumors compressing the brainstem and/or chiasm derives from their sharper penumbra and smaller spot size. Ultimately, clinical data are also needed to confirm this advantage [16].

8.2.2 Meningiomas

Meningiomas are the most common primary intracranial tumors with an incidence rate of 37.6% [17].

There is a range of management options for meningioma from observation for small, asymptomatic, and benign lesions to surgery or radiation options for other patients with meningioma. Surgically accessible meningiomas that can be safely removed have indications of surgical resection, the cornerstone for symptomatic or growing meningioma is the maximal surgical resection minimizing morbidity and preserving neurological functions. However, as happens with skull base tumors located close to the cavernous sinus, total removal is rarely achieved and a planned subtotal resection. Incomplete surgical removal or higher-grade meningioma is associated with an increased risk of progression.

External beam radiotherapy improves local control and new advanced radiation techniques can provide excellent target dose coverage, precise target localization, and accurate dose delivery.

Particle therapy may be offered to patients with meningioma as an alternative to photon therapy [18–23] (Table 8.2).

Fig. 8.2 Example of skull-base chondrosarcoma treated with proton radiotherapy

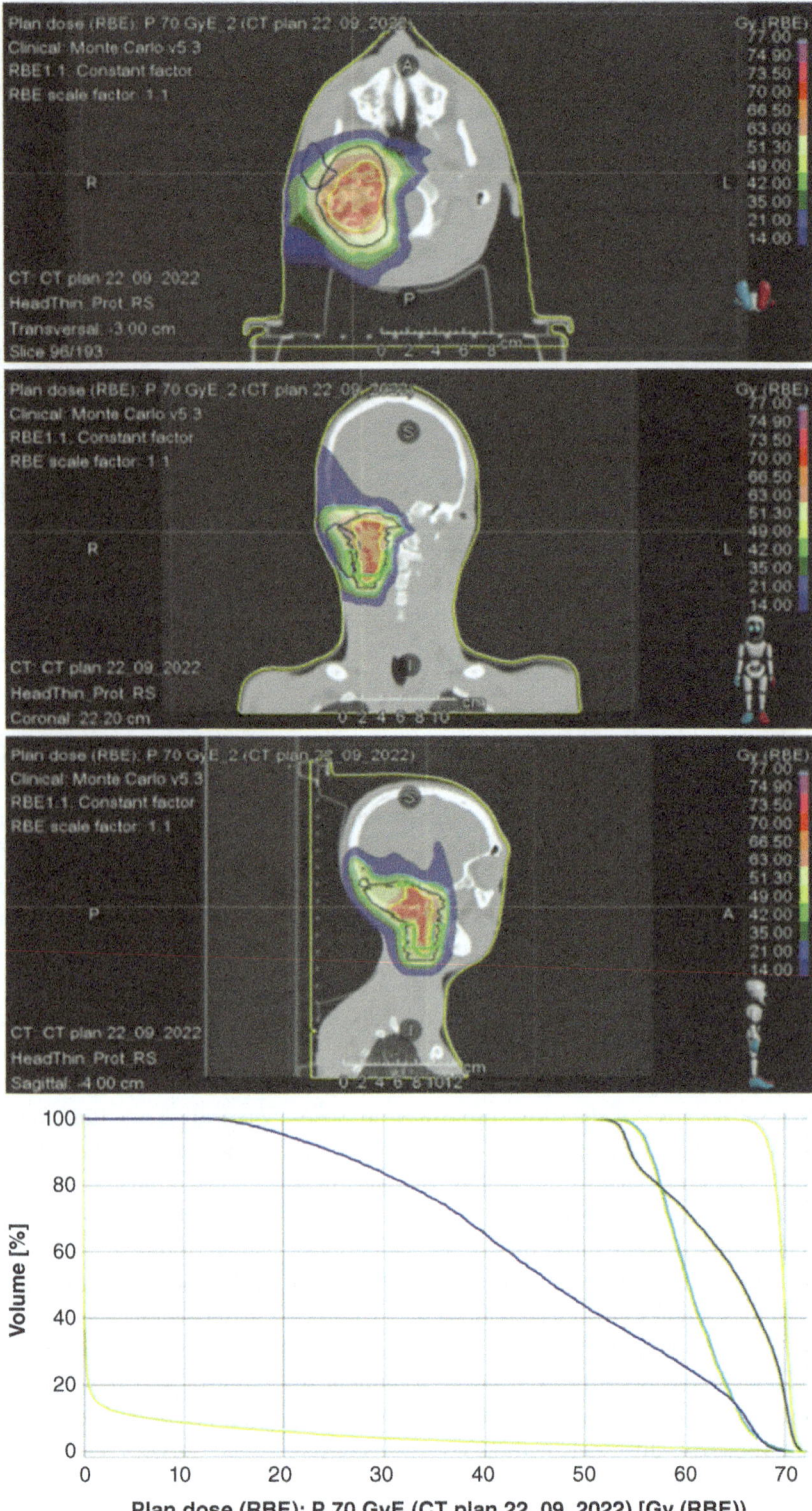

Table 8.1 Patients and treatment description of chordomas and chondrosarcomas irradiated with proton or carbon ion (selected recent series)

Study	Particle	Neoplasia	Patients (number)	Follow-up (months)	RT dose (GyRBE)	LC (%)	OS (%)	Severe late toxicity (%)
Uhl, 2014 [6]	C	Chordoma	155	72 (median)	TD: 60 (median) Dpf: 3	5-y: 72	5-y: 85	0
Weber, 2016 [7]	P	Chordoma	151	50 (mean)	TD: 72.5* (mean) Dpf: 1.8–2	7-y: 70.9		8
Koto, 2020 [9]	C	Chordoma	34	108 (median)	TD: 60.8 (median) Dpf: 3.8 (median)	5-y: 77	5-y: 93	11
Iannalfi, 2020 [10]	P	Chordoma	135		TD: 74 (median) Dpf: 1.8–2	5-y: 84	5-y: 83	12
Iannalfi, 2020 [10]	C	Chordoma	65		TD: 70.4 Dpf: 4.4	5-y: 71	5-y: 82	12
Mattke, 2022 [11]	P	Chordoma	36	36 (median)	TD: 74 (median) Dpf: 1.8–2	5-y: 61	5-y: 92	
Mattke, 2022 [11]	C	Chordoma	111	52 (median)	TD: 66	5-y: 65	5-y: 83	
Weber, 2016 [12]	P	Chondrosarcoma	77	69.2 (mean)	TD: 70.0 (mean) Dpf: 1.8–2	8-y: 89.7	8-y: 93.5	8
Mattke, 2018 [13]	P	Chondrosarcoma	22	30.7 (median)	70 (median)	4-y: 100	4-y: 100	0
Mattke, 2018 [13]	C	Chondrosarcoma	79	43.7 (median)	60 (median)	4-y: 90.5	4-y: 92.9	0
Riva, 2021 [14]	P	Chondrosarcoma	32	31 (median)	TD: 74 (median) Dpf: 2	3-y LC: 100%	–	6
Riva, 2021 [14]	C	Chondrosarcoma	16	66 (median)	70.4 Dpf: 4.4	Dpf: 4.4 3-y LC: 94%	–	12

P proton, *C* carbon ion, *RT* radiotherapy, *TD* total dose, *Dpf* dose per fraction, *LC* local control, *y* years, *OS* overall survival

Table 8.2 Patients and treatment description of meningiomas irradiated with proton and/or carbon ion (selected recent series)

Study	WHO grade	Particle	Patients (number)	Follow-up (months)	RT dose (GyRBE)	LC (%)	OS (%)	Severe late toxicity
Halasz, 2011 [18]	50 (G1)	P	50	32 (median)	TD: 13 Dpf: 13	3-y: 94	/	/
Weber, 2012 [19]	23 (G1) 9 (G2) 2 (G3) 5 (U)	P	39	54.8 (median)	TD: 56 (median) Dpf: 1.8–2	5-y: 84.6	5-y: 82	Late toxicity (any grade): 41% Severe late toxicity: 13%
Combs, 2013 [20]	71 (G1) 36 (G2–3)	P ± C boost	107	12 (median)	TD P: 52.2–57.6 TD C: 18	LC at the end of FUP WHO G1: 100 2-y WHO G2–3: 33	3-y: 100	/
Vlachogiannis, 2017 [21]	170 (G1)	P	170	84	TD: 14–46 Dpf: 3–8	5-y: 93	/	Late toxicity (any grade): 9%
Murray, 2017 [22]	61 (G1) 35 (G2–3)	P	96	56.9 (median)	TD WHO G1: 54 (median) TD WHO G2–3: 62 Dpf: 1.8–2	5-y WHO G1: 95 5-y WHO G2: 69	5-y WHO G1: 92 5-y WHO G2: 80	Late toxicity (any grade): 45% Severe late toxicity: 10%
El Shafie, 2018 [23]	60 (G1) 7 (G2) 1 (G3) 42 (U)	P ± C boost	110	46.8 (median)	TD P: 54 TD P + C: 50P + 18C	5-y: 96.6	5-y: 96.2	Severe late toxicity: 3.6%

G grading according to WHO classification, *U* unknown, *P* proton, *C* carbon ion, *RT* radiotherapy, *TD* total dose, *Dpf* dose per fraction, *LC* local control, *y* years, *OS* overall survival

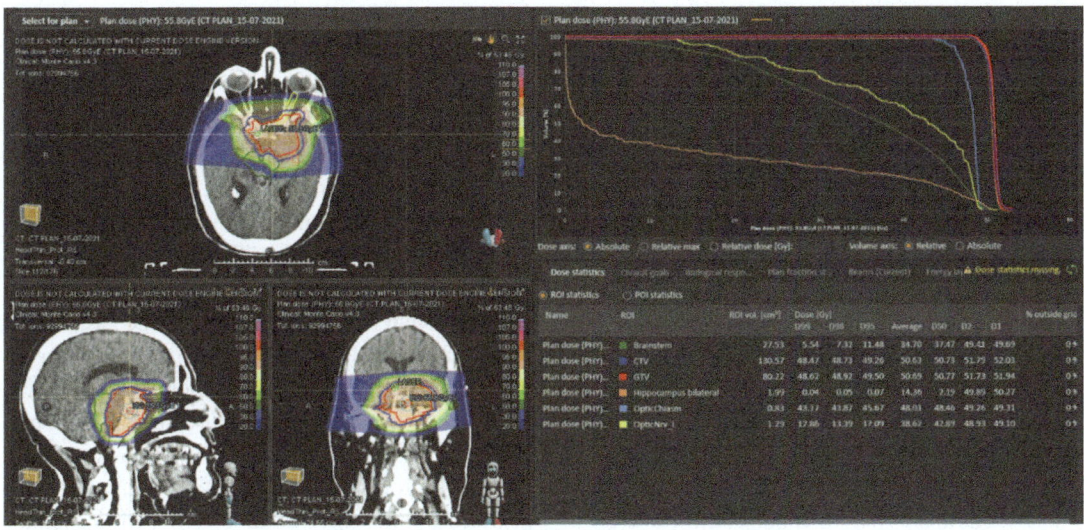

Fig. 8.3 Example of proton radiotherapy treatment plan of skull base meningioma

The rationale of proton therapy consists in minimization of treatment-related side effects is of high importance, including neurocognitive sequelae, in younger patients or, in general, in patients with long-term survival expectancy. On the other hand, in the smaller portion of patients presenting higher grade types meningiomas, higher dose levels are required in order to obtain better rate of local control and particle therapy can be useful for the achievement of the most favorable ratio between optimal coverage of treatment volume with therapeutic higher dose and the sparing of tolerance dose to critical structures [22, 24, 25].

Furthermore, particle therapy can obtain very encouraging outcomes in patients with recurrence disease previously irradiated of aggressive meningiomas, even in case of large recurrent lesions (also volumes more than 70 cm³: median progression-free survival rates) reaching about 25 months in WHO-2 and WHO-3 grades and median overall survival of 60 months were described [26, 27] (Fig. 8.3).

8.2.3 Pituitary Adenoma

Pituitary adenomas are benign tumors arising in the pituitary gland with an incidence of 3.9–7.4 cases per 100,000 [28]. Most new cases diag-nosed annually are nonfunctioning pituitary adenomas prolactinomas. Increased availability of MRI has led to an increase in incidentally found small pituitary lesions.

The most recent classification of pituitary gland tumors (WHO Classification of Endocrine and Neuroendocrine Tumors 5th ed. 2022) [29] distinguishes the anterior lobe (adeno-hypophysis) from posterior lobe (neuro-hypophysis) and hypothalamic tumors. In the anterior lobe, tumors are well-differentiated adenohypophyseal forms that are now classified as pituitary neuroendocrine tumors (PitNETs; formerly known as pituitary adenomas). The immunohistochemistry analysis for pituitary transcription factors (PIT1, TPIT, SF1, GATA3, and ERa) is included in this classification. The "null cell" tumor is reserved for PitNETs with no evidence of adenohypophyseal lineage differentiation. The term "metastatic PitNET" is advocated to replace the previous terminology of "pituitary carcinoma" [29].

Following surgical management of pituitary adenoma, watchful waiting, medical therapy or irradiation can be considered. In daily clinical practice, radiation therapy is not always applied in adjuvant settings but is rather reserved for recurrent or progressive diseases in which no surgical intervention is possible or accepted by the patient. Although slow regrowth is common, the natural evolution of untreated tumors is variable.

Data on proton therapy for pituitary adenomas are available both with the schemes of conventional fractionation at a median dose of 54 Gy (RBE) [30] and with single-session stereotactic approach at a median dose of 20 Gy [31].

Ronson et al. reported outcomes of 100% of local control with 29.3% partial tumor regression and 24.4% complete tumor regression at last follow-up, while 85.7% had normalized or decreased hormone levels at last follow-up. In this series, seven patients developed minor visual deficits and two patients developed major visual deficits (new quadrantanopsia and bilateral optic nerve atrophy) [30].

Wattson et al. reported that in 165 mixed functional adenomas, 98% of local control and 59% of 5-year hormonal normalization rates [31].

Nowadays, the proton therapy in the treatment of pituitary adenomas can find a real perspective of clinical application as an alternative of photon therapy when conventional fractionated dose schedule is required: in cases with larger sized/giant tumor volumes and cases with tumor with very close proximity or involving optic pathways by abutting or compressing.

8.2.4 Craniopharyngioma

Craniopharyngioma is a rare neuroepithelial tumor arising from the embryological remnants of the primitive craniopharyngeal duct or Rathke's pouch. Craniopharyngiomas present two subtypes in adults: adamantinomatous and papillary. In children, adamantinomatous form is nearly total. The overall incidence is reported as 0.13–0.16 in 100,000, constituting 5–10% of pediatric and 1–4% of adult brain tumors, respectively [32].

The treatment of craniopharyngioma is based on surgical management with transcranial approaches or endoscopic endonasal surgery eventually followed by radiotherapy.

Radiotherapy is usually indicated after incomplete or debulking surgery, at the time of first diagnosis, or at progression. Proton therapy in craniopharyngioma is recommended for several reasons. Craniopharyngioma is a benign tumor arising mainly in children and young adults with a long life expectancy of survivors. The incidence of radiation-induced tumors is expected to be reduced using proton therapy given its significant reduction in integral dose.

In addition, because of the dose distribution of proton therapy with pencil-beam delivery, organs at risk (OAR) should receive a reduced dose compared to 3DRT, IMRT, and passively scattered proton therapy [33, 34].

Fractionated radiation regimens are more commonly employed as proximity of tumor to the optic apparatus often renders radiosurgical modalities unsafe [35–38]. Recently Jimenez et al. published a series on 77 pediatric patients affected by craniopharyngioma and treated with proton radiotherapy (2002–2018) with a median dose of 52.2 Gy [36]. At a median of 4.8 years from radiotherapy, six local failures were observed and the 5-year local failure estimate was 9.9%, while the 5-year OS was 97.7%. Only 4% developed any acute G3 toxicity. The authors observed no patients with new cases of visual impairment after radiotherapy and the majority (68%) of baseline visual deficits presented stability with 10% improving and 10% worsening. New endocrinopathies were reported in 7%, among pre-existing cases worsened in 47%, stable in 49%, and improved in 4%. Concerning cognitive function, scores were stable and did not significantly change.

The potential range of application for proton radiotherapy in adult patients is more selective. Rutenberg et al. reported a series of 14 patients with 3-year LC and OS rates were 100%. There were no G3 or greater acute or late radiotherapy-related side effects. There was no RT-related vision loss or optic neuropathy. No patients required intervention or treatment replanning due to tumor changes during RT [37].

8.2.5 Gliomas

Gliomas are the most frequent primary brain malignancies, ranging from indolent (WHO Grade 1 pilocytic astrocytoma) to very aggressive forms such as glioblastoma (WHO grade 4) [39]. Radiotherapy is an integral part of modern multimodal therapy for brain cancers.

8.2.5.1 Low-Grade Glioma

Low-grade glioma (LGG) is a rare primary intracranial tumor (incidence around 1 per 100,000 per year) with an infiltrative and slow growth pattern. LGG accounts for 20% of all gliomas and typically occur in young patients and adults [40, 41].

LGG usually has a good prognosis with an increasing proportion of patients that are long-term survivors.

The first-line treatment is maximal tumor resection, studies have shown that the extent of resection is directly correlated with overall survival. Post-operative therapies (radiotherapy and chemotherapy) are generally recommended for high-risk patients.

So, the risk of long-term side effects with a possible detrimental impact on a patient's life must be taken into account. The most important late effects regard neurocognitive domains, quality of life, and the risk of radio-induced cancer.

The impact of radiotherapy dose parameters on neurocognitive function reported in literature support that reduction of radiation dose-volume relationships to hippocampi and brain volume can actually positively affect the preservation of neurocognitive functions.

Particle radiotherapy, due to peculiar physical properties of charged particles, permits precise targeting of the tumor minimizing healthy tissue exposure and may be an alternative to conventional photon-based radiotherapy.

Proton therapy permits to significantly reduce radiation dose-volume delivery to nearby OARs. These areas include the hippocampi and subventricular zones, hearing and visual apparatus, and pituitary gland [4, 39].

Consequently, this dosimetric advantage can determine better outcomes in terms of neurocognitive sparing as supported also by normal tissue complication probability (NTCP) modeling studies [2].

Large clinical series of patients affected by low-grade gliomas treated with proton therapy have reported tumor regression or stability in 60% and estimated 5 year overall survival (OS) accounted for 85% [42] with preservation of cognitive function [41, 43, 44] (Fig. 8.4).

8.2.5.2 High-Grade Glioma

High-grade gliomas (HGGs) are the most frequent primary brain malignancies, accounting for approximately 47% of all malignant brain tumors. The features of HGGs are a highly infiltrative growth pattern and a rapid progression. HGGs mainly consist of glioblastoma multiforme, anaplastic astrocytoma, or oligodendroglioma [45].

Despite the aggressive standard of care, including gross total resection, radiotherapy, and chemotherapy, the prognosis remains poor and the recurrence rate is high [45].

For patients with recurrence, unfortunately, treatment options are limited [46].

Dosimetry studies have demonstrated an improved dose distribution of particle therapy compared with photon-RT for glioma. In addition to particles' physical characteristics, carbon ions have higher LET, which inflicts more damage through direct DNA double-strand breaks. The RBE of carbon-ion beams is 3–5 for glioblas-

Fig. 8.4 Brainstem low-grade glioma treated with proton radiotherapy. MRI imaging at baseline and 17 months after treatment

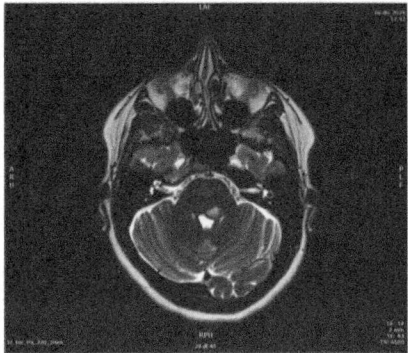
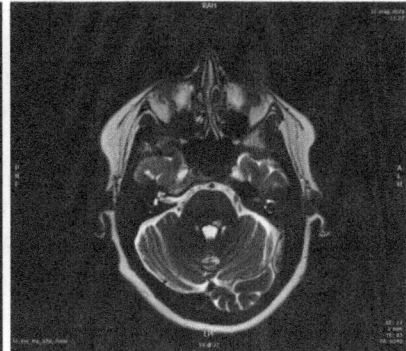

toma cells. The results from in-vitro studies have revealed greater cell-kill efficiency by carbon-ion radiotherapy compared with low LET (photon X and proton) beams. CIRT is also potentially more effective in killing cancerous cells in a hypoxic microenvironment [47].

A particle beam could provide good target coverage, and it seems to reduce dose exposure to near OARs significantly.

The use of particle radiotherapy seems to be effective with acceptable adverse effects when used either alone or as a boost. To date, no adequate evidence validates which protocol is much more effective. Regarding survival outcomes, carbon ion boost is superior to proton boost concerning biological effects. In terms of toxicity, the side effects could be acceptable.

Is worthy of attention to the risk of developing brain radionecrosis with the dose-escalation, despite the improving survival rates.

Furthermore, high-quality RCTs should be conducted in the future. Moreover, systemic therapy options combined with charged particles are necessary [45].

8.3 Particle Therapy for Pediatric Tumors

Pediatric brain tumor is the most common among pediatric solid malignancies. Radiotherapy plays an important role in the treatment of pediatric brain malignancies, because obtaining a sufficient surgical margin is often unfeasible [48].

Current proton therapy is mainly administered with the schedule to that of photon radiotherapy for all brain pediatric tumors such as glioma, medulloblastoma, ependymoma, germinoma, and craniopharyngioma. Based on studies with short follow-ups and a small number of patients, proton therapy seems to have an equivalent therapeutic effect to that of photon radiotherapy.

However, in consideration of the better dose conformation of protons (especially in the case of large treatment volumes) and the life expectancy of pediatric patients treated for some brain tumors, the topic of late toxicities and second tumors plays an important role in the choice of

the type of treatment (protons vs photons) and an increasing consensus has been developed in last decades about the role of proton radiotherapy for the treatment of pediatric patients [49–52].

Radiation sensitivity in children is higher than in adults and toxicities related to impairment of growth and development are also significant problems in growing children, and intelligence retardation is related to the irradiation dose, age at irradiation, time since irradiation, and the mean dose to normal brain [53, 54].

Growth hormone is the most susceptible to irradiation among hypothalamic-pituitary hormones.

Also, a relatively small critical normal organ, such as the cochlea can be preserved in proton therapy when not adjacent to the primary tumor volume.

These advantages can result in preservation of cognitive function, endocrine function, and hearing.

In the literature, there are many studies based on dose-volume histogram (DVH) analyses that indicate that protons can reduce the risk of late toxicity and secondary cancer [33, 34, 55]. In 2008, Merchant et al. suggested that, although the differences in the volume receiving highest doses (40–60 Gy) are negligible, protons, when compared to photons, consistently lower the distribution of low (0–20 Gy) and intermediate (20–40 Gy) doses to portions of the brain in children irradiated for intracranial tumors [55].

Predictive NTCP models have also supported superiority of protons in the treatment of pediatric tumors [56].

The superior capability of protons compared with photons in terms of sparing cognitive function and quality of life has been largely evidenced also in clinical series [57–60]. A supplementary discussion is necessary for medulloblastoma and for radiotherapy treatment volumes needed. Medulloblastoma is a common malignant pediatric brain tumor that arises in the posterior fossa. This tumor is characterized by its propensity for leptomeningeal spread. Therefore, current treatment strategies include maximal safe resection of the primary lesion followed by craniospinal irradiation (CSI) with concurrent and adjuvant chemotherapy.

While there is no evidence that proton therapy is related to better disease control, proton beam properties allow complete or near-complete organ sparing compared with photons of many organs, including bowel with lower rate of acute gastrointestinal toxicity (nausea and vomiting accompanied by anorexia).

The treatment volume of CSI is large and the risk of late toxicity and secondary cancer is higher than for other irradiation fields.

Intracranial toxicities are a significant problem in whole brain irradiation and posterior fossa boost, abundant data correlate medulloblastoma treatment with a decline in neurocognitive function with increased risk of memory impairment [61].

As brain irradiation, radiation therapy for medulloblastoma can damage the pituitary gland and hypothalamus, resulting in endocrine defects. Growth hormone deficiency is the most common endocrinopathy in these patients, resulting in short stature as a common sequela [61].

Moreover, children who receive standard photon CSI are also at risk for cardiac toxicities including coronary artery disease, left ventricular scarring and dysfunction, valvular damage, and atherosclerosis [62].

Secondary malignancies are among the most serious long-term toxicity in children treated for childhood brain tumors especially when CSI is performed. The relative risk for secondary malignancies in medulloblastoma has been calculated between 4.59 and 20 without decline after 10 years [63, 64]. Children treated for medulloblastoma may experience a variety of secondary malignancies including leukemias and solid tumors of the urinary or digestive tracts, thyroid, and CNS [63].

According to Zhang and colleagues, the calculated total lifetime risk for second cancer after proton is much lower than that after photon radiotherapy, with a lifetime risk ratio of 0.18 [65]. In conclusion, there is a large benefit in using protons, especially for CSI, based on sufficient evidence to support the argument that all children with medulloblastoma should be offered proton therapy [66, 67].

8.4 Cost-Effectiveness Consideration

Particle therapy is an expensive anti-cancer treatment, with a cost factor of approximately 2.5, when compared to modern radiation treatment techniques, with some differences from country to country, depending on insurance/national reimbursement policies [68].

This is certainly due to the considerable investment costs but also related to the high operation and maintenance costs. But this has been done in the last decade and a lot more is yet to be done to reduce cost. The costs are even higher for a multi-ion facility, such as the Heidelberg Ion Therapy (HIT) Center in Germany, the Hyogo Ion Beam Medical Centre (HIBMC) in Japan, and the Centro Nazionale di Adroterapia Oncologica (CNAO) in Italy where patients are currently treated either with protons or carbon ions. For example, to reach the same depth, the magnetic rigidity of carbon ions is 2.5 times greater compared to protons, demanding corresponding more powerful and larger magnets for beam bending and steering.

The capital cost of particle therapy facilities is still relatively high compared with photon therapy, mostly dominated by construction and technology component costs. The costs are drastically reduced for "small-scale" (compact proton cyclotron, single room) centers, but the business plan is probably not as attractive as a large-scale facility, where the investment will be compensated by relatively high reimbursement [69].

The construction of new treatment centers raises the question of how many centers are needed to treat patients who can potentially benefit from particle therapy and there is an ongoing debate on the value of particle therapy and its cost-effectiveness.

In literature, four publications on cost-effectiveness of proton therapy in brain tumors could be identified, comparing proton vs photon therapy [70–73]. All investigators have shown that proton therapy is cost-effective with regard to long-term risk of radiation side-effects.

Lundkvist et al. from the Karolinska Institute evaluated the cost-effectiveness of proton beam vs. photon beam therapy in the management of pediatric medulloblastoma by using a Markov simulation model [70]. When the investigators included all the adverse effects that the treated children were at risk for developing following irradiation, they discovered that proton beam therapy was associated with a $23,600 reduction in costs and 0.68 additional quality-adjusted life years per patient compared with photons. Such reduction in dose deposition in normal tissues obtained with particle therapy is expected to reduce the need for medical procedures to treat the side effects from unnecessary irradiation of uninvolved tissue, reduce the risk of developing secondary malignancy, and the subsequent need to treat radiation-induced cancer, and even potentially improve local control in selected patients.

Most insurances reimburse the costs of particle therapy for brain tumors listed above. Nevertheless, patients may experience expenses to cover costs for housing and traveling during multi-week treatment, special food, and potentially lost wages. For some patients, these out-of-pocket payments can cause substantial financial distress that adversely affects a patient's quality of life, treatment choice, treatment compliance, and treatment outcome. Treatment-related financial distress can be just as toxic as the effects of chemotherapy or radiation and was therefore defined as a treatment-related financial toxicity.

References

1. Florijn MA, Sharfo AWM, Wiggenraad RGJ, van Santvoort JPC, Petoukhova AL, Hoogeman MS, Mast ME, Dirkx MLP. Lower doses to hippocampi and other brain structures for skull-base meningiomas with intensity modulated proton therapy compared to photon therapy. Radiother Oncol. 2020;142:147–53. https://doi.org/10.1016/j.radonc.2019.08.019.
2. Dutz A, Lühr A, Troost EGC, Agolli L, Bütof R, Valentini C, Baumann M, Vermeren X, Geismar D, Timmermann B, Krause M, Löck S. Identification of patient benefit from proton beam therapy in brain tumour patients based on dosimetric and NTCP analyses. Radiother Oncol. 2021;160:69–77. https://doi.org/10.1016/j.radonc.2021.04.008.
3. Arvold ND, Niemierko A, Broussard GP, Adams J, Fullerton B, Loeffler JS, Shih HA. Projected second tumor risk and dose to neurocognitive structures after proton versus photon radiotherapy for benign meningioma. Int J Radiat Oncol Biol Phys. 2012;83(4):e495–500. https://doi.org/10.1016/j.ijrobp.2011.10.056.
4. Harrabi SB, Bougatf N, Mohr A, Haberer T, Herfarth K, Combs SE, Debus J, Adeberg S. Dosimetric advantages of proton therapy over conventional radiotherapy with photons in young patients and adults with low-grade glioma. Strahlenther Onkol. 2016;192(11):759–69. https://doi.org/10.1007/s00066-016-1005-9.
5. Brown E, Hug EB, Weber AL. Chondrosarcoma of the skull base. Neuroimaging Clin N Am. 1994;4(3):529–41.
6. Uhl M, Mattke M, Welzel T, Roeder F, Oelmann J, Habl G, Jensen A, Ellerbrock M, Jäkel O, Haberer T, Herfarth K, Debus J. Highly effective treatment of skull base chordoma with carbon ion irradiation using a raster scan technique in 155 patients: first long-term results. Cancer. 2014;120(21):3410–7. https://doi.org/10.1002/cncr.28877.
7. Weber DC, Malyapa R, Albertini F, Bolsi A, Kliebsch U, Walser M, Pica A, Combescure C, Lomax AJ, Schneider R. Long term outcomes of patients with skull-base low-grade chondrosarcoma and chordoma patients treated with pencil beam scanning proton therapy. Radiother Oncol. 2016;120(1):169–74. https://doi.org/10.1016/j.radonc.2016.05.011.
8. Fung V, Calugaru V, Bolle S, Mammar H, Alapetite C, Maingon P, De Marzi L, Froelich S, Habrand JL, Dendale R, Noël G, Feuvret L. Proton beam therapy for skull base chordomas in 106 patients: a dose adaptive radiation protocol. Radiother Oncol. 2018;128(2):198–202. https://doi.org/10.1016/j.radonc.2017.12.017.
9. Koto M, Ikawa H, Kaneko T, Hagiwara Y, Hayashi K, Tsuji H. Long-term outcomes of skull base chordoma treated with high-dose carbon-ion radiotherapy. Head Neck. 2020;42(9):2607–13. https://doi.org/10.1002/hed.26307.
10. Iannalfi A, D'Ippolito E, Riva G, Molinelli S, Gandini S, Viselner G, Fiore MR, Vischioni B, Vitolo V, Bonora M, Ronchi S, Petrucci R, Barcellini A, Mirandola A, Russo S, Vai A, Mastella E, Magro G, Maestri D, Ciocca M, Preda L, Valvo F, Orecchia R. Proton and carbon ion radiotherapy in skull base chordomas: a prospective study based on a dual particle and a patient-customized treatment strategy. Neuro Oncol. 2020;22(9):1348–58. https://doi.org/10.1093/neuonc/noaa067.
11. Mattke M, Ohlinger M, Bougatf N, Harrabi S, Wolf R, Seidensaal K, Welzel T, Röder F, Gerum S, Ellerbrock M, Jäkel O, Haberer T, Herfarth K, Uhl M, Debus J. Proton and carbon ion beam treatment with active raster scanning method in 147 patients with skull base chordoma at the Heidelberg Ion Beam Therapy Center—a single-center experience.

Strahlenther Onkol. 2022; https://doi.org/10.1007/s00066-022-02002-4.

12. Weber DC, Badiyan S, Malyapa R, Albertini F, Bolsi A, Lomax AJ, Schneider R. Long-term outcomes and prognostic factors of skull-base chondrosarcoma patients treated with pencil-beam scanning proton therapy at the Paul Scherrer Institute. Neuro Oncol. 2016;18(2):236–43. https://doi.org/10.1093/neuonc/nov154.

13. Mattke M, Vogt K, Bougatf N, Welzel T, Oelmann-Avendano J, Hauswald H, Jensen A, Ellerbrock M, Jäkel O, Haberer T, et al. High control rates of proton- and carbon-ion–beam treatment with intensity-modulated active raster scanning in 101 patients with skull base chondrosarcoma at the Heidelberg Ion Beam Therapy Center. Cancer. 2018;124:2036–44. https://doi.org/10.1002/cncr.31298.

14. Riva G, Cavallo I, Gandini S, Ingargiola R, Pecorilla M, Imparato S, Rossi E, Mirandola A, Ciocca M, Orlandi E, Iannalfi A. Particle radiotherapy for skull base chondrosarcoma: a clinical series from Italian National Center for Oncological Hadrontherapy. Cancers (Basel). 2021;13(17):4423. https://doi.org/10.3390/cancers13174423.

15. Amichetti M, Amelio D, Cianchetti M, Enrici RM, Minniti G. A systematic review of proton therapy in the treatment of chondrosarcoma of the skull base. Neurosurg Rev. 2010;33(2):155–65. https://doi.org/10.1007/s10143-009-0235-z.

16. Hug EB, Pelak M, Frank SJ, Fossati P. A review of particle therapy for skull base tumors: modern considerations and future directions. Int J Part Ther. 2021;8(1):168–78.

17. Goldbrunner R, Stavrinou P, Jenkinson MD, et al. EANO guideline on the diagnosis and management of meningiomas. Neuro Oncol. 2021;23(11):1821–34. https://doi.org/10.1093/neuonc/noab150.

18. Halasz LM, Bussière MR, Dennis ER, Niemierko A, Chapman PH, Loeffler JS, Shih HA. Proton stereotactic radiosurgery for the treatment of benign meningiomas. Int J Radiat Oncol Biol Phys. 2011;81(5):1428–35. https://doi.org/10.1016/j.ijrobp.2010.07.1991.

19. Weber DC, Schneider R, Goitein G, Koch T, Ares C, Geismar JH, Schertler A, Bolsi A, Hug EB. Spot scanning-based proton therapy for intracranial meningioma: long-term results from the Paul Scherrer Institute. Int J Radiat Oncol Biol Phys. 2012;83(3):865–71. https://doi.org/10.1016/j.ijrobp.2011.08.027.

20. Combs SE, Kessel K, Habermehl D, Haberer T, Jäkel O, Debus J. Proton and carbon ion radiotherapy for primary brain tumors and tumors of the skull base. Acta Oncol. 2013;52(7):1504–9. https://doi.org/10.3109/0284186X.2013.818255.

21. Vlachogiannis P, Gudjonsson O, Montelius A, Grusell E, Isacsson U, Nilsson K, Blomquist E. Hypofractionated high-energy proton-beam irradiation is an alternative treatment for WHO grade I menin-

giomas. Acta Neurochir. 2017;159(12):2391–400. https://doi.org/10.1007/s00701-017-3352-4.

22. Murray FR, Snider JW, Bolsi A, Lomax AJ, Walser M, Kliebsch U, Schneider RA, Weber DC. Long term clinical outcomes of pencil beam scanning proton therapy for benign and non-benign intracranial meningiomas. Int J Radiat Oncol Biol Phys. 2017;99(5):1190–8. https://doi.org/10.1016/j.ijrobp.2017.08.005.

23. El Shafie RA, Czech M, Kessel KA, Habermehl D, Weber D, Rieken S, Bougatf N, Jäkel O, Debus J, Combs SE. Clinical outcome after particle therapy for meningiomas of the skull base: toxicity and local control in patients treated with active rasterscanning. Radiat Oncol. 2018;13(1):54. https://doi.org/10.1186/s13014-018-1002-5.

24. Wu A, Jin MC, Meola A, Wong HN, Chang SD. Efficacy and toxicity of particle radiotherapy in WHO grade II and grade III meningiomas: a systematic review. Neurosurg Focus. 2019;46(6):E12. https://doi.org/10.3171/2019.3.FOCUS1967.

25. Coggins WS, Pham NK, Nguyen AV, Branch DW, Guillet JY, Korst G, Lall RR. A systematic review of ion radiotherapy in maintaining local control regarding atypical and anaplastic meningiomas. World Neurosurg. 2019;132:282–91. https://doi.org/10.1016/j.wneu.2019.08.149.

26. El Shafie RA, Czech M, Kessel KA, Habermehl D, Weber D, Rieken S, Bougatf N, Jäkel O, Debus J, Combs SE. Evaluation of particle radiotherapy for the re-irradiation of recurrent intracranial meningioma. Radiat Oncol. 2018;13(1):86. https://doi.org/10.1186/s13014-018-1026-x.

27. Imber BS, Neal B, Casey DL, Darwish H, Lin AL, Cahlon O, Chon B, Tsai H, Hug E, Yamada Y, Yang TJ. Clinical outcomes of recurrent intracranial meningiomas treated with proton beam reirradiation. Int J Part Ther. 2019;5(4):11–22. https://doi.org/10.14338/IJPT-18-00045.1.

28. Daly AF, Beckers A. The epidemiology of pituitary adenomas. Endocrinol Metab Clin N Am. 2020;49(3):347–55.

29. Asa SL, Mete O, Perry A, Osamura RY. Overview of the 2022 WHO classification of pituitary tumors. Endocr Pathol. 2022;33(1):6–26. https://doi.org/10.1007/s12022-022-09703-7.

30. Ronson BB, Schulte RW, Han KP, Loredo LN, Slater JM, Slater JD. Fractionated proton beam irradiation of pituitary adenomas. Int J Radiat Oncol Biol Phys. 2006;64:425–34.

31. Wattson DA, Tanguturi SK, Spiegel DY, Niemierko A, Biller BM, Nachtigall LB, Bussiere MR, Swearingen B, Chapman PH, Loeffler JS, Shih HA. Outcomes of proton therapy for patients with functional pituitary adenomas. Int J Radiat Oncol Biol Phys. 2014;90:532–9.

32. Momin AA, Recinos MA, Cioffi G, Patil N, Soni P, Almeida JP, Kruchko C, Barnholtz-Sloan JS, Recinos PF, Kshettry VR. Descriptive epidemiology of craniopharyngiomas in the United States. Pituitary.

2021;24(4):517–22.   https://doi.org/10.1007/
s11102-021-01127-6.

33. Boehling NS, Grosshans DR, Bluett JB, Palmer MT, Song X, Amos RA, Sahoo N, Meyer JJ, Mahajan A, Woo SY. Dosimetric comparison of three-dimensional conformal proton radiotherapy, intensity-modulated proton therapy, and intensity-modulated radiotherapy for treatment of pediatric craniopharyngiomas. Int J Radiat Oncol Biol Phys. 2012;82(2):643–52. https://doi.org/10.1016/j.ijrobp.2010.11.027.

34. Beltran C, Roca M, Merchant TE. On the benefits and risks of proton therapy in pediatric craniopharyngioma. Int J Radiat Oncol Biol Phys. 2012;82(2):e281–7. https://doi.org/10.1016/j.ijrobp.2011.01.005.

35. Bishop AJ, Greenfield B, Mahajan A, Paulino AC, Okcu MF, Allen PK, Chintagumpala M, Kahalley LS, McAleer MF, McGovern SL, Whitehead WE, Grosshans DR. Proton beam therapy versus conformal photon radiation therapy for childhood craniopharyngioma: multi-institutional analysis of outcomes, cyst dynamics, and toxicity. Int J Radiat Oncol Biol Phys. 2014;90(2):354–61. https://doi.org/10.1016/j.ijrobp.2014.05.051.

36. Jimenez RB, Ahmed S, Johnson A, Thomas H, Depauw N, Horick N, Tansky J, Evans CL, Pulsifer M, Ebb D, Butler WE, Fullerton B, Tarbell NJ, Yock TI, MacDonald SM. Proton radiation therapy for pediatric craniopharyngioma. Int J Radiat Oncol Biol Phys. 2021;110(5):1480–7. https://doi.org/10.1016/j.ijrobp.2021.02.045.

37. Rutenberg MS, Rotondo RL, Rao D, Holtzman AL, Indelicato DJ, Huh S, Morris CG, Mendenhall WM. Clinical outcomes following proton therapy for adult craniopharyngioma: a single-institution cohort study. J Neurooncol. 2020;147(2):387–95. https://doi.org/10.1007/s11060-020-03432-9.3.

38. Ajithkumar T, Mazhari AL, Stickan-Verfürth M, Kramer PH, Fuentes CS, Lambert J, Thomas H, Müller H, Fleischhack G, Timmermann B. Proton therapy for craniopharyngioma—an early report from a single European centre. Clin Oncol (R Coll Radiol). 2018;30(5):307–16.   https://doi.org/10.1016/j.clon.2018.01.012.

39. Adeberg S, Harrabi SB, Verma V, et al. Treatment of meningioma and glioma with protons and carbon ions. Radiat Oncol. 2017;12(1):193. https://doi.org/10.1186/s13014-017-0924-7.

40. Thurin E, Nyström PW, Smits A, et al. Proton therapy for low-grade gliomas in adults: a systematic review. Clin Neurol Neurosurg. 2018;174:233–8. https://doi.org/10.1016/j.clineuro.2018.08.003.

41. Tabrizi S, Yeap BY, Sherman JC, et al. Long-term outcomes and late adverse effects of a prospective study on proton radiotherapy for patients with low-grade glioma. Radiother Oncol. 2019;137:95–101. https://doi.org/10.1016/j.radonc.2019.04.027.

42. Eichkorn T, Lischalk JW, Hörner-Rieber J, Deng M, Meixner E, Krämer A, Hoegen P, Sandrini E, Regnery S, Held T, Harrabi S, Jungk C, Herfarth K, Debus J, König L. Analysis of safety and efficacy of proton

radiotherapy for IDH-mutated glioma WHO grade 2 and 3. J Neurooncol. 2023; https://doi.org/10.1007/s11060-022-04217-y.

43. Shih HA, Sherman JC, Nachtigall LB, Colvin MK, Fullerton BC, Daartz J, Winrich BK, Batchelor TT, Thornton LT, Mancuso SM, Saums MK, Oh KS, Curry WT, Loeffler JS, Yeap BY. Proton therapy for low-grade gliomas: results from a prospective trial. Cancer. 2015;121(10):1712–9. https://doi.org/10.1002/cncr.29237.

44. Sherman JC, Colvin MK, Mancuso SM, Batchelor TT, Oh KS, Loeffler JS, Yeap BY, Shih HA. Neurocognitive effects of proton radiation therapy in adults with low-grade glioma. J Neurooncol. 2016;126(1):157–64. https://doi.org/10.1007/s11060-015-1952-5.

45. Wang Y, Liu R, Zhang Q, Dong M, Wang D, Chen J, Ou Y, Luo H, Yang K, Wang X. Charged particle therapy for high-grade gliomas in adults: a systematic review. Radiat Oncol. 2023;18(1):29. https://doi.org/10.1186/s13014-022-02187-z.

46. Goff KM, Zheng C, Alonso-Basanta M. Proton radiotherapy for glioma and glioblastoma. Chin Clin Oncol. 2022;11(6):46. https://doi.org/10.21037/cco-22-92.

47. Kong L, Wu J, Gao J, et al. Particle radiation therapy in the management of malignant glioma: early experience at the Shanghai Proton and Heavy Ion Center. Cancer. 2020;126(12):2802–10. https://doi.org/10.1002/cncr.32828.

48. Mizumoto M, Oshiro Y, Yamamoto T, Kohzuki H, Sakurai H. Proton beam therapy for pediatric brain tumor. Neurol Med Chir (Tokyo). 2017;57(7):343–55.

49. Hess CB, Indelicato DJ, Paulino AC, Hartsell WF, Hill-Kayser CE, Perkins SM, Mahajan A, Laack NN, Ermoian RP, Chang AL, Wolden SL, Mangona VS, Kwok Y, Breneman JC, Perentesis JP, Gallotto SL, Weyman EA, Bajaj BVM, Lawell MP, Yeap BY, Yock TI. An update from the Pediatric Proton Consortium Registry. Front Oncol. 2018;8:165. https://doi.org/10.3389/fonc.2018.00165.

50. Huynh M, Marcu LG, Giles E, Short M, Matthews D, Bezak E. Current status of proton therapy outcome for paediatric cancers of the central nervous system—analysis of the published literature. Cancer Treat Rev. 2018;70:272–88. https://doi.org/10.1016/j.ctrv.2018.10.003.

51. Huynh M, Marcu LG, Giles E, Short M, Matthews D, Bezak E. Are further studies needed to justify the use of proton therapy for paediatric cancers of the central nervous system? A review of current evidence. Radiother Oncol. 2019;133:140–8. https://doi.org/10.1016/j.radonc.2019.01.009.

52. Indelicato DJ, Merchant T, Laperriere N, Lassen Y, Vennarini S, Wolden S, Hartsell W, Pankuch M, Brandal P, Law CK, Taylor R, Laskar S, Okcu MF, Bouffet E, Mandeville H, Björk-Eriksson T, Nilsson K, Nyström H, Constine LS, Story M, Timmermann B, Roberts K, Kortmann RD. Consensus report from the Stockholm Pediatric Proton Therapy Conference. Int J Radiat Oncol Biol Phys. 2016;96(2):387–92. https://doi.org/10.1016/j.ijrobp.2016.06.2446.

53. Pearce MS, Salotti JA, Little MP, et al. Radiation exposure from CT scans in childhood and subsequent risk of leukaemia and brain tumours: a retrospective cohort study. Lancet. 2012;380:499–505.

54. Dennis M, Spiegler BJ, Hetherington CR, Greenberg ML. Neuropsychological sequelae of the treatment of children with medulloblastoma. J Neurooncol. 1996;29:91–101.

55. Merchant TE, Hua CH, Shukla H, Ying X, Nill S, Oelfke U. Proton versus photon radiotherapy for common pediatric brain tumors: comparison of models of dose characteristics and their relationship to cognitive function. Pediatr Blood Cancer. 2008;51:110–7.

56. Stokkevåg CH, Indelicato DJ, Herfarth K, Magelssen H, Evensen ME, Ugland M, Nordberg T, Nystad TA, Hægeland A, Alsaker MD, Ulven K, Dale JE, Engeseth GM, Boer CG, Toussaint L, Kornerup JS, Pettersen HES, Brydøy M, Brandal P, Muren LP. Normal tissue complication probability models in plan evaluation of children with brain tumors referred to proton therapy. Acta Oncol. 2019;58(10):1416–22. https://doi.org/10.1080/0284186X.2019.1643496.

57. Pulsifer MB, Duncanson H, Grieco J, Evans C, Tseretopoulos ID, MacDonald S, Tarbell NJ, Yock TI. Cognitive and adaptive outcomes after proton radiation for pediatric patients with brain tumors. Int J Radiat Oncol Biol Phys. 2018;102(2):391–8. https://doi.org/10.1016/j.ijrobp.2018.05.069.

58. Gross JP, Powell S, Zelko F, Hartsell W, Goldman S, Fangusaro J, Lulla RR, Smiley NP, Chang JH, Gondi V. Improved neuropsychological outcomes following proton therapy relative to X-ray therapy for pediatric brain tumor patients. Neuro Oncol. 2019;21(7):934–43. https://doi.org/10.1093/neuonc/noz070.

59. Kahalley LS, Peterson R, Ris MD, Janzen L, Okcu MF, Grosshans DR, Ramaswamy V, Paulino AC, Hodgson D, Mahajan A, Tsang DS, Laperriere N, Whitehead WE, Dauser RC, Taylor MD, Conklin HM, Chintagumpala M, Bouffet E, Mabbott D. Superior intellectual outcomes after proton radiotherapy compared with photon radiotherapy for pediatric medulloblastoma. J Clin Oncol. 2020;38(5):454–61. https://doi.org/10.1200/JCO.19.0170.

60. Greenberger BA, Pulsifer MB, Ebb DH, MacDonald SM, Jones RM, Butler WE, Huang MS, Marcus KJ, Oberg JA, Tarbell NJ, Yock TI. Clinical outcomes and late endocrine, neurocognitive, and visual profiles of proton radiation for pediatric low-grade gliomas. Int J Radiat Oncol Biol Phys. 2014;89(5):1060–8. https://doi.org/10.1016/j.ijrobp.2014.04.053.

61. Christopherson KM, Rotondo RL, Bradley JA, Pincus DW, Wynn TT, Fort JA, Morris CG, Mendenhall NP, Marcus RB Jr, Indelicato DJ. Late toxicity following craniospinal radiation for early-stage medulloblastoma. Acta Oncol. 2014;53(4):471–80.

62. Cacciotti C, Chordas C, Valentino K, Allen R, Lenzen A, Burns K, Nagarajan R, Manley P, Pillay-Smiley N. Cardiac dysfunction in medulloblastoma survivors treated with photon irradiation. Neurooncol Pract. 2022;9(4):338–43. https://doi.org/10.1093/nop/npac030.

63. Strodtbeck K, Sloan A, Rogers L, Fisher PG, Stearns D, Campbell L, et al. Risk of subsequent cancer following a primary CNS tumor. J Neurooncol. 2013;112:285–95.

64. Goldstein AM, Yuen J, Tucker MA. Second cancers after medulloblastoma: population-based results from the United States and Sweden. Cancer Cause Control. 1997;8:865–71.

65. Zhang R, Howell RM, Giebeler A, Taddei PJ, Mahajan A, Newhauser WD. Comparison of risk of radiogenic second cancer following photon and proton craniospinal irradiation for a pediatric medulloblastoma patient. Phys Med Biol. 2013;58:807–23.

66. Uemura S, Demizu Y, Hasegawa D, Fujikawa T, Inoue S, Nishimura A, Tojyo R, Nakamura S, Kozaki A, Saito A, Kishimoto K, Ishida T, Mori T, Koyama J, Kawamura A, Akasaka Y, Yoshida M, Fukumitsu N, Soejima T, Kosaka Y. The comparison of acute toxicities associated with craniospinal irradiation between photon beam therapy and proton beam therapy in children with brain tumors. Cancer Med. 2022;11(6):1502–10.

67. Johnstone PA, McMullen KP, Buchsbaum JC, Douglas JG, Helft P. Pediatric CSI: are protons the only ethical approach? Int J Radiat Oncol Biol Phys. 2013;87:228–30.

68. Goitein M, Jermann M. The relative costs of proton and X-ray radiation therapy. Clin Oncol (R Coll Radiol). 2003;15:S37–50.

69. Loeffler JS, Durante M. Charged particle therapy—optimization, challenges and future directions. Nat Rev Clin Oncol. 2013;10(7):411–24. https://doi.org/10.1038/nrclinonc.2013.79.

70. Lundkvist J, Ekman M, Ericsson SR, Jönsson B, Glimelius B. Cost-effectiveness of proton radiation in the treatment of childhood medulloblastoma. Cancer. 2005;103:793–801. https://doi.org/10.1002/cncr.20844.

71. Mailhot Vega RB, Kim J, Bussière M, Hattangadi J, Hollander A, Michalski J, et al. Cost effectiveness of proton therapy compared with photon therapy in the management of pediatric medulloblastoma. Cancer. 2013;119:4299–307. https://doi.org/10.1002/cncr.28322.

72. Hirano E, Fuji H, Onoe T, Kumar V, Shirato H, Kawabuchi K. Cost-effectiveness analysis of cochlear dose reduction by proton beam therapy for medulloblastoma in childhood. J Radiat Res. 2014;55:320–7. https://doi.org/10.1093/jrr/rrt112.

73. Mailhot Vega R, Kim J, Hollander A, Hattangadi-Gluth J, Michalski J, Tarbell NJ, et al. Cost effectiveness of proton versus photon radiation therapy with respect to the risk of growth hormone deficiency in children. Cancer. 2015;121:1694–702. https://doi.org/10.1002/cncr.29209.

New Radiopharmaceuticals for Brain Tumors Imaging

Adrien Holzgreve and Nathalie L. Albert

9.1 Introduction

The standard imaging modality for brain tumors is magnetic resonance imaging (MRI). However, MRI has relevant limitations for adequate evaluation of brain tumors in multiple clinical scenarios. Therefore, positron emission tomography (PET) imaging has evolved as an established companion to MRI over the last decades and adds valuable information beyond conventional imaging for the assessment of brain tumors, e.g., with regard to differential diagnosis, treatment planning, or treatment response assessment [1, 2].

The brain has a high physiological glucose turnover. As a consequence, a possibly altered glucose metabolism associated with brain lesions, including brain tumors, is difficult to demarcate from surrounding healthy brain tissue. Therefore, unlike for most other oncologic entities, radiolabeled glucose (2-[^{18}F]fluoro-2-deoxy-D-glucose, [^{18}F]FDG) is generally not recommended for the imaging of brain tumors [3]. Instead, other radiopharmaceuticals have emerged as the standard PET tracers for distinct brain tumor groups. In gliomas and brain metastases, radiolabeled amino acid analogs are now well-established for PET imaging and recommended for a variety of clinical indications. These tracers include O-(2-[^{18}F]-fluoroethyl)-L-tyrosine ([^{18}F]FET), [^{11}C]-methyl-L-methionine ([^{11}C]MET), and 3,4-dihydroxy-6-[^{18}F]-fluoro-L-phenylalanine ([^{18}F]DOPA) [4]. Meningiomas, on the other hand, are primarily susceptible to imaging with somatostatin receptor (SSTR)-targeting PET tracers, these typically include [^{68}Ga]DOTA-Tyr3-octreotide ([^{68}Ga]DOTA-TOC) and [^{68}Ga]DOTA-D-Phe1-Tyr-3-octreotide ([^{68}Ga]DOTA-TATE) [5, 6]. SSTR-based PET/computed tomography (CT) has now become an established tool for meningioma imaging and is increasingly recommended, especially in cases with equivocal CT or MRI findings [7].

The previously mentioned tracers can be considered as well-established for the distinct brain tumor groups, and PET imaging with these tracers is now a widely accepted technique for the management of brain tumor patients in clinical routine, at least in Europe. However, neurooncological nuclear medicine is a dynamic field and multiple additional targets can be addressed in brain tumors with the use of innovative PET tracers. In this chapter, we briefly review selected developments on new radiopharmaceuticals for brain tumor imaging.

A. Holzgreve · N. L. Albert (✉)
Department of Nuclear Medicine, University Hospital, LMU Munich, Munich, Germany
e-mail: Adrien.Holzgreve@med.lmu.de;
Nathalie.Albert@med.uni-muenchen.de

© The Author(s), under exclusive license to Springer Nature Switzerland AG 2024
E. Lopci, L. Mansi (eds.), *Advanced Imaging and Therapy in Neuro-Oncology*,
https://doi.org/10.1007/978-3-031-59341-3_9

9.2 Why to Address Other Targets and Mechanisms Beyond the Established PET Radiopharmaceuticals in Brain Tumors?

The previous and currently established PET imaging of brain tumors mainly focused on the detection and delineation of vital tumor tissue and has thus helped to reduce an unmet clinical need compared to conventional imaging with CT and MRI alone. A typical indication for amino acid PET in patients with glioblastoma or brain metastasis is, for example, the differentiation of vital tumor tissue in terms of a local tumor recurrence/progression after irradiation from post-therapeutic changes in terms of a radiation necrosis/pseudoprogression. While MRI may show comparably increased contrast enhancement in both cases, the absence of increased amino acid uptake on PET here would strongly advocate against the presence of a recurrence and may thus prevent the patient from undergoing unnecessary and potentially dangerous consequential procedures such as surgery or a further line of tumor-directed systemic treatment [8]. Although the clinical benefit of such applications is intuitive, they rely on a rather simplistic biological view to enable straightforward clinical decision-making (vital tumor tissue: yes or no). However, brain tumors are by far more complex and the rationale for imaging cannot be reduced to the question of whether or not vital tumor tissue is present. That alone is shown by the fact that in pre-treated cases not always binary statements regarding the presence of vital tumor tissue are possible but there are also borderline cases with a certain range of interpretation. Also in untreated glioma cases, amino acid tracers may show a relevant intra-tumoral uptake heterogeneity [9, 10] and also an inter-individual uptake variety, the latter even facilitating prognostic stratification within distinct neuropathological tumor types based on PET-derived parameters [11].

Instead, it is precisely this heterogeneity and complexity of brain tumors that holds a presumed key to overcoming their pertinent treatment resistance, especially with regard to the poor prognosis of malignant brain tumors. Several underlying

(patho-)physiological processes, including those involved in the tumor growth initiation, the tumor infiltration in surrounding brain structures, the related immunological landscape, or the tumor-host interaction in general, for instance, are susceptible to PET imaging. Both processes within the tumor core such as those linked to apoptosis or hypoxia and at the tumor/brain infiltration zone such as those linked to the host immune response can be selectively captured using PET imaging. Another intriguing perspective lies in the identification and visualization of potentially druggable pathways in a therapeutic frame and/or theranostic approaches.

In a nutshell, PET imaging is a versatile tool with great potential to comprehensively and non-invasively characterize brain tumors using a wide range of diverse PET tracers. Here, new radiopharmaceuticals are a key driver for the advancement of PET imaging in neuro-oncology and therefore deserve to be considered in more detail.

9.3 Gliomas

Even though amino acid PET is well established, new amino acid radiopharmaceuticals continue to be developed, e.g., N-(2-[^{18}F]-fluoropropionyl)-L-glutamate has recently been proposed for imaging glioma [12]. The mode of action however is rather comparable to the existing tracers and so far, no clinically relevant progress is to be expected here yet. As another mode of action, PET tracers can selectively depict areas of high proliferation. An increased proliferation rate is a key defining characteristic of malignant neoplasms such as brain tumors. 3'-deoxy-3'-[^{18}F] fluorothymidine ([^{18}F]FLT) is the most common PET tracer for proliferation imaging and has been applied in brain tumors for nearly 20 years [13, 14]. Prior to that, 2-[^{11}C]thymidine has also been used as a proliferation marker, although largely abandoned due to the short half-life of ^{11}C and unfavorable chemical properties [15]. Attempts to optimize [^{18}F]FLT through radiopharmaceutical modifications remained partly unsatisfactory [16]. As a limitation, the utility of [^{18}F]FLT to depict increased phosphorylation by thymidine kinase-1 in brain tumors seems to depend on the integrity of the blood-brain-barrier (BBB), and therefore the use of [^{18}F]FLT has been questioned in non-enhancing gliomas [17]. Also, [^{18}F]FLT is thought only to reflect parts of the DNA synthesis [18]. New proliferation-targeted radiopharmaceuticals with minor structural differences to [^{18}F]FLT try to overcome some of these issues [12, 19]. Here, however, 4′-[methyl-^{11}C]thiothymidine ([^{11}C]-4DST) has been shown to be non-superior to [^{18}F]FLT in a direct comparison in gliomas [20].

Perfusion PET imaging has been applied in glioma especially using [^{15}O]H$_2$O and [^{13}N]NH$_3$ as radiopharmaceuticals and principally enables to generate scientifically interesting insights, e.g., it has been shown that perfusion and metabolism are coupled in recurrent gliomas in a dual tracer approach with [^{18}F]FDG [21]. However, perfusion values were incongruent compared to MRI perfusion in a multi-modal brain tumor study including gliomas, meningiomas, and cerebral metastasis [22], and [^{15}O] requires highly demanding logistic circumstances due to its half-life of only 2 min. These and other limitations currently prevent a broader clinical implementation of perfusion PET data in brain tumor patients.

Several PET tracers have been applied to address angiogenesis in gliomas, especially in high-grade gliomas, as they tend to be highly vascularized. Targets mainly include integrin $\alpha_v\beta_3$ and the vascular endothelial grow factor (VEGF) receptor. RGD-based radiopharmaceuticals used in glioma include [^{18}F]Galacto-RGD [23], [^{68}Ga] NOTA-PRGD2 [24], and [^{18}F]FPPRGD2 [25]. As drugs exist to target both VEGF (bevacizumab) and $\alpha_v\beta_3$ (cilengitide), the corresponding PET tracers are interesting also with regard to treatment response evaluation or potentially even prediction, which may be of interest for patient selection. Further PET radiopharmaceuticals for imaging of angiogenesis are being developed, e.g., an apelin-based radiotracer ([^{68}Ga] Ga-AP747) was recently designed to specifically target the APJ receptor, which is heavily involved in angiogenesis [26].

Hypoxia in glioma is known to favor several pathophysiological processes such as the stimulation of stem-like cellular properties linked to treatment resistance [27]. Consequently, hypoxia is an interesting target for PET imaging in glioma, the most common radiopharmaceutical used in this perspective is [^{18}F]fluoromisonidazole ([^{18}F]FMISO) [28]. Further PET tracers for hypoxia which have been used in glioma include [^{18}F]fluoroazomycinarabinoside ([^{18}F]FAZA), [^{18}F]fluoroerythronitroimidazole ([^{18}F]FETNIM) but also compounds targeted with other radionuclides than ^{18}F such as [^{64}Cu][Cu(ATSM)] [29, 30]. Newer developments involve adjusted scan protocols for [^{18}F]FMISO imaging [31].

One of the currently most dynamic fields regarding innovative PET tracers for brain tumor imaging focuses on the tumor microenvironment and immune-mediated processes. Here, especially tracers directed against the mitochondrial 18-kDa translocator protein (TSPO) are extensively studied and include [^{11}C]PBR28, [^{18}F]PBR111, [^{11}C] PK11195, [^{18}F]DPA-714, and [^{18}F]GE-180 [32]. An intriguing aspect here is that both tumor-associated microglia/macrophages and tumor cells overexpress TSPO and can be visualized by means of PET. While increased tumoral TSPO expression is commonly associated with increased malignancy [33] (see Fig. 9.1 for an example), it is still unclear whether or at what stage the immunologically driven component of the TSPO radioligand uptake in PET may be protective or rather have pro-tumoral effects [34, 35].

Alternative targets beyond TSPO are continuously explored and harbor the potential to depict a more in-depth insight such as different states of microglia activation, but the corresponding tracers have not yet reached a successful transition into human application, including cyclooxygenase-targeting radiopharmaceuticals such as [^{11}C]MC1 [36, 37]. Other cell entities of the tumor microenvironment can be selectively targeted and further enhance the understanding of the in vivo composition of the tumor microenvironment of glioma, e.g., a new marker for reactive astrogliosis, [^{18}F]F-DED, has recently been applied in human glioma [38].

One of the most recent and iconic developments in nuclear medicine in this regard is the imaging of fibroblasts with radioligands inhibit-

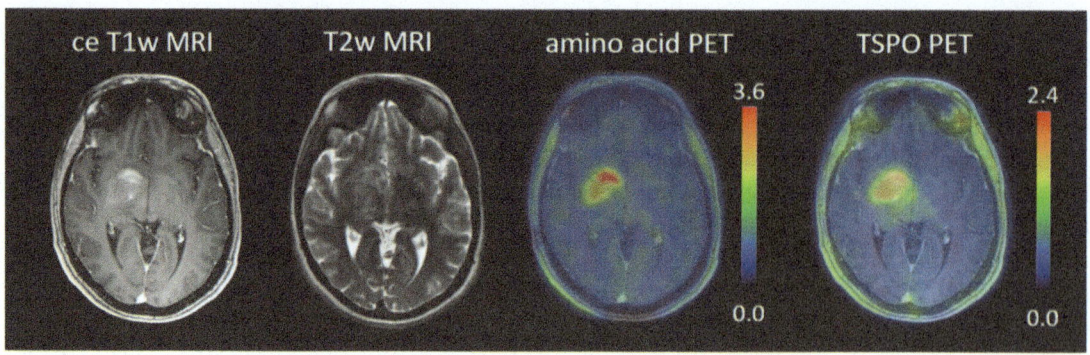

Fig. 9.1 Multimodal imaging with contrast-enhanced MRI, amino acid PET using [18F]FET and TSPO PET using [18F]GE-180 in a patient with a glioma-suspicious lesion in the right basal ganglia shows inhomogeneous contrast-enhancement and intense tracer signal in both, amino acid and TSPO PET. The high TSPO signal points to a highly aggressive tumor biology, subsequent stereotactic biopsy confirmed the neuropathological diagnosis of a glioblastoma, *IDH*-wildtype

ing the fibroblast activation protein (FAP) which has also been applied in gliomas with interesting preliminary results [39].

Further, less common targets are explored in glioma PET imaging including for instance transforming growth factor-β (TGF-β), pyruvate kinase M2 (PKM2), or human copper transporter 1 (hCtr1) [40–42]. An overview of some selected uncommon PET targets in glioma imaging can be found in Table 2 in Laudicella et al. [43].

In particular, the combinatorial use of several of the tracers discussed seems valuable if one aims to comprehensively and non-invasively assess a glioma and its microenvironment [44, 45].

9.4 Meningiomas

68Ga-labeled radioligands constitute the mainstay for SSTR-based PET/CT imaging in meningioma. Typical representatives of this class are [68Ga]DOTA-Tyr3-octreotide ([68Ga]DOTA-TOC), [68Ga]1-Nal3-octreotide ([68Ga]DOTA-NOC) and [68Ga]DOTA-D-Phe1-Tyr-3-octreotide ([68Ga]DOTA-TATE) [5, 6]. A recent development is the clinical implementation of 18F-labeled SSTR radioligands, which is associated with tremendous logistical advantages, partly given the longer half-life of 18F compared to 68Ga [46]. Such new radiopharmaceuticals have preliminarily also been applied in meningioma with prom-

ising results and further data in larger meningioma cohorts are expected to be published soon [47].

Other radiopharmaceuticals than SSTR-based radioligands have sporadically been used in meningioma. Uptake on [18F]FLT PET has been found to be a predictor of meningioma progression [48]. Few case reports illustrate the use of FAPI PET/CT in meningioma with partially increased uptake [49]. Although rarely performed in this indication, [18F]FET has also been shown to provide additional information for the grading of meningiomas and possibly for discrimination in challenging cases [50]. The approach deserves further consideration.

9.5 A Brief Outlook on New Radiopharmaceutical Targets for Brain Tumors Imaging in a Theranostic Perspective

Theranostic approaches are on the rise in nuclear medicine. In 2022, both the FDA and EMA approved prostate-specific membrane antigen (PSMA)-radioligand therapy for advanced prostate cancer owing to its significant treatment success [51]. Peptide receptor radionuclide therapy (PRRT) had previously been approved for use in gastro-entero-pancreatic neuroendocrine tumors [52]. The underlying principles are simple: A tumor-associated target structure (in this case PSMA or SSTR) is addressed by means of a carrier substance. In the first step, a diagnostic nuclide, e.g., ^{68}Ga or ^{18}F, is coupled to this carrier to visualize on PET imaging whether the target structure is expressed to a sufficient extent in the tumor. In the second step, a therapeutic nuclide, e.g., ^{177}Lu or ^{90}Y, is coupled to the carrier, which now allows the tumor to be irradiated selectively and precisely with therapeutic intent.

As meningiomas overexpress SSTR and show a high uptake of diagnostic SSTR-radioligands on PET—comparable to neuroendocrine tumors—they can be likewise addressed by the theranostic concept of PRRT. Initial experiences with ^{177}Lu-DOTA-TATE PRRT in meningioma patients were promising, but the overall published experience is still limited [53, 54]. In view of the promising preliminary results, several prospective multicenter trials are currently ongoing to substantiate the efficacy of PRRT in meningioma. Furthermore, an innovative ^{64}Cu/^{67}Cu-based SSTR-targeted theranostic approach has recently been proposed for meningioma treatment and showed promise [55].

In gliomas, a variety of targets and new radiopharmaceuticals have been investigated or are currently under investigation with an aim to perform radioligand therapy. These innovative approaches include the targets PSMA, tenascin, the epidermal growth factor receptor (EGFR), SSTR, C-X-C chemokine receptor type 4 (CXCR4), and several others [56–61]. A prominent further, envisaged "pan-tumor" theranostic target is FAP. Data on the theranostic use of FAPI-radiopharmaceuticals in brain tumors are to be expected.

In the era of precision oncology, in addition to nuclear medicine theranostic concepts, innovative PET tracers may also be used to select patients for non-radiopharmaceutical targeted therapies. In brain metastases, for instance, HER2 constitutes a relevant target for a variety of agents such as trastuzumab, pertuzumab, and lapatinib, and HER2 expression can be visualized using PET imaging [62]. Likewise, EGFR is a relevant target in brain metastases of lung cancer or breast cancer as well as in glioma, since EGFR-targeted treatments such as osimertinib and afatinib are available. Here, EGFR-targeted immune-PET using ^{89}Zr-Pertuzumab or comparable new radiopharmaceuticals may be useful [63]. Multiple further targets are currently under investigation.

9.6 Conclusion/Summary

In sum, a broad range of new radiopharmaceuticals for brain tumor imaging has been developed or is currently investigated, and further innovations are to be expected both for the diagnostics and the treatment of gliomas, meningiomas, and brain metastases. A major advantage of PET imaging is the ability to image selective biological processes and thus gain comprehensive knowledge of the tumor in a non-invasive manner. PET results can support the decision to target therapies, either non-radioactive or radioactive as part of a theranostic approach. Neuro-oncological nuclear medicine remains a vibrant field and could make a relevant contribution to a better understanding of brain tumors as well as to improved management of affected patients.

Acknowledgments Adrien Holzgreve is a member of the European Organization for the Research and Treatment of Cancer (EORTC) brain tumor group and the EORTC imaging committee. Nathalie Albert is the current chair of the Nuclear Medicine committee of the EORTC brain tumor group. Adrien Holzgreve is a member of the PET committee of the German Society of Nuclear Medicine (DGN). Nathalie Albert is a member of the neuroimaging committee of the DGN as well as the European Association of Nuclear Medicine (EANM). Nathalie Albert has received honoraria for consultation or advisory board participation from Novartis, Advanced Accelerator Applications, Servier and Telix Pharmaceuticals, speakers honoraria from OncLive and Telix Pharmaceuticals, and research funding from Novocure.

Ethics Approval The image examples originate from the Department of Nuclear Medicine, University Hospital, LMU Munich, Munich, Germany. The local ethics Committee waives additional approval for case reports.

References

1. Albert NL, Weller M, Suchorska B, et al. Response Assessment in Neuro-Oncology working group and European Association for Neuro-Oncology recommendations for the clinical use of PET imaging in gliomas. Neuro Oncol. 2016;18:1199–208.
2. Holzgreve A, Albert NL, Galldiks N, et al. Use of PET imaging in neuro-oncological surgery. Cancers. 2021;13(9):2093.
3. Law I, Albert NL, Arbizu J, et al. Joint EANM/EANO/RANO practice guidelines/SNMMI procedure standards for imaging of gliomas using PET with radiolabelled amino acids and [(18)F]FDG: version 1.0. Eur J Nucl Med Mol Imaging. 2019;46:540–57.
4. Galldiks N, Lohmann P, Fink GR, et al. Amino acid PET in neurooncology. J Nucl Med. 2023;64:693–700.
5. Bashir A, Larsen VA, Ziebell M, et al. Improved detection of postoperative residual meningioma with [(68)Ga]Ga-DOTA-TOC PET imaging using a high-resolution research tomograph PET scanner. Clin Cancer Res. 2021;27:2216–25.
6. Rachinger W, Stoecklein VM, Terpolilli NA, et al. Increased 68Ga-DOTATATE uptake in PET imaging discriminates meningioma and tumor-free tissue. J Nucl Med. 2015;56:347–53.
7. Galldiks N, Albert NL, Sommerauer M, et al. PET imaging in patients with meningioma-report of the RANO/PET Group. Neuro Oncol. 2017;19:1576–87.
8. Galldiks N, Stoffels G, Filss CP, et al. Role of O-(2-(18)F-fluoroethyl)-L-tyrosine PET for differentiation of local recurrent brain metastasis from radiation necrosis. J Nucl Med. 2012;53:1367–74.
9. Kunz M, Thon N, Eigenbrod S, et al. Hot spots in dynamic (18)FET-PET delineate malignant tumor parts within suspected WHO grade II gliomas. Neuro Oncol. 2011;13:307–16.
10. Wyss MT, Hofer S, Hefti M, et al. Spatial heterogeneity of low-grade gliomas at the capillary level: a PET study on tumor blood flow and amino acid uptake. J Nucl Med. 2007;48:1047–52.
11. Li Z, Holzgreve A, Unterrainer LM, et al. Combination of pre-treatment dynamic [(18)F]FET PET radiomics and conventional clinical parameters for the survival stratification in patients with IDH-wildtype glioblastoma. Eur J Nucl Med Mol Imaging. 2023;50:535–45.
12. Sun A, Liu S, Tang X, et al. N-(2-(18) F-fluoropropionyl)-l-glutamate as a potential oncology tracer for PET imaging of glioma. Appl Radiat Isot. 2021;168:109530.
13. Choi SJ, Kim JS, Kim JH, et al. [18F]3′-deoxy-3′-fluorothymidine PET for the diagnosis and grading of brain tumors. Eur J Nucl Med Mol Imaging. 2005;32:653–9.
14. Shields AF, Grierson JR, Dohmen BM, et al. Imaging proliferation in vivo with [F-18]FLT and positron emission tomography. Nat Med. 1998;4:1334–6.
15. Eary JF, Mankoff DA, Spence AM, et al. 2-[C-11] thymidine imaging of malignant brain tumors. Cancer Res. 1999;59:615–21.
16. Brickute D, Beckley A, Allott L, et al. Synthesis and evaluation of 3′-[(18)F]fluorothymidine-5′-squaryl as a bioisostere of 3′-[(18)F]fluorothymidine-5′-monophosphate. RSC Adv. 2021;11:12423–33.
17. Muzi M, Spence AM, O'sullivan F, et al. Kinetic analysis of 3′-deoxy-3′-18F-fluorothymidine in patients with gliomas. J Nucl Med. 2006;47:1612–21.
18. Rasey JS, Grierson JR, Wiens LW, et al. Validation of FLT uptake as a measure of thymidine kinase-1 activity in A549 carcinoma cells. J Nucl Med. 2002;43:1210–7.
19. Takami Y, Yamamoto Y, Ueno M, et al. Correlation of 4′-[methyl-(11)C]-thiothymidine uptake with human equilibrative nucleoside transporter-1 and thymidine kinase-1 expressions in patients with newly diagnosed gliomas. Ann Nucl Med. 2018;32:634–41.
20. Toyota Y, Miyake K, Kawai N, et al. Comparison of 4′-[methyl-(11)C]thiothymidine ((11)C-4DST) and 3′-deoxy-3′-[(18)F]fluorothymidine ((18)F-FLT) PET/CT in human brain glioma imaging. EJNMMI Res. 2015;5:7.
21. Khangembam BC, Karunanithi S, Sharma P, et al. Perfusion-metabolism coupling in recurrent gliomas: a prospective validation study with 13N-ammonia and 18F-fluorodeoxyglucose PET/CT. Neuroradiology. 2014;56:893–902.
22. Lüdemann L, Warmuth C, Plotkin M, et al. Brain tumor perfusion: comparison of dynamic contrast enhanced magnetic resonance imaging using T1, T2, and T2* contrast, pulsed arterial spin labeling, and H2(15)O positron emission tomography. Eur J Radiol. 2009;70:465–74.
23. Schnell O, Krebs B, Carlsen J, et al. Imaging of integrin alpha(v)beta(3) expression in patients with malignant glioma by [18F] Galacto-RGD positron emission tomography. Neuro Oncol. 2009;11:861–70.
24. Li D, Zhao X, Zhang L, et al. (68)Ga-PRGD2 PET/CT in the evaluation of Glioma: a prospective study. Mol Pharm. 2014;11:3923–9.
25. Iagaru A, Mosci C, Mittra E, et al. Glioblastoma multiforme recurrence: an exploratory study of (18) F FPPRGD2 PET/CT. Radiology. 2015;277:497–506.
26. Louis B, Nail V, Nachar O, et al. Design and preclinical evaluation of a novel apelin-based PET radiotracer targeting APJ receptor for molecular imaging of angiogenesis. Angiogenesis. 2023;26(3):463–75.
27. Harris AL. Hypoxia—a key regulatory factor in tumour growth. Nat Rev Cancer. 2002;2:38–47.
28. Galldiks N, Langen KJ, Albert NL, et al. Investigational PET tracers in neuro-oncology—what's on the horizon? A report of the PET/RANO group. Neuro Oncol. 2022;24:1815–26.
29. Gangemi V, Mignogna C, Guzzi G, et al. Impact of [(64)Cu][Cu(ATSM)] PET/CT in the evaluation of hypoxia in a patient with Glioblastoma: a case report. BMC Cancer. 2019;19:1197.
30. Mapelli P, Callea M, Fallanca F, et al. 18F-FAZA PET/CT in pretreatment assessment of hypoxic status in high-grade glioma: correlation with hypoxia immunohistochemical biomarkers. Nucl Med Commun. 2021;42:763–71.

31. Kobayashi K, Manabe O, Hirata K, et al. Influence of the scan time point when assessing hypoxia in (18) F-fluoromisonidazole PET: 2 vs. 4 h. Eur J Nucl Med Mol Imaging. 2020;47:1833–42.

32. Zinnhardt B, Roncaroli F, Foray C, et al. Imaging of the glioma microenvironment by TSPO PET. Eur J Nucl Med Mol Imaging. 2021;49:174–85.

33. Ammer LM, Vollmann-Zwerenz A, Ruf V, et al. The role of translocator protein TSPO in hallmarks of glioblastoma. Cancers. 2020;12(10):2973.

34. Menevse AN, Ammer LM, Vollmann-Zwerenz A, et al. TSPO acts as an immune resistance gene involved in the T cell mediated immune control of glioblastoma. Acta Neuropathol Commun. 2023;11:75.

35. Quach S, Holzgreve A, Von Baumgarten L, et al. Increased TSPO PET signal after radiochemotherapy in IDH-wildtype glioma-indicator for treatment-induced immune activation? Eur J Nucl Med Mol Imaging. 2022;49:4282–3.

36. Beaino W, Janssen B, Vugts DJ, et al. Towards PET imaging of the dynamic phenotypes of microglia. Clin Exp Immunol. 2021;206:282–300.

37. Janssen B, Vugts DJ, Windhorst AD, et al. PET imaging of microglial activation-beyond targeting TSPO. Molecules (Basel, Switzerland). 2018;23(3):607.

38. Ballweg A, Klaus C, Vogler L, et al. [(18)F]F-DED PET imaging of reactive astrogliosis in neurodegenerative diseases: preclinical proof of concept and first-in-human data. J Neuroinflammation. 2023;20:68.

39. Röhrich M, Loktev A, Wefers AK, et al. IDH-wildtype glioblastomas and grade III/IV IDH-mutant gliomas show elevated tracer uptake in fibroblast activation protein-specific PET/CT. Eur J Nucl Med Mol Imaging. 2019;46:2569–80.

40. Beinat C, Patel CB, Haywood T, et al. Human biodistribution and radiation dosimetry of [(18)F]DASA-23, a PET probe targeting pyruvate kinase M2. Eur J Nucl Med Mol Imaging. 2020;47:2123–30.

41. Den Hollander MW, Bensch F, Glaudemans AW, et al. TGF-β antibody uptake in recurrent high-grade glioma imaged with 89Zr-fresolimumab PET. J Nucl Med. 2015;56:1310–4.

42. Peng F. Recent advances in cancer imaging with (64)CuCl(2) PET/CT. Nucl Med Mol Imaging. 2022;56:80–5.

43. Laudicella R, Quartuccio N, Argiroffi G, et al. Unconventional non-amino acidic PET radiotracers for molecular imaging in gliomas. Eur J Nucl Med Mol Imaging. 2021;48:3925–39.

44. Bailo M, Pecco N, Callea M, et al. Decoding the heterogeneity of malignant gliomas by PET and MRI for spatial habitat analysis of hypoxia, perfusion, and diffusion imaging: a preliminary study. Front Neurosci. 2022;16:885291.

45. Collet S, Guillamo JS, Berro DH, et al. Simultaneous mapping of vasculature, hypoxia, and proliferation using dynamic susceptibility contrast MRI, (18) F-FMISO PET, and (18)F-FLT PET in relation to contrast enhancement in newly diagnosed glioblastoma. J Nucl Med. 2021;62:1349–56.

46. Leupe H, Ahenkorah S, Dekervel J, et al. (18) F-labeled somatostatin analogs as PET tracers for the somatostatin receptor: ready for clinical use. J Nucl Med. 2023;64(6):835–41.

47. Unterrainer M, Lindner S, Beyer L, et al. PET imaging of meningioma using the novel SSTR-targeting peptide 18F-SiTATE. Clin Nucl Med. 2021;46:667–8.

48. Bashir A, Vestergaard MB, Marner L, et al. PET imaging of meningioma with 18F-FLT: a predictor of tumour progression. Brain. 2020;143:3308–17.

49. Denizmen D, Isik EG, Buyukkaya F, et al. 68 Ga-FAPI04 versus 68 Ga-DOTATATE PET/CT in a patient with multiple meningioma. Clin Nucl Med. 2023;48:e244–5.

50. Cornelius JF, Stoffels G, Filß C, et al. Uptake and tracer kinetics of O-(2-(18)F-fluoroethyl)-L-tyrosine in meningiomas: preliminary results. Eur J Nucl Med Mol Imaging. 2015;42:459–67.

51. Anonymous. FDA approves pluvicto/locametz for metastatic castration-resistant prostate cancer. J Nucl Med. 2022;63:13n.

52. Anonymous. FDA approves lutathera for GEP NET therapy. J Nucl Med. 2018;59:9n.

53. Bartolomei M, Bodei L, De Cicco C, et al. Peptide receptor radionuclide therapy with (90)Y-DOTATOC in recurrent meningioma. Eur J Nucl Med Mol Imaging. 2009;36:1407–16.

54. Minczeles NS, Bos EM, De Leeuw RC, et al. Efficacy and safety of peptide receptor radionuclide therapy with [(177)Lu]Lu-DOTA-TATE in 15 patients with progressive treatment-refractory meningioma. Eur J Nucl Med Mol Imaging. 2023;50:1195–204.

55. Bailey DL, Willowson KP, Harris M, et al. (64)Cu treatment planning and (67)Cu therapy with radiolabeled [(64)Cu/(67)Cu]MeCOSar-octreotate in subjects with unresectable multifocal meningioma: initial results for human imaging, safety, biodistribution, and radiation dosimetry. J Nucl Med. 2023;64:704–10.

56. Fiedler L, Kellner M, Gosewisch A, et al. Evaluation of (177)Lu[Lu]-CHX-A″-DTPA-6A10 Fab as a radio-immunotherapy agent targeting carbonic anhydrase XII. Nucl Med Biol. 2018;60:55–62.

57. Holzgreve A, Biczok A, Ruf VC, et al. PSMA expression in glioblastoma as a basis for theranostic approaches: a retrospective, correlational panel study including immunohistochemistry, clinical parameters and PET imaging. Front Oncol. 2021;11: 646387.

58. Jacobs SM, Wesseling P, De Keizer B, et al. CXCR4 expression in glioblastoma tissue and the potential for PET imaging and treatment with [(68)Ga] Ga-Pentixafor/[(177)Lu]Lu-Pentixather. Eur J Nucl Med Mol Imaging. 2022;49:481–91.

59. Li L, Quang TS, Gracely EJ, et al. A Phase II study of anti-epidermal growth factor receptor radioimmunotherapy in the treatment of glioblastoma multiforme. J Neurosurg. 2010;113:192–8.

60. Nemati R, Shooli H, Rekabpour SJ, et al. Feasibility and therapeutic potential of peptide receptor radionuclide therapy for high-grade gliomas. Clin Nucl Med. 2021;46:389–95.

61. Reardon   DA,   Zalutsky   MR,   Bigner
    DD. Antitenascin-C monoclonal antibody radioim-
    munotherapy for malignant glioma patients. Expert
    Rev Anticancer Ther. 2007;7:675–87.
62. Seban RD, Champion L, Bellesoeur A, et al.
    Clinical potential of HER2 PET as a predictive bio-
    marker to guide the use of trastuzumab deruxtecan

in breast cancer patients. J Nucl Med. 2023;64(7):
    1164–5.
63. Ulaner GA, Lyashchenko SK, Riedl C, et al. First-
    in-human human epidermal growth factor receptor
    2-targeted imaging using (89)Zr-pertuzumab PET/
    CT: dosimetry and clinical application in patients with
    breast cancer. J Nucl Med. 2018;59:900–6.

Laszlo Papp, Clemens Spielvogel, David Haberl, and Boglarka Ecsedi

10.1 Introduction

Advancements in artificial intelligence (AI) have been one of the most discussed topics recently, affecting nearly all aspects of our modern lives. A significant portion of focus, dedication, and interdisciplinary engagement had been invested in advancing medical science with AI, which to date, resulted in a wide-range of experiences, including premature enthusiasm, facing the AI uncanny valley, lack of trust, but luckily, a strong and focused scientific persistence as well. Understanding complex AI is challenging for all its stakeholders, including the AI experts themselves. Understanding how the human brain works remains one of the most challenging activities of medical research. In light of the above, deciphering brain disorders—such as neuro-oncological diseases—with one of the most complex AI advancements, appears to be a bold move. Still, the potential benefits outweigh the challenges ahead, thus, rendering neuro-oncological AI research one of the most interesting scientific endeavors one may pursue. Understandably, this process is not without pitfalls, and many of those pitfalls are not due to lack of clinical expertise or technological mediocrity, but rather, due to the non-trivial size of communication and knowledge gap being present between clinicians and AI experts who attempt to advance neuro-oncological AI on their own or together.

To support this process, this book chapter wishes to avoid promoting and detailing any particular radiomics or AI-related approaches from the methodological point of view, as such information has been widely presented and discussed in various contexts [1–4]. Instead, it aims to provide valuable insights for clinicians, written by self-critical AI experts with the intention to help filling up the gap in-between the diverse domains they both represent. Therefore, we aim to provide a comprehensive overview throughout discussing steps of a processing pipeline we see in front of us when dealing with neuro-oncological AI activities. Many of these aspects are generic to all medical AI studies as well.

L. Papp (✉)
Applied Quantum Computing Group, Center for Medical Physics and Biomedical Engineering, Medical University of Vienna, Vienna, Austria
e-mail: laszlo.papp@meduniwien.ac.at

C. Spielvogel · D. Haberl
Division of Nuclear Medicine, Medical University of Vienna, Vienna, Austria

B. Ecsedi
Applied Quantum Computing Group, Center for Medical Physics and Biomedical Engineering, Medical University of Vienna, Vienna, Austria

Georgia Institute of Technology, Atlanta, GA, USA

10.2 Processing Pipeline

While AI expertise can be incorporated into a wide-range of clinical activities, including image acquisition and reconstruction steps, this chapter

© The Author(s), under exclusive license to Springer Nature Switzerland AG 2024
E. Lopci, L. Mansi (eds.), *Advanced Imaging and Therapy in Neuro-Oncology*,
https://doi.org/10.1007/978-3-031-59341-3_10

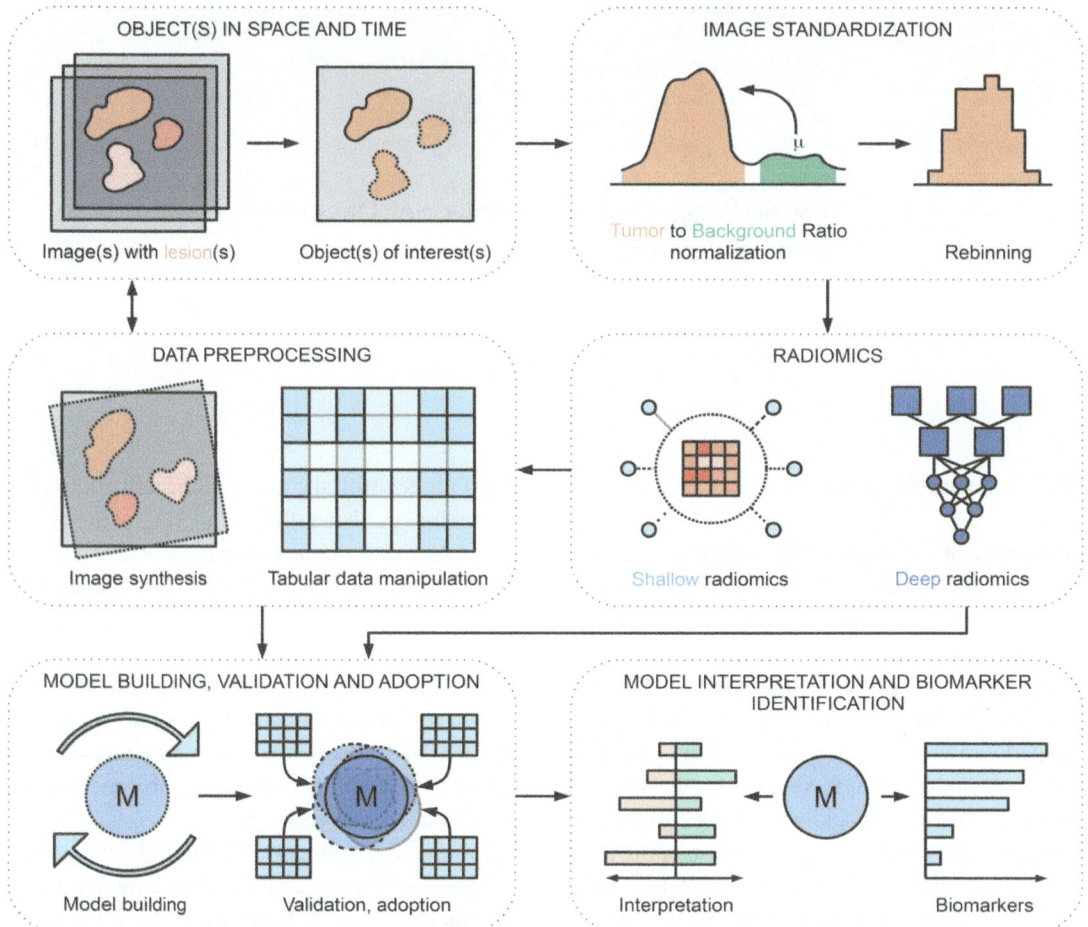

Fig. 10.1 The processing pipeline of artificial intelligence (AI) in neuro-oncological applications. First, objects of interest are defined in medical imaging data. This step often requires consolidating time-series imaging data and multiple lesions to static and singular or aggregated lesion analysis. Image values can be standardized by, e.g., tumor-to-background ratio normalization, followed by binning image intensity values. Radiomics feature extraction may include extracting shallow or deep radiomic features. Data preprocessing can be made both in the image domain (thereby, providing synthetic data for analysis) and in the shallow radiomics feature space, followed by machine learning model building, validation, and adoption. Model interpretation and biomarker identification are essential steps before clinical adoption. This book chapter discusses the above steps according to the six main processing categories and presents potential pitfalls clinicians need to understand and mitigate together with their AI expert

focuses on starting the discussion of AI activities, once imaging and non-imaging data have been collected by standard clinical approaches. Furthermore, while this chapter does not promote any specific delineation approach, them being strongly cohort-specific [5], automated or novel deep-learning-driven approaches have shown promising results when used as an initial delinea-tion to generate, which is then validated and adapted by clinicians if required [6]. Thus, within the realms of this chapter, we consider that such steps have been made together with data collection. Consistently, we identify the main activities as described in Fig. 10.1, and we denote which sections correspond to which of these activities below.

10.3   Object(s) in Space and Time

The disease one wishes to characterize in medical images may either be a singular object (e.g., primary tumor, largest lesion in body) or may be composed of multiple disjunctive objects (e.g., metastatic lesions) within the given image. Furthermore, the acquired image may not be static, but a dynamic one, containing time-series information. Both aspects of single vs. multi-lesion, as well as static vs. dynamic image analysis have similar implications on the radiomic technique being followed (see Sect. 10.5). While there are both multi-lesion radiomic [7, 8] and dynamic radiomic approaches reported [9], these techniques are to date underrepresented and are not yet part of the Imaging Biomarker Standardization Initiative (IBSI) guideline [10], which was presented to standardize how shallow radiomic features are extracted from medical images. Consequently, current research typically falls back to static image analysis, where in the case of dynamic time series, static parametric images are generated for conventional radiomic analysis. In case of multiple lesions, disjunctive regions can be aggregated to one virtual volume of interest (VOI), or only the lesion having the largest metabolic volume may be analyzed. The way of parametric imaging generations and whether to aggregate multiple lesions or to focus on one lesion has to be overseen by clinicians to ensure that clinical relevance remains intact in case the above consolidation step occurs.

10.4   Image Standardization

When one aims to analyze neuro-oncological endpoints by relying on medical imaging data, the first axiom to accommodate is that most imaging protocols are designed to provide images for visual interpretation, and not for radiomics or machine learning (ML) analysis [3, 4, 11]. This means that what the experienced human eye may causally and properly analyze, an ML algorithm may systematically misinterpret. Characteristics, such as physical resolution, signal-to-noise ratio, or quantitativeness shall be understood and be addressed by both ML experts and clinicians as well as the methods they intend to rely on to prepare their data for proper ML analysis. Specifically, value range normalization (a.k.a. rescaling) and binning strategies play an important role in the training and performance of ML models and differ depending on the given data and selected approach.

There is a particularly important aspect of rescaling, which is routinely present in neuro-oncological analyses: tumor-to-background ratio (TBR) normalization [12, 13]. TBR normalization requires a reference region or VOI drawn from a healthy and homogeneous tissue. The given voxel values of the entire image are then divided by the mean of the TBR VOI. There are strong arguments for utilizing TBR normalization in neuro-oncological images. First, images with semi-quantitative values, e.g., Positron Emission Tomography (PET) with standardized uptake value (SUV) units and individual characteristics in metabolic uptake patterns may be counterbalanced by a per-patient reference tissue normalization step. Second, analyzing non-quantitative images (e.g., various MRI sequences such as T2w MRI) after TBR normalization may help to counterbalance patient-specific voxel value range variations that would otherwise result in incorrect analysis. In light of the above, it is crucial to understand that TBR is a per-image normalization step, and hence, any patient-specific variation being present—regardless of the given disease—may be minimized as well. This property may have unwanted effects when one intends to preserve e.g., sex or age-related differences that may be vital for characterizing the given disease. If the TBR reference VOI is affected by such difference, the TBR-normalized radiomic features will be affected by it as well. Consistently, sex-specific variations in, e.g., glioma brain images both in tumors and normal background brain regions have been observed [12]. Therefore, clinicians explicitly need to reflect on the given disease, its sex-specific as well as imaging-specific characteristics, the choice of the reference region for TBR normalization, and whether TBR normalization is an ideal approach to normalize images prior to binning and radiomic analysis at all. Alternatively, assuming that the amount of data is representative and large enough, one may decide not to mix male and female patients in building and utilizing any prediction models at all.

In contrast to normalization, binning shifts and resamples original voxel values to new, standardized value ranges which not only aids noise reduction, but also results in a standardized image intensity scale for analysis [14, 15]. In case the standardized images undergo shallow radiomics (see Sect. 10.5), binning typically results in integer value ranges. This is a technical requirement to ensure that extracted radiomic features conform with respective guidelines, such as the IBSI [10]. In contrast, extracting and analyzing deep radiomic features (see Sect. 10.5) would typically rescale input values in the range of 0.0–1.0 real values, which is mainly a technical reason to support deep learning (DL) training processes converge faster and more stable. In light of the above, it is important to understand, that TBR normalization and binning are not mutually exclusive steps, and they are also not surrogates of each other, however, both may be needed for the given analysis. As such, one may perform TBR normalization, then bin TBR value ranges for appropriate ML/DL analysis. In planning this process, the clinician's presence is imperative.

10.5 Radiomics

The term "radiomics" refers to the approach to extract numerical features from medical images for analysis [1, 4]. At the dawn of adopting this technique in nuclear medicine research, radiomics was associated with extracting hand-crafted features, such as metabolic tumor volume, basic shape features, or textural features. Nevertheless, learning features via deep learning from images can also be considered radiomic features. Recent guidelines systematically separate these two as shallow (a.k.a. hand-crafted) and deep (a.k.a. learnt) radiomic features [5]. Here, we wish to emphasize the underlying issues and characteristics that may help clinicians understanding the implications of whether a shallow or a deep analysis shall be performed on their data, and how

clinical data can be incorporated into their analysis.

Shallow radiomics allows to perform feature ranking and selection (see Sect. 10.6), which not only supports avoiding overfitting of ML models but also supports biomarker identification (see Sect. 10.8). An important recommendation here is to extract IBSI radiomic features having "strong" and "very strong" consensus as of the IBSI standard to support the reproducibility of any findings. While shallow radiomics can be successfully applied to small and representative medical data, it may not be able to properly characterize the underlying disease as it operates with pre-defined sets of markers.

In the field of medical image analysis, the most widely applied deep learning technique to date is the convolutional neural network (CNN) scheme [16, 17]. CNNs are composed of multiple convolutional layers that extract and analyze deep radiomic features from images to predict respective clinical endpoints from them. During the training, both the convolutional kernel values, as well as weights in-between their connected artificial neurons are trained. When certain conditions apply—such as CNNs are trained on whole delineated lesions—the convolutional layers of a CNN can also act as deep radiomic feature extractors. Here, one may utilize both shallow and deep radiomic features to analyze them in one ML model scheme afterward [5], however, this is an emerging field and requires further investigations.

Beyond analyzing imaging-only features, holomics (a.k.a. holistic multi-omics) has been demonstrated as a powerful approach to merge multiple information sources into one holistic database, followed by building holistic ML models [3, 18]. While radiomic feature extraction is primarily driven by ML experts, the collection, preprocessing, and annotation of non-imaging (e.g., patient characteristics, clinical values) data—either for labeling radiomic features or to merge them together with clinical ones—is routinely done by clinicians. While this is a justified approach, many pitfalls may emerge that require careful consideration.

First, clinicians may pre-select and/or delete features they find less descriptive than others, while for an AI approach, those features may prove to be high-ranking. Thus, manual exclusion of features shall only be done based on strong clinical grounds, and not based on personal experience or bias. Second, some features may not be represented as numbers but as strings or qualitative values. When qualitative values are converted to numbers manually, a hidden stratification may mislead subsequent ML analyses that assume a tendency across the numbers within the given feature, while such tendency is not necessarily present on the level of qualitative features. Third, in the process of filling in clinical feature tables, case sensitiveness, invisible spaces after strings or numbers as well as how missing values are denoted shall be carefully investigated and communicated with the ML expert. In particular, missing values shall never be denoted by numbers, especially not numbers that are outliers relative to normal value ranges, as they might misguide the data preprocessing or ML analysis steps (see Sect. 10.6). It is generally not advised to remove complete features or samples manually just because they have missing values unless the amount of them is high in comparison to the total number of features or samples being present in the given database. Missing data imputation typically investigates the distribution of non-missing values in the given features where for example, the median or mean value is imputed. As long as the number of missing values is low compared to the sample size, this simple method often proves to be adequate and safe.

Assuming that the above pitfalls are addressed, the process of merging imaging and non-imaging data together still requires careful considerations. As an example, the radiomic features may not be aggregated but lesion-specific, while the non-imaging ones may be patient-specific. Clinicians shall decide which non-imaging features are allowed to be included in such mixed datasets.

10.6   Data Preprocessing

Data preprocessing (DP) is an often underestimated and overseen step in the processing pipeline of machine learning applications, while in real-life scenarios, the vast majority of time invested into building effective ML models is spent on data pre-

processing [19]. Data preprocessing covers a wide range of specific algorithms, that operate on the basis of purely mathematical or statistical rules and not on domain knowledge. Therefore, the ML expert is the one who analyzes the data and decides what the ideal set and order of DP steps should be for an optimal ML model afterward. Since DP is a highly-complex activity, it also tends to repel clinicians from being appropriately present. Below, potential pitfalls are discussed per the most popular data preprocessing steps that are typically performed by ML experts.

Data augmentation is often considered a step to counterbalance small sample sizes for training ML models. This step is mostly performed for DL applications in the form of image synthesis, and it covers a range of image augmentation techniques, e.g., shifting, rotation, or flipping transformations to generate synthetic images to boost model performance and robustness through enhancing the richness of the training dataset [20]. A similar approach to data augmentation is data synthesis [21, 22] which is often performed as a class imbalance correction step in the radiomic feature domain. The most important aspect of these approaches is that synthetic data can only be added to training subsets in a cross-validation setting. Therefore, clinicians shall get confirmation from their AI experts, where exactly synthetic data was utilized in the processing pipeline.

Outlier removal is a process that identifies if a given sample is significantly different from all other samples. While outlier detection can be performed by relatively straightforward algorithms [23, 24], not all detected samples may be outliers in light of the given disease. Here, clinicians shall ask AI experts to provide them with a list of samples that they detected as outliers to confirm if there are false positives among them.

Redundancy reduction removes highly correlated features and can therefore help to reduce chances for overfitting and improve model explainability (see Sect. 10.8). In contrast, feature ranking and selection rank each feature in correlation to their respective labels to predict. Most redundancy reduction approaches select one feature from redundant clusters having the highest variation [25]. Nevertheless, it is not guaranteed that the feature with the highest variance is the most descriptive in light of the given disease. Recently, the minimum-Redundancy-Maximum-Relevance (mRMR) approach has gained popularity to first identify redundant clusters of features and then select the one that has the highest correlation with the given clinical endpoint to predict [25]. It is imperative to understand that while basic and often used correlation matrix-based redundancy reduction is done without accessing clinical endpoints [19, 26], mRMR does access the labels of the given clinical endpoints to predict. Therefore, while mRMR is a superior approach to identify high-ranking features, it shall only be used on the given training subset when cross-validation is performed.

Collected numerical features (either radiomic or clinical) may be the subjects of artificial feature engineering steps that select two or more features to map them to potentially higher-ranking meta-features [27–29]. In contrast, dimensionality reduction creates meta-features to map high-dimensional data to lower dimensions [30–32]. Here, clinicians have to keep in mind that neither engineered features, nor dimensionally-reduced datasets remain in the original feature space. Therefore, they are challenging to be involved in any biomarker identification step (see Sect. 10.8).

While the above steps pose a challenge and a potential pitfall to result in suboptimal datasets, they are necessary steps to be considered in successful ML projects. Given the high-complexity of data preprocessing, the hyperparameters and the order of these steps are often AI-driven throughout, e.g., automated machine learning [33, 34] or ML-driven data preprocessing [19]. In case ML experts rely on these automated tools, clinicians shall still demand the required amount of transparency to ensure that none of the above issues occur.

10.7 Model Building, Validation, and Adoption

When building prediction models with ML or DL, one of the most important requirements is to build high-performing and generalizable mod-els. In case all the above steps are properly done, the choice of ideal ML approaches and the way of building them shall remain straightforward and mostly reflect on the matter of training sample counts. In this regard, a governing rule clinicians shall keep in mind is that the more hyperparameters (parameters of the model builder) an ML/DL training process has or the more complexity the model has, the more training data is required to avoid over or underfitting the resulted model. Low sample count is in general the Achilles point of any clinical ML research and it is the main reason why DL is challenging to be applied on small medical data. Consistently, DL approaches have been mostly utilized for object detection or delineation of suspicious lesions [35–37], as in these cases a single patient may provide many small training imaging patches for DL [19]. In addition, hyperparameters can be optimized during the training process, by further splitting the training data to train-validate subsets and identifying those parameters that result in the highest-performing models over the internal validation data [38]. Here, clinicians have to ensure that there is enough data to perform train-validate-test splits in a cross-validation setting. In the case of small datasets, one may consider only utilizing train-test splits and low-hyperparameter ML approaches that are also ideal for successfully modeling non-linear relationships in their data. Such approaches are typically based on random forest, or recently on XGBoost methods [39–41], while non-linear support vector machines (SVM) may also result in high-performing and generalizable models [42]. Linear regression or LASSO approaches are ideal candidates for regression ML tasks [43, 44]. Model building is also affected by the given clinician endpoint to utilize. Labeled samples can be used for building supervised ML models, while non-labeled datasets can be utilized for unsupervised ML. Most clinical ML projects suffer from partially labeled datasets. Here, clinicians shall consider semi-supervised learning. In this scenario, labeled datasets may still be subjects of train-test splitting, and the given training subset can be artificially labeled [45, 46].

Validating built ML models is a basic requirement before reporting or using such models in clinical research. Validation in the case of single-center studies has to rely on cross-validation, where a high fold count (e.g., 100) is suggested. Here, either Monte Carlo or a k-fold cross-validation scheme is advised. Regardless, only independent test subset-based predictive performance values shall be reported. In general, not only the average performance values (e.g., sensitivity, specificity) but their confidence intervals (CI) should be reported as well. Analyzing CI across multiple folds can help identifying the stability of the given ML model, and it can also help comparing different ML models. When relying on cross-validation in a classification setting, it is strongly advised to perform random splits that select an equal number of clinical endpoint subgroups for test cases in order to avoid biased performance estimations [19]. Here, clinicians shall compare test sensitivity and specificity values to the given class imbalance of their data, to ensure that no class imbalance-related performance loss occurred. If there is a clear indication that sensitivity-specificity values are correlating with class imbalance, the method of class imbalance correction has to be reconsidered.

In the case of dual or multi-centric projects or when a built model is shared to be utilized on independent data, independent testing can be performed. Here, many vs. a single validation in permutation is advised, as different center-specific cohorts may demonstrate different training and test performances depending on how representative they are of the given disease, regardless of their sample counts. Note that while ComBat is often utilized to harmonize multi-centric radiomic data [47, 48], not all cohorts benefit from such harmonization, and multiple ComBat variants may need to be tested to find the ideal one [49]. In contrast to the above, utilizing federated learning will result in an ensemble average model across multiple centers [50], where multi-center normalizations such as ComBat shall still be investigated. In these scenarios, the performance of the ensemble-averaged federated model is to be evaluated on all center's data that was not part of the federated learning process (hold-out per-center).

Regardless of whether a multi-centric validation or federated learning scheme is utilized, incorporating transfer learning [51, 52]—a method that fine-tunes already trained model parameters to center-specific characteristics—is advised at least to investigate its effect on model performance and generalizability. When estimating the predictive performance of built ML models, sex-specific differences and predictability shall be considered as they are significant contributing factors in neuro-oncological applications [12, 53, 54]. Here, the predictability of female and male independent test cases shall be analyzed.

10.8 Model Interpretation and Biomarker Identification

In the application of ML to medical tasks, interpretability, and explainability present invaluable concepts to support the development and validation of the corresponding models. Interpretability refers to the inherent ability of a model to be interpreted. For example, a decision tree can be easily interpreted by following the simple subsequent decisions it applies to classify a given instance (e.g., a patient). On the other hand, opaque (black-box) models cannot be comprehended as easily and require the assistance of supportive tools to explain the complex procedures carried out by the opaque model. These so-called explainable artificial intelligence (XAI) methods include, for example, global feature importance measures that describe the relative importance of individual features for the decision-making procedures within a given model [55, 56]. Most XAI methods have been developed for tabular data and cannot directly be applied to DL methods based on CNNs. Nevertheless, CNN-specific XAI tools exist and mostly focus on providing information on the importance of individual regions in the input image [57, 58]. Overall, XAI and interpretability methods are understood to be extremely useful for model troubleshooting and ensuring model safety [59]. However, caution has to be exercised when it comes to the usage of XAI tools for clinical decision-making [59].

In the mid 2010s, an important milestone was achieved with the establishment of the Imaging Biomarker Standardization Initiative (IBSI) [10]. Relying on shallow radiomic approaches and IBSI, one may support the process of imaging biomarker identification. When identifying biomarkers that are relevant for ML models is a priority in the given neuro-oncological application, relying on data preprocessing steps such as feature engineering and dimensionality reduction should be avoided. Similarly, DL-learnt features are not directly digestible for human observers; however, learnt DL features may still be correlated with shallow radiomic ones to identify any shallow surrogates for deep features. Identifying relevant (imaging) biomarkers in a particular dataset may be performed directly by feature ranking and selection. Highest-ranking features can be then analyzed in light of the given disease. This shall be an interactive process involving both clinicians and ML experts. Ideally, imaging features are IBSI-conform, where the IBSI definition of each feature provides adequate explanations to understand the essence of imaging patterns of the given disease, which can be translated to clinical relevance by clinicians.

10.9 Ensuring Quality of Medical AI Studies

A variety of guidelines have been published aiding the process of creating high-quality AI publications in the area of medicine and life sciences. Table 10.1 highlights a subset of the most prominent and most commonly employed medical AI guidelines. In addition to the guidelines listed in Table 10.1, there are multiple upcoming guidelines, which represent extensions of existing guidelines that aim to add a set of AI-specific items. These extensions include TRIPOD-AI and PROBAST-AI [60], TRIPOD-ML [61], and STARD-AI [62].

Table 10.1 List of guidelines involving medical artificial intelligence

Name	Guideline type	Number of items	Reference
Checklist for Artificial Intelligence in Medical Imaging (CLAIM)	Reporting	42	[63]
Transparent Reporting of multivariable prediction model for Individual Prognosis or Diagnosis (TRIPOD)	Reporting	22	[64]
Medical algorithmic audit	Model evaluation	–	[65]
Reproducibility standards for machine learning in the life sciences	Reproducibility	7	[66]
Standard Protocol Items: Recommendations for Interventional Trials (SPIRIT-AI)	Clinical trial reporting	15	[67]
Consolidated Standards of Reporting Trials (CONSORT-AI)	Randomized trial reporting	14	[68]
Developmental and Exploratory Clinical Investigations of DEcision support systems driven by Artificial Intelligence (DECIDE-AI)	Reporting guideline	17	[69]

10.10 Summary

The ever-growing realms of medicine and AI already pose a significant level of complexity on their own, which in combination shall be properly handled by a more in-depth collaborative and discussion-oriented approach involving both clinicians and AI experts. In light of this, near-term technological advancements may not be the primary drivers to witness the incremental role and adoption of radiomics in neuro-oncological applications, but a close clinician-AI-expert-driven interdisciplinary engagement will be.

With this chapter, we wished to highlight the most typical potential pitfalls that may occur in neuro-oncological applications if the required level of mutual engagement and communication is not present between the above stakeholders. Demystifying AI is one of the most important aspects of this endeavor, and here, we encourage clinicians to engage their AI experts with questions that are relevant to build interdisciplinary knowledge together. This chapter serves as an ideal base for conducting such collaborative work.

References

1. Aerts HJWL, Velazquez ER, Leijenaar RTH, Parmar C, Grossmann P, Cavalho S, et al. Decoding tumour phenotype by noninvasive imaging using a quantitative radiomics approach. Nat Commun. 2014;5:4006. http://www.nature.com/doifinder/10.1038/ncomms5006.
2. Mayerhoefer ME, Materka A, Langs G, Häggström I, Szczypiński P, Gibbs P, et al. Introduction to radiomics. J Nucl Med. 2020;61(4):488–95. http://jnm.snmjournals.org/lookup/doi/10.2967/jnumed.118.222893.
3. Papp L, Spielvogel CP, Rausch I, Hacker M, Beyer T. Personalizing medicine through hybrid imaging and medical big data analysis. Front Phys. 2018;6:51. https://www.frontiersin.org/article/10.3389/fphy.2018.00051/full.
4. Gillies RJ, Kinahan PE, Hricak H. Radiomics: images are more than pictures, they are data. Radiology. 2016;278(2):563–77. http://pubs.rsna.org/doi/10.1148/radiol.2015151169.
5. Hatt M, Krizsan AK, Rahmim A, Bradshaw TJ, Costa PF, Forgacs A, et al. Joint EANM/SNMMI guideline on radiomics in nuclear medicine. Eur J Nucl Med Mol Imaging. 2023;50(2):352–75. https://link.springer.com/10.1007/s00259-022-06001-6.
6. Poirot MG, Caan MWA, Ruhe HG, Bjørnerud A, Groote I, Reneman L, et al. Robustness of radiomics to variations in segmentation methods in multimodal brain MRI. Sci Rep. 2022;12(1):16712. https://www.nature.com/articles/s41598-022-20703-9.
7. Chang E, Joel MZ, Chang HY, Du J, Khanna O, Omuro A, et al. Comparison of radiomic feature aggregation methods for patients with multiple tumors. Sci Rep. 2021;11(1):9758. https://www.nature.com/articles/s41598-021-89114-6.
8. Zhao M, Kluge K, Papp L, Grahovac M, Yang S, Jiang C, et al. Multi-lesion radiomics of PET/CT for non-invasive survival stratification and histologic tumor risk profiling in patients with lung adenocarcinoma. Eur Radiol. 2022;32(10):7056–67. https://link.springer.com/10.1007/s00330-022-08999-7.
9. Qu H, Shi R, Li S, Che F, Wu J, Li H, et al. Dynamic radiomics: a new methodology to extract quantitative time-related features from tomographic images. Appl Intell. 2022;52(10):11827–45. https://link.springer.com/10.1007/s10489-021-03053-3.
10. Zwanenburg A, Vallières M, Abdalah MA, Aerts HJWL, Andrearczyk V, Apte A, et al. The image biomarker standardization initiative: standardized quantitative radiomics for high-throughput image-based phenotyping. Radiology. 2020;295(2):328–38. http://pubs.rsna.org/doi/10.1148/radiol.2020191145.
11. Hatt M, Tixier F, Pierce L, Kinahan PE, Le Rest CC, Visvikis D. Characterization of PET/CT images using texture analysis: the past, the present… any future? Eur J Nucl Med Mol Imaging. 2017;44(1):151–65. http://link.springer.com/10.1007/s00259-016-3427-0.
12. Papp L, Rasul S, Spielvogel CP, Krajnc D, Poetsch N, Woehrer A, et al. Sex-specific radiomic features of L-[S-methyl-11C] methionine PET in patients with newly-diagnosed gliomas in relation to IDH1 predictability. Front Oncol. 2023;13:986788. https://www.frontiersin.org/articles/10.3389/fonc.2023.986788.
13. Poetsch N, Woehrer A, Gesperger J, Furtner J, Haug AR, Wilhelm D, et al. Visual and semiquantitative 11C-methionine PET: an independent prognostic factor for survival of newly diagnosed and treatment-naïve gliomas. Neuro Oncol. 2018;20(3):411–9. https://academic.oup.com/neuro-oncology/article/20/3/411/4110230.
14. Desseroit M-C, Tixier F, Weber WA, Siegel BA, Cheze Le Rest C, Visvikis D, et al. Reliability of PET/CT shape and heterogeneity features in functional and morphologic components of non-small cell lung cancer tumors: a repeatability analysis in a prospective multicenter cohort. J Nucl Med. 2017;58(3):406–11. http://jnm.snmjournals.org/lookup/doi/10.2967/jnumed.116.180919.
15. Leijenaar RTH, Nalbantov G, Carvalho S, Van Elmpt WJC, Troost EGC, Boellaard R, et al. The effect of SUV discretization in quantitative FDG-PET Radiomics: the need for standardized methodology in tumor texture analysis. Sci Rep. 2015;5(1):11075. http://www.nature.com/articles/srep11075.

16. Suzuki K. Overview of deep learning in medical imaging. Radiol Phys Technol. 2017;10:257–73.
17. Ker J, Wang L, Rao J, Lim T. Deep learning applications in medical image analysis. IEEE Access. 2017;6(1):9375–9. http://www.annualreviews.org/doi/10.1146/annurev-bioeng-071516-044442.
18. Gatta R, Depeursinge A, Ratib O, Michielin O, Leimgruber A. Integrating radiomics into holomics for personalised oncology: from algorithms to bedside. Eur Radiol Exp. 2020;4(1):11. https://eurradiolexp.springeropen.com/articles/10.1186/s41747-019-0143-0.
19. Krajnc D, Spielvogel CP, Grahovac M, Ecsedi B, Rasul S, Poetsch N, et al. Automated data preparation for in vivo tumor characterization with machine learning. Front Oncol. 2022;12:1017911. https://www.frontiersin.org/articles/10.3389/fonc.2022.1017911/full.
20. Hernández-García A, König P. Data augmentation instead of explicit regularization. 2018. http://arxiv.org/abs/1806.03852.
21. Amin A, Anwar S, Adnan A, Nawaz M, Howard N, Qadir J, et al. Comparing oversampling techniques to handle the class imbalance problem: a customer churn prediction case study. IEEE Access. 2016;4:7940–57.
22. Krajnc D, Papp L, Nakuz TS, Magometschnigg HF, Grahovac M, Spielvogel CP, et al. Breast tumor characterization using [18F]FDG-PET/CT imaging combined with data preprocessing and radiomics. Cancers (Basel). 2021;13(6):1249. https://www.mdpi.com/2072-6694/13/6/1249.
23. Liu FT, Ting KM, Zhou Z-H. Isolation forest. In: 2008 Eighth IEEE International Conference on Data Mining. IEEE; 2008. p. 413–22. http://ieeexplore.ieee.org/document/4781136/.
24. Breunig MM, Kriegel H-P, Ng RT, Sander J. LOF. ACM SIGMOD Rec. 2000;29(2):93–104. https://dl.acm.org/doi/10.1145/335191.335388.
25. Ding C, Peng H. Minimum redundancy feature selection from microarray gene expression data. In: Computational Systems Bioinformatics CSB2003 Proceedings of the 2003 IEEE Bioinformatics Conference CSB2003. IEEE Comput. Soc. p. 523–8. http://ieeexplore.ieee.org/document/1227396/.
26. Grahovac M, Spielvogel CP, Krajnc D, Ecsedi B, Traub-Weidinger T, Rasul S, et al. Machine learning predictive performance evaluation of conventional and fuzzy radiomics in clinical cancer imaging cohorts. Eur J Nucl Med Mol Imaging. 2023; https://link.springer.com/10.1007/s00259-023-06127-1.
27. Qiu J, Wu Q, Ding G, Xu Y, Feng S. A survey of machine learning for big data processing. EURASIP J Adv Signal Process. 2016;2016(1):67. https://asp-eurasipjournals.springeropen.com/articles/10.1186/s13634-016-0355-x.
28. Talagala PD, Hyndman RJ, Smith-Miles K. Anomaly detection in high dimensional data. 2019;1–30. http://arxiv.org/abs/1908.04000.
29. Verleysen M, François D. The curse of dimensionality in data mining and time series prediction.
Analysis. 2005;3512:758–70. http://link.springer.com/10.1007/11494669_93.
30. Akhbardeh A, Jacobs MA. Comparative analysis of nonlinear dimensionality reduction techniques for breast MRI segmentation. Med Phys. 2012;39(4):2275–89. http://doi.wiley.com/10.1118/1.3682173.
31. van der Maaten L, Hinton G. Visualizing data using t-SNE. J Mach Learn Res. 2008;9:2579–605.
32. Kickingereder P, Götz M, Muschelli J, Wick A, Neuberger U, Shinohara RT, et al. Large-scale radiomic profiling of recurrent glioblastoma identifies an imaging predictor for stratifying antiangiogenic treatment response. Clin Cancer Res. 2016;22(23):5765–71. https://doi.org/10.1158/1078-0432.CCR-16-0702.
33. Ritter Z, Papp L, Zámbó K, Tóth Z, Dezső D, Veres DS, et al. Two-year event-free survival prediction in DLBCL patients based on in vivo radiomics and clinical parameters. Front Oncol. 2022;12:820136. https://www.frontiersin.org/articles/10.3389/fonc.2022.820136/full.
34. Hasimbegovic E, Papp L, Grahovac M, Krajnc D, Poschner T, Hasan W, et al. A sneak-peek into the physician's brain: a retrospective machine learning-driven investigation of decision-making in TAVR versus SAVR for young high-risk patients with severe symptomatic aortic stenosis. J Pers Med. 2021;11(11):1062. https://www.mdpi.com/2075-4426/11/11/1062.
35. Moe YM, Groendahl AR, Tomic O, Dale E, Malinen E, Futsaether CM. Deep learning-based auto-delineation of gross tumour volumes and involved nodes in PET/CT images of head and neck cancer patients. Eur J Nucl Med Mol Imaging. 2021;48(9):2782–92. https://link.springer.com/10.1007/s00259-020-05125-x.
36. Isensee F, Jaeger PF, Kohl SAA, Petersen J, Maier-Hein KH. nnU-Net: a self-configuring method for deep learning-based biomedical image segmentation. Nat Methods. 2021;18(2):203–11. http://www.nature.com/articles/s41592-020-01008-z.
37. Capobianco N, Meignan MA, Cottereau A-S, Vercellino L, Sibille L, Spottiswoode B, et al. Deep learning FDG uptake classification enables total metabolic tumor volume estimation in diffuse large B-cell lymphoma. J Nucl Med. 2020;62(1):30–6. http://jnm.snmjournals.org/lookup/doi/10.2967/jnumed.120.242412.
38. Feurer M. Hyperparameter optimization. In: Hutter F, Kotthoff L, Vanschoren J, editors. Automated machine learning, The Springer series on challenges in machine learning. Cham: Springer; 2019. p. 3–33. http://link.springer.com/10.1007/978-3-030-05318-5_1.
39. Park DJ, Park MW, Lee H, Kim Y-J, Kim Y, Park YH. Development of machine learning model for diagnostic disease prediction based on laboratory tests. Sci Rep. 2021;11(1):7567. http://www.nature.com/articles/s41598-021-87171-5.
40. Le NQK, Do DT, Chiu F-Y, Yapp EKY, Yeh H-Y, Chen C-Y. XGBoost improves classification of MGMT promoter methylation status in IDH1 wildtype glioblas-

toma. J Pers Med. 2020;10(3):128. https://www.mdpi.com/2075-4426/10/3/128.

41. Chen T, Guestrin C. XGBoost. In: Proceedings of the 22nd ACM SIGKDD International Conference on Knowledge Discovery and Data Mining. New York: ACM; 2016. p. 785–94. https://dl.acm.org/doi/10.1145/2939672.2939785.

42. Ajani TS, Imoize AL, Atayero AA. An overview of machine learning within embedded and mobile devices—optimizations and applications. Sensors. 2021;21(13):4412. https://www.mdpi.com/1424-8220/21/13/4412.

43. Wu S, Zheng J, Li Y, Wu Z, Shi S, Huang M, et al. Development and validation of an MRI-based radiomics signature for the preoperative prediction of lymph node metastasis in bladder cancer. EBioMedicine. 2018;34(22):76–84.

44. Wu Y, Liu B, Wu W, Lin Y, Yang C, Wang M. Grading glioma by radiomics with feature selection based on mutual information. J Ambient Intell Humaniz Comput. 2018;9(5):1671–82. https://doi.org/10.1007/s12652-018-0883-3.

45. Khan H, Liu H, Liu C. Missing label imputation through inception-based semi-supervised ensemble learning. Adv Comput Intell. 2022;2(1):10. https://link.springer.com/10.1007/s43674-021-00015-7.

46. Chapelle O, Scholkopf B, Zien A. Semi-supervised learning. 1st ed. The MIT Press; 2010.

47. Fortin J-P, Parker D, Tunç B, Watanabe T, Elliott MA, Ruparel K, et al. Harmonization of multisite diffusion tensor imaging data. NeuroImage. 2017;161:149–70. https://linkinghub.elsevier.com/retrieve/pii/S1053811917306948.

48. Orlhac F, Boughdad S, Philippe C, Stalla-Bourdillon H, Nioche C, Champion L, et al. A post-reconstruction harmonization method for multicenter radiomic studies in PET. J Nucl Med. 2018;59:1321–8. http://jnm.snmjournals.org/lookup/doi/10.2967/jnumed.117.199935.

49. Horng H, Singh A, Yousefi B, Cohen EA, Haghighi B, Katz S, et al. Generalized ComBat harmonization methods for radiomic features with multi-modal distributions and multiple batch effects. Sci Rep. 2022;12(1):4493. https://www.nature.com/articles/s41598-022-08412-9.

50. Bonawitz K, Eichner H, Grieskamp W, Huba D, Ingerman A, Ivanov V, et al. Towards federated learning at scale: system design. 2019. http://arxiv.org/abs/1902.01046.

51. Hatt M, Tixier F, Visvikis D, Cheze Le Rest C. Radiomics in PET/CT: more than meets the eye? J Nucl Med. 2017;58(3):365–6. http://jnm.snmjournals.org/lookup/doi/10.2967/jnumed.116.184655.

52. Zhuang F, Qi Z, Duan K, Xi D, Zhu Y, Zhu H, et al. A comprehensive survey on transfer learning. Proc IEEE. 2021;109(1):43–76. https://ieeexplore.ieee.org/document/9134370/.

53. Ostrom QT, Coleman W, Huang W, Rubin JB, Lathia JD, Berens ME, et al. Sex-specific gene and pathway modeling of inherited glioma risk. Neuro

Oncol. 2019;21(1):71–82. https://academic.oup.com/neuro-oncology/article/21/1/71/5073373.

54. Massey SC, Whitmire P, Doyle TE, Ippolito JE, Mrugala MM, Hu LS, et al. Sex differences in health and disease: a review of biological sex differences relevant to cancer with a spotlight on glioma. Cancer Lett. 2021;498:178–87. https://linkinghub.elsevier.com/retrieve/pii/S0304383520303876.

55. Yaqub M, Javaid MK, Cooper C, Noble JA. Machine learning in medical imaging. Lect Notes Comput Sci. 2011;7009(4):184–92. http://www.scopus.com/inward/record.url?eid=2-s2.0-80053932755&partnerID=tZOtx3y1.

56. Molnar C. Interpretable machine learning. A guide for making black box models explainable. 2019. https://christophm.github.io/interpretable-ml-book/.

57. Jung H, Oh Y. Towards better explanations of class activation mapping. 2021. http://arxiv.org/abs/2102.05228.

58. Rudin C. Stop explaining black box machine learning models for high stakes decisions and use interpretable models instead. Nat Mach Intell. 2019;1(5):206–15.

59. Ghassemi M, Oakden-Rayner L, Beam AL. The false hope of current approaches to explainable artificial intelligence in health care. Lancet Digit Health. 2021;3(11):e745–50. https://linkinghub.elsevier.com/retrieve/pii/S2589750021002089.

60. Collins GS, Dhiman P, Andaur Navarro CL, Ma J, Hooft L, Reitsma JB, et al. Protocol for development of a reporting guideline (TRIPOD-AI) and risk of bias tool (PROBAST-AI) for diagnostic and prognostic prediction model studies based on artificial intelligence. BMJ Open. 2021;11(7):e048008. https://bmjopen.bmj.com/lookup/doi/10.1136/bmjopen-2020-048008.

61. Collins GS, Moons KGM. Reporting of artificial intelligence prediction models. Lancet. 2019;393(10181):1577–9. https://linkinghub.elsevier.com/retrieve/pii/S0140673619300376.

62. Sounderajah V, Ashrafian H, Golub RM, Shetty S, De Fauw J, Hooft L, et al. Developing a reporting guideline for artificial intelligence-centred diagnostic test accuracy studies: the STARD-AI protocol. BMJ Open. 2021;11(6):e047709. https://bmjopen.bmj.com/lookup/doi/10.1136/bmjopen-2020-047709.

63. Mongan J, Moy L, Kahn CE. Checklist for artificial intelligence in medical imaging (CLAIM): a guide for authors and reviewers. Radiol Artif Intell. 2020;2(2):e200029. http://pubs.rsna.org/doi/10.1148/ryai.2020200029.

64. Collins GS, Reitsma JB, Altman DG, Moons KGM. Transparent Reporting of a multivariable prediction model for Individual Prognosis Or Diagnosis (TRIPOD): the TRIPOD statement. Ann Intern Med. 2015;162(1):55–63. https://www.acpjournals.org/doi/10.7326/M14-0697.

65. Liu X, Glocker B, McCradden MM, Ghassemi M, Denniston AK, Oakden-Rayner L. The medical algorithmic audit. Lancet Digit Health. 2022;4(5):e384–97. https://linkinghub.elsevier.com/retrieve/pii/S2589750022000036.

66. Heil BJ, Hoffman MM, Markowetz F, Lee S-I, Greene CS, Hicks SC. Reproducibility standards for machine learning in the life sciences. Nat Methods. 2021;18(10):1132–5. https://www.nature.com/articles/s41592-021-01256-7.

67. Cruz Rivera S, Liu X, Chan A-W, Denniston AK, Calvert MJ, Ashrafian H, et al. Guidelines for clinical trial protocols for interventions involving artificial intelligence: the SPIRIT-AI extension. Lancet Digit Health. 2020;2(10):e549–60. https://linkinghub.elsevier.com/retrieve/pii/S2589750020302193.

68. Liu X, Cruz Rivera S, Moher D, Calvert MJ, Denniston AK, Chan A-W, et al. Reporting guidelines for clinical trial reports for interventions involving artificial intelligence: the CONSORT-AI extension. Nat Med. 2020;26(9):1364–74. https://www.nature.com/articles/s41591-020-1034-x.

69. Vasey B, Nagendran M, Campbell B, Clifton DA, Collins GS, Denaxas S, et al. Publisher Correction: Reporting guideline for the early-stage clinical evaluation of decision support systems driven by artificial intelligence: DECIDE-AI. Nat Med. 2022;28(10):2218. https://www.nature.com/articles/s41591-022-01951-8.

Antonio Tanzilli, Andrea Pace, Dario Benincasa,
and Antonio Silvani

11.1 Introduction

Primary malignant brain tumors (BTs) are rare in developed countries with an incidence rate of 5.8 (in men) and 4.1 (in women) per 100,000 persons [1]. Despite current multimodality treatment, including surgery, radiotherapy and chemotherapy, and ongoing development of potentially more effective novel therapeutic modalities, the prognosis of such patients still remains poor. High-grade gliomas (HGG) have the worse outcome, with a predicted median survival ranging from 12 to 15 months for glioblastoma and from 2 to 5 years for anaplastic neoplasms [2]. Therefore, Clinicians dealing with patients affected by malignant BTs are frequently involved in providing palliative and supportive care, particularly at the end-of-life (EoL). Palliative and supportive care, are very important for effective management of neurological symptoms and complications directly or indirectly caused by the intracranial lesion. Symptoms observed during the disease trajectory of BTs patients are quite different in respect to those observed in general cancer population. Additionally, disease history and needs of care of BTs, differ from other cancers patients, due to unique trajectory of this disease, rather short life expectancy, high incidence of specific symptoms caused by neurological impairment, frequent psychosocial problems and many general symptoms due to neurological deficits which necessitates tailored palliative strategy and predetermines complexity of supportive care needs [3–6].

While the development of more active therapies is ongoing, physicians caring for BTs patients have the important role of providing effective and adequate supportive care for symptoms and complications that may result directly or indirectly from the tumor (neurologic and/or general symptoms). Supportive care includes problems such as management of peritumoral brain edema, venous thromboembolism (VTE), seizures, rehabilitation, depression, opportunistic infections, psychological support/communication and EoL issues/treatment decisions. The main goal of palliative care in neuro-oncology is the control of symptoms during the disease course and particularly at advanced stages and at EoL. The needs of malignant BTs patients at EoL require specific, multidisciplinary palliative interventions performed by a well-trained neuro-oncological team. These include effective management of pain, confusion, agitation, delirium, and seizure management with the overall aim being to allow the patient to experience a peace-

A. Tanzilli · A. Pace · D. Benincasa
IRCCS Regina Elena National Cancer Institute,
Rome, Italy
e-mail: andrea.pace@ifo.it

A. Silvani (✉)
IRCCS Besta Neurological Institute, Milan, Italy
e-mail: Antonio.Silvani@istituto-besta.it

© The Author(s), under exclusive license to Springer Nature Switzerland AG 2024
E. Lopci, L. Mansi (eds.), *Advanced Imaging and Therapy in Neuro-Oncology*,
https://doi.org/10.1007/978-3-031-59341-3_11

ful death. In this chapter, we will address recent data that may provide a basis for strong clinical recommendations in the field of palliative and EoL care in BTs and the relationship with quality of life (QoL) in these patients.

11.2 Determinants of QoL and Symptoms Management

11.2.1 Seizures

Seizures may be the symptom leading to the diagnosis of glioma but also may signal disease recurrence or progression [7–9]. For 30–50% of patients with BTs, an epileptic seizure is the presenting clinical tumor sign, while 10–30% will develop seizures in the course of disease [7, 10]. Epileptogenesis in patients with BTs is influenced by many factors including tumor histology and location, changes in the peritumoral environment, and genetic factors [8, 9, 11]. Low-grade gliomas (LGG) are the most epileptogenic ones and the incidence of seizures is reported in 60–88% of patients. Slow growing pattern and cortical involvement may account to the high incidence of seizures in LGG [12]. The frequency of seizures decreases significantly to 30–50% in high-grade gliomas (HGG) but seizures may occur from onset to EoL (late-onset seizures) [7]. Recurrent seizures are frequent (50–75%) in patients presenting with a seizure in spite of antiepileptic treatment (AEDs) [7, 13]. Seizure control is a crucial issue in clinical management and supportive care in neuro-oncology. QoL of BTs patients is strongly influenced by the severity of the seizures and by the intensity of Anti-epileptic drugs (AED) treatment. Uncontrolled seizures may result in neurological, cognitive and psychological deficits [13, 14]. The presence of epilepsy is considered the most important risk factor for long-term disability in BTs patients [15, 16]. Good seizure control can significantly improve patient's psychological and relational sphere (i.e., social, personal, and professional) [17]. The selection of an AED therapy must consider not only the drug's efficacy, but also possible side effects on important aspects of the patient's daily life [18].

11.2.2 Edema

The pathogenetic mechanism of peritumoral edema in BTs patients is mainly vasogenic, resulting from the flow of fluid into the extracellular space of the brain parenchyma through an incompetent blood-brain barrier (BBB) [19]. Prolonged treatment with steroids, to control edema, has multiple adverse effects including iatrogenic Cushing syndrome with weight gain and moon facies, glucose intolerance, steroid myopathy, opportunistic infection [particularly Pneumocystis Jirovecii pneumonitis (PJP)], osteoporosis, psychiatric symptoms, and adrenal insufficiency secondary to suppression of the hypothalamopituitary-adrenal (HPA) axis [19–21]. Rapid tapering of steroids may induce a withdrawal syndrome with myalgia/arthralgia and bodily pain requiring a dosage increase [20]. Therapeutic efficacy and side effects of corticosteroid treatment is also related to important interactions with enzyme-inducing AED and other concomitant treatments [22].

11.2.3 Venous Thromboembolism (VTE)

Malignant glioma patients seem to represent the second highest risk of developing VTE among all cancer patients, with a range of 16–28% in the first year from diagnosis [23–25]. A recent meta-analysis estimated that BTs were associated with the second greatest risk of VTE (48 per 1000 person-years) among average-risk cancer patients after cancer of pancreas [26]. Direct secretion of pro-coagulants from the tumor and/or dysregulation of thrombogenic factors are much likely involved in the pathogenesis of VTE in this high-risk population. Surgical resection, age greater than 75, and glioblastomas are the most important risk factors for VTE in malignant glioma patients [25]. The use of low molecular weight heparin (LMWH) for the treatment of symptomatic VTE and the prevention of recurrent VTE is recommended, however, there is uncertainty on the benefits of primary prophylaxis for VTE [27, 28]. The risk of VTE associated with newer antiangiogenic therapies such as bevacizumab in these patients remains unclear. When VTE occurs in this patient population, concern regarding the potential for intracranial hemorrhage complicates management decisions regarding anticoagulation, and these patients have a worse prognosis than their VTE-free counterparts.

11.2.4 Fatigue

Between 25% and 90% of all patients with primary BTs report fatigue, which can occur at any time during the disease course [29]. The biological mechanisms leading to cancer-related fatigue have not yet been fully elucidated. The potential mechanisms involve increased blood concentrations of inflammatory cytokines, influencing neuroendocrine function, and decreased concentrations of glutamine and tryptophan in the brain, with or without disturbance of circadian rhythms. Management of fatigue can be non-pharmacological (e.g., physical exercise) or pharmacological. Despite this, no evidence suggests that modafinil, armodafinil, methylphenidate, or donepezil confer a significant beneficial effect on fatigue in patients with stable BTs.

11.2.5 Mood and Behavioral Disorders

Mood and behavioral disorders represent important comorbidities for BTs patients. The 6-month prevalence of clinical depression is in the order of 20% and personality change might affect up to 60% of patients [30]. Although the management of such disorders in patients with cancer has been reviewed [31], guidance specific to BTs patients is required because they present with neurological disease together with cancer. Diagnosing depression can be challenging because symptoms that may suggest depression could be related to the effects of the tumor or its treatment. In these patients, depression is often associated with functional impairment, cognitive dysfunction, and reduced QoL. A clear link between developing depression and tumor location has never been established. Aetiological hypotheses focus on a neurochemical imbalance and the destructive effect of glioma or surgery on critical emotional pathways. Others see depression as a psychological response to disease stress. Currently, there is no high-quality trial evidence to help clinicians decide whether to prescribe antidepressants to glioma patients [32]. The use of antidepressants in people with BTs should be considered on an individual basis. Given the lack of data from large trials, the choice of which agent to prescribe must necessarily be based on data on the efficacy of antidepressants in the general population, considering possible drug interactions and the possible impact on the incidence of seizures [31]. When choosing a medication for these patients, physicians should consider selective serotonin reuptake inhibitors (SSRIs) or Serotonin and norepinephrine reuptake inhibitors (SNRIs), particularly sertraline, citalopram, mirtazapine, reboxetine, paroxetine, fluoxetine, escitalopram, fluvoxamine, venlafaxine, and duloxetine.

11.2.6 Cognition

Cognitive impairment is a common symptom in BTs patients, even before treatment [33]. It is associated with poor prognosis and hurts the QoL of patients and their families. Patients with gliomas may be suffering from significant deficits in attention, mental speed and flexibility, abstract thinking and memory, and a higher number of symptoms of anxiety and depression compared with healthy people. In BTs patients, cognitive abilities might be threatened by the disease in terms of disruption of local and distant neurocognitive networks, but also by patient characteristics (age and educational level, tumor characteristics, tumor treatment, supportive medication, and psychological distress). Depending on the definition of cognitive disturbances, type of outcome measure used, and extent of cognitive functions examined, up to 91% of BTs patients can have cognitive disturbances before treatment, which only moderately correlate with cognitive complaints [34, 35]. Unfortunately, cognitive impairment is often underestimated in a more complex clinical picture. Neuropsychological assessment is often delegated to the Mini-Mental State Examination (MMSE). The MMSE has several limitations when applied to these patients. More detailed structured tests have the disadvantage of being time-consuming to administer. They are also often poorly tolerated by patients outside of clinical trials. Many glioma patients are aware of their cognitive difficulties. The worst perceived problems were related to neuropsychological deficits [36]. This awareness does not automatically mean good QoL, but the patient needs to improve this aspect to be more involved in assessments and treatments. A clear idea of the patient's level of awareness is essential for sharing clinical decisions.

Medical treatment to prevent cognitive decline in patients with BTs has been shown to be unsuccessful, while few randomized studies [37–39] assessed the effect of cognitive rehabilitation to improve cognitive functioning.

11.2.7 Work Ability

Work is one of the factors contributing to Health-related Quality of Life (HRQoL) for tumor survivors. One outcome parameter also sought to be applied in BTs patients is the return to work, understood as a return to normalcy. Unfortunately, the percentage of patients who return to work after 6 months is minimal in glioblastoma. Glioblastoma patients who are considered long-term survivors at 5 years, experience significant symptoms, signs and need to care for themselves. The situation is better for patients with grade 2 glioma. Approximately 50% of these patients return to work. In the first 2 years after diagnosis, the treatment burden has been shown to affect work capacity. Frequent financial difficulties further complicate day-to-day management. Survivors of stable glioma who are not receiving active treatment continue to be significantly affected by direct medical, non-medical, and indirect costs associated with the BTs and its treatment [40]. The negative impact on work is constant and independent of histology, treatment, and income level [41, 42]. There is a direct and consistent relationship between loss of employment and the financial impact of a BTs diagnosis. This is ubiquitous across tumor subtypes, particularly in patients with lower levels of education and poorer performance status [41]. In terms of direct expenditure and its impact, there are obvious differences between countries, reflecting the organization of the health service and the coverage it can provide.

11.3 Management of Symptoms at EoL

11.3.1 Headache

It is difficult to assess the incidence of pain in the last hours of life, but the presence of agitation and restlessness with moaning and grimacing is often interpreted as physical pain, requiring appropriate treatment [43]. Literature reports that headache may be present in a large proportion of patients. In the large majority of patients, headache is mild, intermittent, due to increased intracranial pressure, and usually responding to steroid treatment. In some cases, headache may be severe and requires a high dose of steroids and pain medication (opioid or non-opioid). In patients with meningeal syndrome, both for neoplastic meningitis from systemic cancer and for meningeal spread from primary BTs, pain treatment requires multidrug approach with steroids, opioids, and neuropathic pain relievers (gabapentin, pregabalin).

11.3.2 Dysphagia

Dysphagia is reported to be one of the more frequent symptoms in the EoL phase. Loss of the ability to swallow may induce pulmonary inhalation and may affect nutrition and hydration. Moreover, the patients' difficulty in the oral intake of drugs, liquids, and food requires appropriate modification of treatment and discussion with families and the home care team of issues concerning nutrition and hydration. In patients presenting dysphagia in the last weeks of life, anticonvulsant therapy needs to be modified by changing oral treatment to other routes of administration [43].

11.3.3 Death Rattle

The death rattle may be very distressing for the family and home care professionals and it is caused by changes in breathing patterns with an accumulation of bronchial secretions especially in the last hours of life in comatose dying patients. However, it is important to explain to the relatives of a patient with decreased level of consciousness that death rattle is unlikely to be distressing for the patient.

Anticholinergic drugs (natural belladonna alkaloids: just like atropine and scopolamine) may reduce the production of secretions and mild dehydration may help to control this symptom [44]. There are also non pharmacological treatments of death rattle which include gentle suction in the nasopharynx and trachea and postural drainage.

11.3.4 Alterations of Consciousness

Drowsiness and gradual loss of consciousness have been reported in up to 90% of BTs patients at the EoL [45]. Confusion, somnolence, and sleep inversion may be early symptoms of such alterations and steadily progress up to deep irreversible coma. While increased doses of steroids may decelerate development of this dysfunction, such treatment may be complicated by increased confusion and agitation, negatively affecting the process of peaceful dying. On the other hand, reducing doses of steroids may result in control of agitation.

Occurrence of severe confusion, agitation, or delirium with preserved consciousness may be very distressing for both the patients and their relatives, and may require palliative (or terminal) sedation, which is defined as the monitored use of medications to induce a state of decreased or absent awareness in order to relieve the burden of otherwise intractable suffering in a manner that is ethically acceptable to the patient, family, and healthcare providers [46]. Administration of neuroleptics, opioids, and/or benzodiazepins may be required in the last hours of life not only because of severe agitation or uncontrolled delirium, but also for control of refractory seizures and death rattle. It is not aimed on shortening of the patient life and suffering, but on management of refractory symptoms. Nevertheless, very limited data are available about role of such strategy in cases of BTs at the terminal disease stage.

11.3.5 Delirium

Besides reduced consciousness due to progressive tumor growth leading to increased intracranial pressure, alterations in consciousness and reduced awareness and inattention might be part of the complex neuropsychiatric syndrome of delirium. The underlying causes and risk factors of delirium are multifactorial. For example, commonly prescribed agents in the palliative care setting, such as benzodiazepines, corticosteroids, or opioids, are associated with an increased risk of delirium. In patients receiving palliative care, delirium represents the third most frequent symptom near death and appears in up to 90% of patients in the dying phase [47, 48]. Olanzapine, risperidone, aripiprazole, and haloperidol were found to be equally effective for the treatment of delirium. Extrapyramidal symptoms are frequently reported in patients treated with haloperidol, whereas sedative effects predominately occur during treatment with olanzapine [49].

Palliative sedation of BTs patients to relieve delirium was reported in up to 30% of cases [47]. This treatment option is frequently required for refractory delirium during the EoL phase [50].

11.3.6 Nutrition, Hydration, and Respiration

In the last weeks or days of life, BTs patients often have difficulty swallowing because of dysphagia and decreased consciousness. Losing the ability to swallow might induce pulmonary aspiration and hamper nutrition, hydration, and oral administration of drugs.

Treatment decisions about nutrition and hydration in the EoL phase are among the most important and ethically relevant issues in BTs patients. Ethical and legal approaches to withdrawal and withholding of nutrition and hydration in terminally ill patients vary widely among different countries and cultures. However, there is consensus about the futility of artificial nutrition and hydration at the EoL in comatose patients with glioma.

11.3.7 Organization of Care in the EoL Phase

The availability of palliative care services varies within and between countries and, consequently, the place of death of BTs patients also varies. Moreover, place of death was found to be independently associated with good quality of care, as was effective symptom control, and satisfaction with the type of information received [51]. Factors associated with a low probability of dying at home included repeated admission to the emergency room, prolonged duration as a hospital inpatient, low involvement of general practitioners and few home visits, and accessibility of acute care beds.

Physical and cognitive dysfunctions in BTs patients, with changes in behavior and impairment in communication, might affect dignity and expose patients and relatives to stress [52, 53] and can influence the organization of care, such as place of care, place of death, and decisions about EoL. Dying with dignity was significantly correlated with the absence of communication deficits, good communication with physicians, fewer transitions between health-care settings, and dying at the preferred place of death [52]. Reasons for admission to hospital more frequently include social issues and neurological deficits for BTs patients than for other patients in need of palliative care. Generally, patients are only referred to palliative care services in the last stage of disease. However, an earlier and integrative approach was found to have a positive effect on the quality of EoL and was recommended by several studies [52, 53].

11.4 Influence of Treatment on HRQOL in Glioma's Patients

BTs and their treatments have a significant impact on the QoL of patients; Glioma patients experience both general cancer-related symptoms such as fatigue, anxiety, depression, and neurological specific symptoms such as seizures, cognitive deficits, motor dysfunction, and symptoms caused by elevated intracranial pressure, which may impair their HRQoL. Particularly, Neurocognitive impairments are common in patients with current or previously treated brain tumors, and such impairments can negatively affect patient outcomes including QoL.

11.5 Impact of Surgery on HRQOL

The incidence of post-surgical morbidity in BTs patients after first or repeated surgery is variable in the literature and may depend on tumor grade and brain location. However, tumor mass reduction may alleviate neurological symptoms and cognitive deficits, with a favorable impact on patient's QoL. Surgery is the most radical tumor treatment but may cause neurological and cognitive deficits, harming normal surrounding tissue [33]. Neurological deficits due to surgery may result in a lower perceived QoL even though they're often transient. Patients who undergo gross-total resection generally show both a longer survival duration and better HRQOL than patients who only undergo biopsy [54].

11.6 Impact of Radiotherapy on HRQOL

Radiotherapy may also negatively impact on HRQOL in BTs patients. Patients treated with high-dose radiation had a more compromised HRQOL following treatment than those on low-dose radiation, whereas overall survival did not significantly differ [55]. However, one of the most disabling effect is a long term decrease in cognitive functioning and, consequently, in

HRQOL, due to post radiation leucoencephalopathy, particularly evident in long-term survivors [56, 57]. Radiotherapy has been shown to negatively influence cognitive outcomes in patients with BTs but study results are controversial and in some cases mixed results and improvements in cognition following radiotherapy have been reported.

The benefit of radiotherapy is well established in the treatment of HGG patients, with a significant effect on progression free survival and, overall survival. By stabilizing disease and delaying progression, QoL may be maintained. No clear negative effects of radiotherapy on HRQoL are observed in anaplastic oligodendroglioma patients and in patients with glioblastoma multiforme with a good performance status.

In the elderly population (age >70 years), a moderate survival benefit from radiotherapy has been established for patients who have a good performance status at the beginning of the treatment. However, the role of radiotherapy for patients >70 years of age, is still debated due to the risk of relevant neurocognitive deterioration. Conventional radiotherapy (60 Gy over 6 weeks), particularly in frail patients, seems to be less appropriate than hypofractionated schedules [58].

The impact of re-irradiation, specifically on HRQOL, has been evaluated in a small study with a median follow-up of 9 months [59]. The majority of patients (80%) judged their general health status after re-irradiation to be stable or even improved, compared with before treatment; in 20% of patients, their perceived general health status declined.

11.7 Impact of Chemotherapy on HRQOL

The standard treatment for malignant gliomas after surgery, according to the existing guidelines, is based on concurrent chemo-radiotherapy with temozolomide followed by adjuvant temozolomide chemotherapy (Stupp's protocol) with a significantly longer survival time in HGG patients with newly diagnosed glioblastoma multiforme than in patients treated with radiotherapy alone [60].

Data on the impact of treatment with temozolomide on HRQOL show that during treatment and follow-up, HRQOL domains remain stable in both treatment-group during the first year of follow-up. However, during temozolomide treatment, the patients in the combination treatment group show more side effects (nausea, vomiting, appetite loss, and constipation) than those treated with radiotherapy alone. It can be concluded that the addition of temozolomide during and after radiotherapy produces a significantly longer survival time without a long-lasting negative effect on HRQOL. Data from the Nordic and the NOA-08 trials support the assumption that temozolomide is generally safe also in elderly population of HGG, showing a functional improvement also in term of QoL, and cognitive function [61, 62]. This result demonstrates that effective treatment can be achieved without significant functional loss and temozolomide seems tolerable in also elderly patients with low Karnofsky Performance Status and should not be withheld, especially in patients with hypermethylated *MGMT* promoter.

Other chemotherapy regimens utilized in the treatment of HGG include procarbazine, lomustine, and vincristine (PCV) and Regorafenib. The positive impact of chemotherapy of progression free survival and overall survival result in a delay of neurological deterioration with stable HRQoL, while adverse effects of chemotherapy may result in a deterioration of QoL due to symptoms such as nausea/vomiting, appetite loss, and drowsiness during treatment.

Regorafenib is a small-molecule multi-kinase inhibitor recently introduced in the treatment of recurrent glioiblastoma as second line therapy. In a phase II trial evaluating the efficacy and safety profile compared to lomustine, the final results of the health-related quality of life (HRQoL) assessment showed that regorafenib did not negatively affect HRQoL in patients with recurrent glioblastoma [63].

11.8   Effect of Supportive Treatment on HRQOL

Supportive treatment in BTs patients includes symptomatic medications with AEDs and steroids. Recent studies reported that AEDs use may be associated with concurrent depression, anxiety, behavior alteration or subjective cognitive impairment in glioma patients [64]. Also the occurrence of seizures may reduce patients' HRQOL. In addition to causing morbidity, seizures negatively affect independence and QoL in other ways, for example, by leading to loss of driving privileges. Antiepileptic drugs are known to be associated with cognitive decline, particularly the older antiepileptic medications, however most evidence supports a role for AEDs use (and, to a lesser extent, seizure burden) in adverse cognitive outcomes. The cognitive deficits can primarily be ascribed to the use of AEDs, particularly when multiple drugs are prescribed and the intensity of the epilepsy treatment seems to be a more relevant contributor to cognitive deficits than the occurrence of seizures [15].

Corticosteroids are regularly used in the treatment of BTs to reduce swelling from cerebral edema. Dexamethasone is the cornerstone of anti-edema supportive treatment and is prescribed to alleviate neurological symptoms, thereby improving QoL. Steroid prolonged treatment has been shown to induce also cognitive, psychiatric, and behavioral dysfunction, and some data indicate that their effects on attention, concentration, and memory are relate to neurotoxic effect on the hippocampal and prefrontal areas However, common side effects are myopathy, gastrointestinal complications, hyperglycemia, sleep alteration and psychiatric complications (mainly agitation or depression). The correct administration and dosage of steroid treatment is still controversial and given the well-known adverse effects, the prescribed dosage, steroids should be tapered or maintained at the lowest effective dose [19].

11.9   PROMs in Neuro-Oncology

The use of patient-reported outcome measures (PROMs) in neuro-oncology has significantly grown in recent years [65, 66]. Such increase is due to the possibility to emphasize patients' perspective without clinicians or care-givers interpretation.

The main areas of neuro-oncology in which PROMs are mostly used concern: HRQoL, symptom burden, cognitive function, coping style, needs, and other topics related to daily living.

Information provided by PROMs represent an important integration in research field and in clinical decision-making process. This is because they help to clarify aspects such as disease and treatment-related symptoms, social and working functioning and other aspects related to QoL that do not directly concern survival or treatment response.

Despite their importance and the increase in the use of PROMs in neuro-oncology, some critical issues concern this topic.

A first issue is that only a small number of these tools is brain-tumor specific (19%), while the majority is generic, other cancer specific or designed for different indications [67].

Among BTs-specific PROMs, most frequently used measure are the European Organization for Research and Treatment of Cancer Quality of Life Questionnaire—Brain Cancer 20 (EORTC QLQ-BN20) and the Functional Assessment of Cancer Therapy-Brain (FACT-Br).

The European Organization for Research and Treatment of Cancer Quality of Life Questionnaire—Core 30 (EORTC QLQ-C30), the generic EuroQoL five-dimensional instruments (EQ-5D), the generic Medical Outcomes Study SF-36 ($n = 52$) and the National Comprehensive Cancer Network distress thermometer and problem list (NCCN DT + PL), are the most utilized cancer-specific PROMs.

About symptom-specific questionnaires, the most representative are the Functional Assessment of Chronic Illness Therapy-Fatigue (FACIT-F), the Functional Assessment of Cancer Therapy—Cognitive Function (FACT-Cog) and the MD Anderson Symptom Inventory-Brain Tumor (MDASI-BT).

The Hospital Anxiety and Depression Scale (HADS) the generic Beck Depression Inventory (BDI/BDI-II) are frequently used to assess, respectively, anxiety and depression, and depression only in patients with BTs.

Secondarily, the high number of available PROMs and the lack of information about the timing of assessment increase variability in scientific reports and reduce findings homogeneity and comparability. Indeed, even the most used instruments are included in a small percentage of studies. As reported in the systematic review by Dirven et al., the majority of PROMs measures (70%) are used in one or few literature reports, regardless of the observational or intervention-evaluation design of the studies.

Another relevant issue is that most of the instruments are indifferently used in patients with various histologies and, at present, it is not possible to recommend specific instruments for each tumor type.

Furthermore, future research is needed to clarify if the PROMs exhibit good measurement properties (i.e., content validity, sensitivity to known group comparisons, reliability and responsiveness) and a specific project will investigate these issues (RANO-PRO working plan).

Finally, the use of a high number of tools could constitute a load for patients and provide redundant information. In this sense, a set of symptoms and constructs that are characteristic of neuro-oncological patients has recently been proposed [68], which should always be evaluated. The following topics constitute this core set: Symptoms Pain, Difficulty communicating, Perceived cognition, Seizures, Symptomatic adverse events, Physical functioning and Role functioning while, further and specific measures, depending on the setting or research purposes, could complete the evaluation according to needs.

In conclusion PROMs represent useful tools in neuro-oncology since they emphasize subjective perspective and patient-centered approach. Despite this, an effort to improve their specificity and homogeneity is needed.

11.10 QoL Differences Between HGG and LGG

As expected, the majority of newly diagnosed HGG patients have a significantly impaired level of HRQOL, compared with healthy controls [20, 21]. Systematic pretreatment evaluation of HRQOL in clinical trials emphasize that the disease itself has a major negative impact and that treatment may improve HRQOL [69, 70]. However, the side effects of treatment may seriously hamper QoL, especially in long-term survivors without active disease.

HRQOL studies of LGG patients have employed small samples with a mix of tumor grades, or have employed study-specific HRQOL measures that hinder comparison of studies results [71, 72]. Despite methodological limitations, the studies suggest that many survivors of LGG suffer from cognitive deficits, assessed both objectively and subjectively, and compromised HRQOL and show increased fatigue or depression [73, 74]. Lower HRQOL in long-term LGG survivors is related to the extent of cognitive deficit and the severity of epilepsy [15].

HGG patients experience the same level of HRQOL as those with other neurological diseases of the central and peripheral nervous system [75]. When comparing HGG patients with other cancer patients, such as those with lung cancer, similar QoL results are found [76].

Several tumor-related factors in HGG patients can have an impact on perceived HRQOL. Patients with HGG experience worse QoL than patients who have LGG [77].

The most effective follow-up protocol (including duration, frequency, and type of examinations) after treatment for glioma patients has yet to be well known [78]. However, we must remember that most BTs patients will have active follow-ups throughout their lives. Sometimes, imaging schedules for following up on glioma are pragmatic rather than evidence-based and the prescriptive attitude of the single physician often conditions it. No studies tell whether follow-up is necessary and whether this practice affects patients' prognoses. In the guidelines of scientific societies, indications are given for follow-ups that are routinely designed according to tumor grading. (EANO, AINO) Follow-up can be a time of great stress for the patient. While some patients wait for periodic check-ups and continue to demand and expect them throughout the duration of the disease, for other ones every follow-up appointment is destabilizing.

References

1. Wen PY, Kesari S. Malignant gliomas in adults. N Engl J Med. 2008;359:492–507.
2. Stupp R, Hegi ME, Mason WP, van den Bent MJ, Taphoorn MJ, Janzer RC, Ludwin SK, Allgeier A, Fisher B, Belanger K, Hau P, Brandes AA, Gijtenbeek J, Marosi C, Vecht CJ, Mokhtari K, Wesseling P, Villa S, Eisenhauer E, Gorlia T, Weller M, Lacombe D, Cairncross JG, Mirimanoff RO. Effects of radiotherapy with concomitant and adjuvant temozolomide versus radiotherapy alone on survival in glioblastoma in a randomised phase III study: 5-year analysis of the EORTC-NCIC trial. Lancet Oncol. 2009;10:459–66.
3. Catt S, Chalmers A, Fallowfield L. Psychosocial and supportive-care needs in high-grade glioma. Lancet Oncol. 2008;9:884–91.
4. Ostgathe C, Gaertner J, Kotterba M, Klein S, Lindena G, Nauck F, Radbruch L, Voltz R. Differential palliative care issues in patients with primary and secondary brain tumours. Support Care Cancer. 2010;18:1157–63.
5. Philip J, Collins A, Brand CA, Gold M, Moore G, Sundararajan V, Murphy MA, Lethborg C. Health care professionals' perspectives of living and dying with primary malignant glioma: implications for a unique cancer trajectory. Palliat Support Care. 2015;13:1519–27.
6. Sizoo EM, Pasman HR, Dirven L, Marosi C, Grisold W, Stockhammer G, Egeter J, Grant R, Chang S, Heimans JJ, Deliens L, Reijneveld JC, Taphoorn MJ. The end-of-life phase of high-grade glioma patients: a systematic review. Support Care Cancer. 2014;22:847–57.
7. Hildebrand J, Lecaille C, Perennes J, et al. Epileptic seizures during follow-up of patients treated for primary brain tumors. Neurology. 2005;65:212–5.
8. Scott GM, Gibberd FB. Epilepsy and other factors in the prognosis of gliomas. Acta Neurol Scand. 1980;61:227–39.

9. Wrensch M, Minn Y, Chew T, et al. Epidemiology of primary brain tumors: current concepts and review of the literature. Neuro Oncol. 2002;4:278–99.
10. Sizoo EM, Braam L, Postma TJ, et al. Symptoms and problems in the end-of-life phase of high-grade glioma patients. Neuro Oncol. 2010;12:1162–6.
11. Lee JW, Wen PY, Hurwitz S, et al. Morphological characteristics of brain tumors causing seizures. Arch Neurol. 2010;67:336–42.
12. Rudà R, Trevisan E, Soffietti R. Epilepsy and brain tumors. Curr Opin Oncol. 2010;22:611–20.
13. Glantz MJ, Cole BF, Forsyth PA, et al. Practice parameter: anticonvulsant prophylaxis in patients with newly diagnosed brain tumors. Report of the Quality Standards Subcommittee of the American Academy of Neurology. Neurology. 2000;54:1886–93.
14. Glantz MJ, Cole BF, Friedberg MH, et al. A randomized, blinded, placebo-controlled trial of divalproex sodium prophylaxis in adults with newly diagnosed brain tumors. Neurology. 1996;46:985–91.
15. Klein M, Engelberts NH, van der Ploeg HM, et al. Epilepsy in low-grade gliomas: the impact on cognitive function and quality of life. Ann Neurol. 2003;54:514–20.
16. Taillibert S, Laigle-Donadey F, Sanson M. Palliative care in patients with primary brain tumors. Curr Opin Oncol. 2004;16:587–92.
17. Maschio M, Dinapoli L. Patients with brain tumor-related epilepsy. J Neurooncol. 2012;109:1–6.
18. van Breemen MS, Wilms EB, Vecht CJ. Epilepsy in patients with brain tumours: epidemiology, mechanisms, and management. Lancet Neurol. 2007;6:421–30.
19. Kaal EC, Vecht CJ. The management of brain edema in brain tumors. Curr Opin Oncol. 2004;16:593–600.
20. Kountz DS, Clark CL. Safely withdrawing patients from chronic glucocorticoid therapy. Am Fam Physician. 1997;55:521–5, 529–30.
21. Weissman DE, Dufer D, Vogel V, et al. Corticosteroid toxicity in neuro-oncology patients. J Neurooncol. 1987;5:125–8.
22. Gattis WA, May DB. Possible interaction involving phenytoin, dexamethasone, and antineoplastic agents: a case report and review. Ann Pharmacother. 1996;30:520–6.
23. Brandes AA, Scelzi E, Salmistraro G, et al. Incidence of risk of thromboembolism during treatment high-grade gliomas: a prospective study. Eur J Cancer. 1997;33:1592–6.
24. Kayser-Gatchalian MC, Kayser K. Thrombosis and intracranial tumors. J Neurol. 1975;209:217–24.
25. Marras LC, Geerts WH, Perry JR. The risk of venous thromboembolism is increased throughout the course of malignant glioma: an evidence-based review. Cancer. 2000;89:640–6.
26. Horsted F, West J, Grainge MJ. Risk of venous thromboembolism in patients with cancer: a sys-

tematic review and meta-analysis. PLoS Med. 2012;9:e1001275.

27. Gerber DE, Grossman SA, Streiff MB. Management of venous thromboembolism in patients with primary and metastatic brain tumors. J Clin Oncol. 2006;24:1310–8.

28. Lyman GH. Thromboprophylaxis with low-molecularweight heparin in medical patients with cancer. Cancer. 2009;115:5637–50.

29. Grant R, Brown PD. Fatigue randomized controlled trials—how tired is "too tired" in patients undergoing glioma treatment? Neuro Oncol. 2016;18:759–60.

30. Rooney AG, McNamara S, Mackinnon M, et al. Frequency, clinical associations, and longitudinal course of major depressive disorder in adults with cerebral glioma. J Clin Oncol. 2011;29:4307–12.

31. Ostuzzi G, Matcham F, Dauchy S, Barbui C, Hotopf M. Antidepressants for the treatment of depression in people with cancer. Cochrane Database Syst Rev. 2015;6:Cd011006.

32. Rooney AG, Brown PD, Reijneveld JC, Grant R. Depression in glioma: a primer for clinicians and researchers. J Neurol Neurosurg Psychiatry. 2014;85(2):230–5.

33. Taphoorn MJ, Klein M. Cognitive deficits in adult patients with brain tumours. Lancet Neurol. 2004;3:159–68.

34. Tucha O, Smely C, Preier M, Lange KW. Cognitive deficits before treatment among patients with brain tumors. Neurosurgery. 2000;47:324–33.

35. Gehring K, Taphoorn MJ, Sitskoorn MM, Aaronson NK. Predictors of subjective versus objective cognitive functioning in patients with stable grades II and III glioma. Neurooncol Pract. 2015;2:20–31.

36. Giovagnoli AR, Meneses RF, Paterlini C, Silvani A, Boiardi A. Cognitive awareness after treatment for high-grade glioma. Clin Neurol Neurosurg. 2021;210:106953.

37. Gehring K, Sitskoorn MM, Gundy CM, et al. Cognitive rehabilitation in patients with gliomas: a randomized, controlled trial. J Clin Oncol. 2009;27:3712–22.

38. Yang S, Chun MH, Son YR. Effect of virtual reality on cognitive dysfunction in patients with brain tumor. Ann Rehabil Med. 2014;38:726–33.

39. Zucchella C, Capone A, Codella V, et al. Cognitive rehabilitation for early post-surgery inpatients affected by primary brain tumor: a randomized, controlled trial. J Neurooncol. 2013;114:93–100.

40. Kumthekar P, Stell BV, Jacobs DI, Helenowski IB, Rademaker AW, Grimm SA, Bennett CL, Raizer JJ. Financial burden experienced by patients undergoing treatment for malignant gliomas. Neurooncol Pract. 2014;1(2):71–6. https://doi.org/10.1093/nop/npu002. Epub 2014 May 5. PMID: 26034619; PMCID: PMC4371162.

41. Haider SA, Asmaro K, Kalkanis SN, Lee IY, Bazydlo M, Nerenz DR, Salloum RG, Snyder J, Walbert T. The economic impact of glioma survivorship: the cost of care from a patient perspective. Neurology. 2020;95(11):e1575–81. https://doi.org/10.1212/WNL.0000000000010263. Epub 2020 Jul 9. PMID: 32646959.

42. Paiva ALC, Vitorino-Araujo JL, Lovato RM, Costa GHFD, Veiga JCE. An economic study of neuro-oncological patients in a large developing country: a cost analysis. Arq Neuropsiquiatr. 2022;80(11):1149–58. https://doi.org/10.1055/s--0042-1758649. Epub 2022 Dec 28. PMID: 36577414; PMCID: PMC9797276.

43. Pace A, Di Lorenzo C, Guariglia L, et al. End of life issues in brain tumor patients. J Neurooncol. 2009;91:39–43.

44. Kompanje EJ. 'Death rattle' after withdrawal of mechanical ventilation: practical and ethical considerations. Intensive Crit Care Nurs. 2006;22:214–9.

45. Ford E, Catt S, Chalmers A, Fallowfield L. Systematic review of supportive care needs in patients with primary malignant brain tumors. Neuro Oncol. 2012;14:392–404.

46. Bonito V, Caraceni A, Borghi L, Marcello N, Mori M, Porteri C, Casella G, Causarano R, Gasparini M, Colombi L, Defanti CA. The clinical and ethical appropriateness of sedation in palliative neurological treatments. Neurol Sci. 2005;26:370–85.

47. Breitbart W, Alici Y. Evidence-based treatment of delirium in patients with cancer. J Clin Oncol. 2012;30:1206–14.

48. Agar M, Lawlor P. Delirium in cancer patients: a focus on treatment-induced psychopathology. Curr Opin Oncol. 2008;20:360–6.

49. Boettger S, Jenewein J, Breitbart W. Haloperidol, risperidone, olanzapine and aripiprazole in the management of delirium: a comparison of efficacy, safety, and side effects. Palliat Support Care. 2015;13:1079–85.

50. Bush SH, Leonard MM, Agar M, et al. End-of-life delirium: issues regarding recognition, optimal management, and the role of sedation in the dying phase. J Pain Symptom Manag. 2014;48:215–30.

51. Koekkoek JA, Dirven L, Reijneveld JC, et al. End of life care in high-grade glioma patients in three European countries: a comparative study. J Neurooncol. 2014;120:303–10.

52. Sizoo EM, Taphoorn MJ, Uitdehaag B, et al. The end-of-life phase of high-grade glioma patients: dying with dignity? Oncologist. 2013;18:198–203.

53. Pace A, Villani V, Di Pasquale A, et al. Home care for brain tumor patients. Neurooncol Pract. 2014;1:8–12.

54. Brown PD, Maurer MJ, Rummans TA, et al. A prospective study of quality of life in adults with newly diagnosed high-grade gliomas: the impact of the extent of resection on quality of life and survival. Neurosurgery. 2005;57:495–504.

55. Kiebert GM, Curran D, Aaronson NK, et al. Quality of life after radiation therapy of cerebral low-grade gliomas of the adult: results of a randomised phase III

trial on dose response (EORTC trial 22844). EORTC Radiotherapy Co-operative Group. Eur J Cancer. 1998;34:1902–9.

56. Klein M, Heimans JJ, Aaronson NK, et al. Effect of radiotherapy and other treatment-related factors on mid-term to long-term cognitive sequelae in low-grade gliomas: a comparative study. Lancet. 2002;360:1361–8.

57. Douw L, Klein M, Fagel SS, et al. Cognitive and radiological effects of radiotherapy in patients with low-grade glioma: long-term follow-up. Lancet Neurol. 2009;8:810–8.

58. Perry JR, Laperriere N, O'Callaghan CJ, Brandes AA, Menten J, Phillips C, Fay M, Nishikawa R, Cairncross JG, Roa W, Osoba D, Rossiter JP, Sahgal A, Hirte H, Laigle-Donadey F, Franceschi E, Chinot O, Golfinopoulos V, Fariselli L, Wick A, Feuvret L, Back M, Tills M, Winch C, Baumert BG, Wick W, Ding K, Mason WP, Trial Investigators. Short-course radiation plus temozolomide in elderly patients with glioblastoma. N Engl J Med. 2017;376(11):1027–37. https://doi.org/10.1056/NEJMoa1611977. PMID: 28296618.

59. Ernst-Stecken A, Ganslandt O, Lambrecht U, et al. Survival and quality of life after hypofractionated stereotactic radiotherapy for recurrent malignant glioma. J Neurooncol. 2007;81:287–94.

60. Stupp R, Mason WP, van den Bent MJ, et al. Radiotherapy plus concomitant and adjuvant temozolomide for glioblastoma. N Engl J Med. 2005;352:987–96.

61. Wick W, Platten M, Meisner C, Felsberg J, Tabatabai G, Simon M, Nikkhah G, Papsdorf K, Steinbach JP, Sabel M, Combs SE, Vesper J, Braun C, Meixensberger J, Ketter R, Mayer-Steinacker R, Reifenberger G, Weller M, NOA-08 Study Group of Neuro-oncology Working Group (NOA) of German Cancer Society. Temozolomide chemotherapy alone versus radiotherapy alone for malignant astrocytoma in the elderly: the NOA-08 randomised, phase 3 trial. Lancet Oncol. 2012;13(7):707–15. https://doi.org/10.1016/S1470-2045(12)70164-X. Epub 2012 May 10. PMID: 22578793.

62. Malmström A, Grønberg BH, Marosi C, Stupp R, Frappaz D, Schultz H, Abacioglu U, Tavelin B, Lhermitte B, Hegi ME, Rosell J, Henriksson R, Nordic Clinical Brain Tumour Study Group (NCBTSG). Temozolomide versus standard 6-week radiotherapy versus hypofractionated radiotherapy in patients older than 60 years with glioblastoma: the Nordic randomised, phase 3 trial. Lancet Oncol. 2012;13(9):916–26. https://doi.org/10.1016/S1470-2045(12)70265-6. Epub 2012 Aug 8. PMID: 22877848.

63. Lombardi G, De Salvo GL, Brandes AA, Eoli M, Rudà R, Faedi M, Lolli I, Pace A, Daniele B, Pasqualetti F, Rizzato S, Bellu L, Pambuku A, Farina M, Magni G, Indraccolo S, Gardiman MP, Soffietti R, Zagonel V. Regorafenib compared with lomustine in patients with relapsed glioblastoma (REGOMA): a multicentre, open-label, randomised, controlled, phase 2 trial. Lancet Oncol. 2019;20(1):110–9. https://doi.org/10.1016/S1470-2045(18)30675-2. Epub 2018 Dec 3. PMID: 30522967.

64. van der Meer PB, Dirven L, Fiocco M, Vos MJ, Kouwenhoven MCM, van den Bent MJ, Taphoorn MJB, Koekkoek JAF. First-line antiepileptic drug treatment in glioma patients with epilepsy: levetiracetam vs valproic acid. Epilepsia. 2021;62(5):1119–29. https://doi.org/10.1111/epi.16880. Epub 2021 Mar 18. PMID: 33735464; PMCID: PMC8251728.

65. Basch E. Patient-reported outcomes: an essential component of oncology drug development and regulatory review. Lancet Oncol. 2018;19(5): 595–7.

66. Dirven L, Armstrong TS, Taphoorn MJ. Health-related quality of life and other clinical outcome assessments in brain tumor patients: challenges in the design, conduct and interpretation of clinical trials. Neurooncol Pract. 2015;2(1):2–5.

67. Dirven L, Vos ME, Walbert T, Armstrong TS, Arons D, van den Bent MJ, Blakeley J, Brown PD, Bulbeck H, Chang SM, Coens C, Gilbert MR, Grant R, Jalali R, Leach D, Leeper H, Mendoza T, Nayak L, Oliver K, Reijneveld JC, Le Rhun E, Rubinstein L, Weller M, Wen PY, Taphoorn MJB. Systematic review on the use of patient-reported outcome measures in brain tumor studies: part of the Response Assessment in Neuro-Oncology Patient-Reported Outcome (RANO-PRO) initiative. Neurooncol Pract. 2021;8(4):417–25. https://doi.org/10.1093/nop/npab013. PMID: 34277020; PMCID: PMC8278354.

68. Armstrong TS, Dirven L, Arons D, et al. Glioma patient-reported outcome assessment in clinical care and research: a response assessment in neuro-oncology collaborative report. Lancet Oncol. 2020;21(2):e97–e103.

69. Taphoorn MJ, Stupp R, Coens C, et al. Health-related quality of life in patients with glioblastoma: a randomised controlled trial. Lancet Oncol. 2005;6:937–44.

70. Taphoorn MJ, van den Bent MJ, Mauer ME, et al. Health-related quality of life in patients treated for anaplastic oligodendroglioma with adjuvant chemotherapy: results of a European Organisation for Research and Treatment of Cancer randomized clinical trial. J Clin Oncol. 2007;25:5723–30.

71. Mackworth N, Fobair P, Prados MD. Quality of life self-reports from 200 brain tumor patients: comparisons with Karnofsky performance scores. J Neurooncol. 1992;14:243–53.

72. Sachsenheimer W, Piotrowski W, Bimmler T. Quality of life in patients with intracranial tumors on the basis of Karnofsky's performance status. J Neurooncol. 1992;13:177–81.

73. Reijneveld JC, Sitskoorn MM, Klein M, et al. Cognitive status and quality of life in patients with suspected versus proven low-grade gliomas. Neurology. 2001;56:618–23.

74. Struik K, Klein M, Heimans JJ, et al. Fatigue in low-grade glioma. J Neurooncol. 2009;92:73–8.

75. Giovagnoli AR. Quality of life in patients with stable disease after surgery, radiotherapy, and chemotherapy for malignant brain tumour. J Neurol Neurosurg Psychiatry. 1999;67:358–63.

76. Klein M, Taphoorn MJ, Heimans JJ, et al. Neurobehavioral status and health-related quality of life in newly diagnosed high-grade glioma patients. J Clin Oncol. 2001;19:4037–47.

77. Salo J, Niemelä A, Joukamaa M, et al. Effect of brain tumour laterality on patients' perceived quality of life. J Neurol Neurosurg Psychiatry. 2002;72:373–7.

78. Silvaggi F, Silvani A, Lamperti EA, Leonardi M. Pathways of follow-up care in an Italian center: retrospective study on patients with gliomas II and III. Neurol Sci. 2022;43(2):1303–10. https://doi.org/10.1007/s10072-021-05415-8. Epub 2021 Jul 8. PMID: 34235605.

The manufacturer's authorised representative in the EU is Springer
Nature Customer Service Centre GmbH, Europaplatz 3, 69115 Heidelberg,
Germany. If you have any concerns regarding our products, please
contact ProductSafety@springernature.com

Printed and bound by CPI Group (UK) Ltd, Croydon, CR0 4YY
27/04/2026
02097573-0017